TOXICITY OF HEAVY METALS IN THE ENVIRONMENT

HAZARDOUS AND TOXIC SUBSTANCES
A Series of Reference Books and Textbooks

Series Editor: Seymour S. Block
University of Florida
Department of Chemical Engineering
Gainesville, Florida

1. Highly Hazardous Materials Spills and Emergency Planning, J. E. Zajic and W. A. Himmelman

2. Toxicity of Heavy Metals in the Environment (in two parts), edited by Frederick W. Oehme

Other volumes in preparation

TOXICITY OF HEAVY METALS IN THE ENVIRONMENT

IN TWO PARTS

Part 2

EDITED BY
Frederick W. Oehme
Comparative Toxicology Laboratory
Kansas State University
Manhattan, Kansas

MARCEL DEKKER, INC.   *New York and Basel*

Library of Congress Cataloging in Publication Data   (Revised)
  Main entry under title:

  Toxicity of heavy metals in the environment.

    (Hazardous and toxic substances ; 2)
    Includes index.
    1. Heavy metals--Toxicology. 2. Heavy metals--
Environmental aspects. 3. Veterinary toxicology.
I. Oehme, Frederick W. II. Series.
RA1231.M52T69   615.9'2   78-14758
  ISBN 0-8247-6719-5 (p. 2)

Chapter 24 appeared in Clinical Toxicology 6(3) 1973. Chapter 31
appeared in Clinical Toxicology 5(2) June 1972.

MARCEL DEKKER, INC.
270 Madison Avenue, New York, New York 10016

Current printing (last digit):
10 9 8 7 6 5 4 3 2 1

PRINTED IN THE UNITED STATES OF AMERICA

PREFACE

The environment is here to stay and, chemically and biologically, the heavy
metals fall in the same category. Their persistence and their hazard and
toxicity to human and animal life has been one of the prime impulses behind
the development of this publication. Through a careful selection of authors,
each with a specific expertise and knowledge, an effort has been made to
present an overview of the toxicology associated with heavy metal chemicals
as they occur in the environment of all animals, including humans. Hence,
most of the contributors have adopted a comparative approach in discussing
their assigned topics. This was deliberately requested since much of the
information available has been derived from animals; occasionally, human
instances of environmental toxicity have stimulated the conduct of experiments in laboratory or domestic animals.

This book has been organized by first discussing the basic concepts
and principles of heavy metal pollution, how the heavy metals enter the
environment and animal or human food chain, and the fundamental principles
and mechanisms of toxicity due to heavy metal chemicals. The more common
toxic heavy metals are then described together with their biochemistry and
clinical syndromes. This is followed by an excursion into the area of
trace heavy metals and the interactions of specific metallic compounds. The
concluding chapters deal with quantitative assay of environmental metallic
contaminants and some concepts of chelation therapy. Although printing time
introduces a lag factor, every attempt has been made to provide the most
current material available. The diligence of the contributors in maintaining this objective is greatly appreciated.

It is hoped that this publication will serve two functions: (1) To
provide a review and discussion of the current information on comparative
heavy metal toxicity; and (2) to further demonstrate that comparative

studies involving scientists with diverse backgrounds, training, and spe-
cialty-disciplines provide a well-balanced fuel with which a specific effort can rapidly and accurately arrive at its objective. The contributors
are commended for their cooperation and enthusiasm in responding to this
undertaking. Appreciation is given to the publisher for his interest and
continual guidance in seeing this book through to its fulfillment. The
product is one which the readers can best evaluate; their comments and
suggestions are welcomed.

Frederick W. Oehme

CONTENTS

PREFACE   iii
CONTRIBUTORS TO PART 2   vii
CONTENTS OF PART 1   ix

23. EFFECTS OF FLUORIDES IN DOMESTIC AND WILD ANIMALS   517

     James L. Shupe, Arland E. Olson, and Raghubir P. Sharma

24. TOXICITY OF BERYLLIUM AND OTHER ELEMENTS IN MISSILE
     PROPELLANTS   541

     Farrel R. Robinson

25. THE LESSER METALS   547

     Robert P. Beliles

26. TERATOGENICITY OF HEAVY METALS   617

     Francis L. Earl and Theodore J. Vish

27. INTERACTIONS OF TRACE ELEMENTS   641

     Eric J. Underwood

28. REGULATORY ASPECTS OF TRACE ELEMENTS IN THE ENVIRONMENT   669

     William A. Rader and John E. Spaulding

29. BENEFICIAL EFFECTS OF TRACE ELEMENTS   689

     Raymond J. Shamberger

30. QUANTITATIVE ANALYSIS FOR ENVIRONMENTAL AND
     BIOLOGICAL CONCENTRATIONS OF HEAVY METALS   797

     Clifton E. Meloan

31. BRITISH ANTILEWISITE (BAL), THE CLASSIC HEAVY METAL ANTIDOTE   945

     Frederick W. Oehme

Index, Parts 1 and 2   953

BELILES, ROBERT P., Ph.D., Director, Department of Toxicology,
    Litton Bionetics, Inc., Kensington, Maryland

EARL, FRANCIS L., D.V.M., Facility Manager, Beltsville Research Facility,
    Metabolism Branch, Division of Toxicology, Bureau of Foods, Food and
    Drug Administration, Department of Health, Education and Welfare,
    Washington, D.C.

MELOAN, CLIFTON E., Ph.D., Professor, Department of Chemistry, Kansas State
    University, Manhattan, Kansas

OEHME, FREDERICK W., D.V.M., Ph.D., Professor of Toxicology, Medicine, and
    Physiology, and Director, Comparative Toxicology Laboratory, Kansas
    State University, Manhattan, Kansas

OLSON, ARLAND E., M.S., Research Associate, Department of Animal, Dairy,
    and Veterinary Sciences, Utah State University, Logan, Utah

RADER, WILLIAM A., D.V.M.,[1] Toxicologist, Residue Evaluation and Planning
    Staff, U.S. Department of Agriculture, Washington, D.C.

ROBINSON, FARREL R.,[2] D.V.M., M.S., Ph.D., Lt. Col., U.S. Air Force, VC,
    Veterinary Pathology Division, Armed Forces Institute of Pathology,
    Washington, D.C.

SHAMBERGER, RAYMOND J., M.S., Ph.D., Staff, Department of Biochemistry,
    The Cleveland Clinic Foundation, Cleveland, Ohio

SHARMA, RAGHUBIR P., B.V.Sc., Ph.D., Associate Professor, Department of
    Animal, Dairy, and Veterinary Sciences, Utah State University, Logan,
    Utah

SHUPE, JAMES L., D.V.M., Professor, Department of Animal, Dairy, and
    Veterinary Sciences, Utah State University, Logan, Utah

Present Title:

[1]Consultant, 4638 Bayshore Road, Sarasota, Florida

Present Affiliation:

[2]Professor, Toxicology-Pathology, Purdue University School of Veterinary
Medicine, West Lafayette, Indiana

SPAULDING, JOHN E.,[3] D.V.M., M.S., Chief Staff Officer, Residue Evaluation
    and Planning Staff, U.S. Department of Agriculture, Meat and Poultry
    Inspection Program, Food Safety and Quality Service, Washington, D.C.

UNDERWOOD, ERIC J., Ph.D., Honorary Research Fellow, Department of Animal
    Science and Production, University of Western Australia, Nedlands,
    Western Australia

VISH, THEODORE J., B.S., Research Biologist, Beltsville Research Facility,
    Metabolism Branch, Division of Toxicology, Bureau of Foods, Food and
    Drug Administration, Department of Health, Education and Welfare,
    Washington, D.C.

Present Affiliation:

[3]Acting Director, Residue Evaluation and Surveillance Division, U.S. Department of Agriculture, Food Safety and Quality Service, Washington, D.C.

CONTENTS OF PART 1

1. PERSISTENCE VERSUS PERSEVERANCE

   Frederick W. Oehme

2. HEAVY METALS IN FOODS OF ANIMAL ORIGIN

   Leon H. Russell, Jr.

3. TRACE ELEMENTS IN PLANT FOODSTUFFS

   Hansford T. Shacklette, James A. Erdman,
   Thelma F. Harms, and Clara S. E. Papp

4. MECHANISMS OF HEAVY METAL INORGANIC TOXICITIES

   Frederick W. Oehme

5. METABOLISM AND METABOLIC ACTION OF LEAD AND OTHER HEAVY METALS

   Paul B. Hammond

6. LEAD AND THE NERVOUS SYSTEM

   Gary A. Van Gelder

7. LEAD POISONING

   Vernon A. Green, George W. Wise, and John Corrie Callenbach

8. EPIDEMIOLOGY OF LEAD POISONING IN ANIMALS

   Gary D. Osweiler, Gary A. Van Gelder, and William B. Buck

9. OUTBREAKS OF PLUMBISM IN ANIMALS ASSOCIATED WITH
   INDUSTRIAL LEAD OPERATIONS

   Arthur L. Aronson

10. LEAD INTOXICATION IN URBAN DOGS

    Bernard C. Zook

11. THE USE OF ANIMAL MODELS FOR COMPARATIVE
    STUDIES OF LEAD POISONING

    Nancy N. Scharding and Frederick W. Oehme

12. POLLUTION BY CADMIUM AND THE ITAI-ITAI DISEASE IN JAPAN
    Jun Kobayashi

13. METHYL MERCURY POISONING DUE TO ENVIRONMENTAL
    CONTAMINATION ("MINAMATA DISEASE")
    Masazumi Harada

14. TOXICITY OF INORGANIC AND ORGANIC MERCURY COMPOUNDS
    IN ANIMALS
    Delmar Ronald Cassidy and Allan Furr

15. TOXICITY AND RESIDUAL ASPECTS OF ALKYLMERCURY
    FUNGICIDES IN LIVESTOCK
    Fred C. Wright, Jayme C. Riner, Maurice Haufler,
    J. S. Palmer, and R. L. Younger

16. TOXICITY OF INORGANIC AND ALIPHATIC ORGANIC ARSENICALS
    William B. Buck

17. TOXICITY OF ORGANIC ARSENICALS IN FEEDSTUFFS
    Arlo E. Ledet and William B. Buck

18. BIOLOGICAL EFFECTS OF SELENIUM
    James R. Harr

19. THE RELATIONSHIP OF DIETARY SELENIUM CONCENTRATION,
    CHEMICAL CANCER INDUCTION, AND TISSUE CONCENTRATION
    OF SELENIUM IN RATS
    James R. Harr, Jerry H. Exon, Paul H. Weswig,
    and Philip D. Whanger

20. EFFECT OF DIETARY SELENIUM ON $\underline{N}$-2-FLUORENYL-ACETAMIDE
    (FAA)-INDUCED CANCER IN VITAMIN E-SUPPLEMENTED,
    SELENIUM-DEPLETED RATS
    James R. Harr, Jerry H. Exon, Philip D. Whanger,
    and Paul H. Weswig

21. TOXICOLOGY AND ADVERSE EFFECTS OF MINERAL IMBALANCE
    WITH EMPHASIS ON SELENIUM AND OTHER MINERALS
    Richard C. Ewan

22. COPPER/MOLYBDENUM TOXICITY IN ANIMALS
    William B. Buck

TOXICITY OF HEAVY METALS
IN THE ENVIRONMENT

EFFECTS OF FLUORIDES IN DOMESTIC AND WILD ANIMALS

James L. Shupe, Arland E. Olson, and Raghubir P. Sharma
Utah State University
Logan, Utah

Fluorine is the most electronegative of all known elements and the most active of the halogen group. Rarely does it occur free in nature, but combines chemically to form fluorides. Fluoride-containing minerals have been known since the middle ages. The name is derived from their characteristic property of acting as a flux, i.e., to promote the fusion of other metals. Fluorine was first isolated by Moissan in 1886 [1].

Free fluorine plays little or no part in toxicology because it reacts immediately to form fluoride compounds. It occurs in various amounts in soils, water, the atmosphere, vegetation, and animal tissues. Organic fluorides, i.e., compounds in which fluorine is bound to carbon, occur in nature and in certain commercial products, but have not to date been implicated with fluoride toxicosis in animals.

Animals normally ingest small amounts of fluoride without adverse effects. One part per million of fluoride (1 ppm F) in water is essential for optimal health in man and fluorides in small amounts may also be beneficial to animals. Fluorides are harmful, however, when ingested in excessive amounts.

HISTORICAL BACKGROUND

Fluoride toxicosis in sheep was apparently observed about the year 1000 A.D. in Iceland. Its occurrence was correlated with volcanic eruptions [2]. The disease has played a role in the welfare and economy of Iceland by hampering agricultural progress. In many areas along the coastal plains of North Africa, animals and man have been troubled for centuries by a serious, often painful, deterioration of the teeth called darmous caused by excessive fluoride ingestion [3,4].

In 1803 an Italian chemist, Dominico Morichini, demonstrated the presence of fluorine in a fossil elephant tooth that was found outside the city of Rome, Italy. About the year 1846 George Wilson, a Scottish chemist, showed that fluorine is widespread in nature, in springs and seawater, in vegetable ash, and in the blood and milk of animals.

The toxic properties of fluorine compounds were studied for the first time in animal experiments by Rabuteau in 1867 [5]. In 1901, J. M. Eager, M.D., surgeon, U.S. Public Health Service, while stationed in Naples, Italy, described a dental peculiarity among the inhabitants of the Italian littoral known as denti di Chiaie or Chiaie teeth, which was later identified as dental fluorosis [3]. The first observation of mottled enamel most probably was recorded by C. Kuhns in 1888 [6].

A disease in cattle resembling osteomalacia was observed in 1912 by Bartolucci. The affected animals were located adjacent to an Italian superphosphate factory and Bartolucci expressed the opinion that the etiology might be connected with the fluorine content in the waste products from the factory. During World War I a similar disease broke out endemically in the neighborhood of a Swiss aluminum factory. Horses that ingested fluoride-contaminated hay from the same area showed distinct deformations of the leg bones and thickening of the bones of the skull. Roholm identified a domestic animal disease (gaddur), long known in Iceland, as a poisoning by fluorine compounds [2]. Hupka and Gotze in 1931 reported osteodystrophic symptoms in cattle in the vicinity of both chemical and superphosphate factories [7]. In 1934 Slagsvold described chronic fluorine intoxication among herbivora in the vicinity of Norwegian aluminum factories [8].

During the 1920s the use of feed supplements containing excessive fluoride increased the incidence of fluoride toxicosis in animals. With the expansion of certain industries into agricultural areas, especially during and following World War II, fluoride toxicosis in livestock and wildlife became an important and significant problem. With increased knowledge and awareness of the disease, the institution of governing federal and state laws, and the implementation of preventive measures to control industrial pollutants, the problem has been reduced or eliminated in some areas. Enforcement of additional regulatory and educational measures will further alleviate the problem.

Detailed experimental studies and extensive epidemiological work have established the relationship of the biologic responses of animals to fluoride dosage and to other factors that influence fluoride physiologic and anatomic response.

TABLE 1. Effect of Air Temperature on Recommended Fluoride Limits in Drinking Water[a]

Annual Average of Maximum Daily Air Temperatures (°F)[b]	Recommended Control Limits (fluoride concentrations in mg/l)		
	Lower	Optimum	Upper
50.0-53.7	0.9	1.2	1.7
53.8-58.3	0.8	1.1	1.5
58.4-63.8	0.8	1.0	1.3
63.9-70.6	0.7	0.9	1.2
70.7-79.2	0.7	0.8	1.0
79.3-90.5	0.6	0.7	0.8

[a]Reprinted by permission from Ref. 17.

[b]Based on temperature data obtained for a minimum of 5 years.

The question, "Is fluorine an essential element?" has naturally been raised. Until recently it had not been possible to find a definite answer because it is difficult to produce a practical research environment and a practical and adequate diet that is fluorine-free. There are indications, however, that traces of fluoride are necessary for normal mineralization of some tissue. In particular, an adequate fluoride supply is evidently essential for the formation of a caries-resistant enamel [3,9,10].

Researchers have reported impairment of fertility [11] in laboratory mice. Mice born to laboratory animals on a fluoride-deficient diet exhibited severe anemia [12]. Better growth patterns in rats were observed when small amounts of fluoride were added to controlled diets [13]. In addition, the ability of fluoride to improve the mineralization of bone logically suggests that this element might be useful in preventing and treating some cases of osteoporosis [14-16].

Most beneficial effects occur if the fluoride level in the drinking water is about 1 ppm. This level may be altered somewhat by the annual average air temperature (Table 1) [17].

SOURCES OF FLUORIDE TO DOMESTIC AND WILD ANIMALS

The principal source of fluoride for animals (particularly livestock) is from mineral ores. In certain industrial operations, where the ores are ground or heated to high temperatures, fluorides may escape and, unless measures are taken to control them, they are emitted into the atmosphere.

Such compounds ultimately settle on the vegetation around the processing operations, and these contaminated forages are often ingested by herbivores and other animals [18,19].

In spite of the high level of fluorides in certain soils, most plants usually do not translocate dangerous levels of fluorides from them. Those that do, do not constitute a considerable hazard to animals. However, plants growing on soils high in fluoride content may be contaminated by rain splash or dust storms, and then these plants may be grazed or mechanically harvested for forage. One study of such conditions reported forage samples with as much as 300 ppm F on a dry-weight basis [20]. Animals and livestock grazing such vegetation ingest large amounts of fluorides. Chemical analyses of 107 alfalfa hay samples from nonindustrial areas in the United States ranged from 0.8 to 36.5 ppm F with a mean of 3.6 ppm and a median of 2 ppm [21]. Animals grazing close to the ground are also liable to ingest quantities of high-fluoride soils.

Factors that can influence the fluoride content in unwashed vegetation samples include the length of time the plant has been growing, frequency and amount of precipitation, amount of wind, amount of fluoride in soil and in ambient air, plant type or species, and the portion of the plant sampled.

Fluorides also may be dissolved into surface and/or underground water. High-fluoride water is another source of fluoride to animals. Fluoride contents of 2.5, 8.0, 12.5, and 28.0 ppm have been present in water where studies have been conducted.

A number of fluororganic compounds are used in industry and medicine. Such compounds, however, contain fluorine in a tight covalent binding, so that physiologically the fluoride is not readily available to animals exposed to them.

DISTRIBUTION OF FLUORIDE IN THE BODY

After ingestion, most fluorides are absorbed in the stomach and intestines. The gastrointestinal absorption of fluorides is markedly influenced by dietary composition. The presence of large amounts of certain ions in the diet, particularly calcium, aluminum, and magnesium, which form less soluble complexes with fluoride, decrease the amount of absorbable fluoride (Fig. 1).

Following absorption, fluorides are distributed throughout the body, the concentration in most soft tissues being roughly equal to that in the

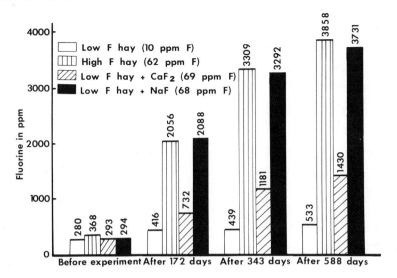

FIG. 1. Influence of dietary fluoride in hay and as calcium and sodium fluoride salts on the absorption and concentration of fluorine in the bones of cattle.

plasma [9]. The tissues where fluorides are selectively accumulated are skeletal, dental, and mineralizing tissue. Deposition of fluorides in the bone serves as an excellent example of a cumulative element. Approximately 98% of the fluoride in the body is deposited in bones, and such accumulation normally continues throughout life. However, an individual on a long-time, constant, elevated fluoride intake does tend to reach a state of equilibrium in which the amount of fluoride retained by the body is reduced and the amount excreted in the urine is increased [23]. In both dental and skeletal tissues, the deposition of fluoride is related to the metabolism of the tissue; for example, the forming teeth and bone will accumulate the fluoride ion more readily [9,24-26]. The fluoride ion is incorporated in the hydroxyapatite crystal of bone forming fluorapatite. In this form it remains incorporated until remodeling resorption of the bone mineral complex. Fluoride thus incorporated has been reported to increase the apatite crystal size, to stabilize the unit cell, and to decrease the mineral solubility [27].

Fluoride ions are also found in fetal tissues. Fetal blood fluoride concentration is approximately equal to that of the maternal blood. In the fetus, fluoride is selectively deposited in the teeth and bones, but not in high enough levels to cause demonstrable pathologic changes [9,28].

A large fraction of ingested fluoride is excreted in the urine, and urinary fluoride levels provide a relative index of current fluoride intake [29]. Human urinary fluoride concentrations depend upon and, in fact, are nearly equal to the drinking water concentrations [3,9].

SOURCES OF INFORMATION IN THE PRESENT REPORT

The observations described here are based on clinical and necropsy data collected from controlled long-term studies in animals (which were published in detail earlier [22,28-30], clinical and necropsy information from domestic animals, and necropsy data from various wildlife species obtained from areas of endemic fluorosis [31-33]. The animals on controlled experiments were fed various levels and types of fluorides [22,29,30,34]. The other animals came from areas of industrial fluoride contamination and from places where water sources were high in fluoride content. Primary emphasis in this report is placed on the lesions in teeth and bones obtained from such animals because these tissues are major sites of fluoride accumulation and subsequent pathological changes [10,35-38].

FLUORIDE TOXICOSIS

Excessive fluoride ingestion can induce either an acute or a chronic disease [24]. The latter condition has been called fluoride toxicosis, chronic fluoride toxicity, or fluorosis. Although specific conditions such as osteofluorosis and dental fluorosis are definable, the general term fluorosis does not lend itself to a clear-cut definition; therefore the term fluoride toxicosis is used to describe the conditions that result when excess fluorides are ingested. An understanding of the clinical signs and a thorough awareness of the pathogenesis and lesions of fluoride toxicosis are essential for correct diagnosis and accurate evaluation of the disease [31].

Acute Fluoride Toxicosis

Acute fluoride toxicosis has not been studied as extensively and elucidated as well as chronic fluoride toxicosis because it is relatively rare [9,24,39-41]. Acute fluoride toxicosis most often results from accidental ingestion of high levels of fluoride compounds [24,42,43]. The sources of such poisonings in livestock have been sodium fluorosilicate, used as a rodenticide, and sodium fluoride, used as an ascaricide in swine.

Accidental and experimentally induced acute responses have been reviewed by Cass [44]. The distinction between acute and chronic fluoride toxicosis is not always possible, however, because of the complex situations involved.

The responses seen in acute fluoride toxicosis are varied and depend on many factors. Clinically the following signs may be observed: restlessness, stiffness, nausea and vomiting, excessive salivation, severe depression, incontinence of urine and feces, clonic convulsions, and cardiac failure. Chemical analyses reveal a high fluoride content in the urine and blood.

Chronic Fluoride Toxicosis

Chronic fluoride toxicosis is the type of fluoride poisoning most often observed in livestock [31,35,36,45-47]. The development and onset of this condition is usually gradual and may be insidious. Some signs of the disease may be confused with other chronic debilitating diseases, such as osteoarthritis or some trace element poisonings or deficiencies [48]. The point at which the ingested fluoride becomes detrimental to the animal may vary in individual cases and can be influenced by the following factors: (1) amount of fluoride ingested, (2) duration of fluoride ingestion, (3) solubility of the ingested fluoride, (4) fluctuations in fluoride ingestion levels, (5) species, (6) age at time of ingestion, (7) level of nutrition, (8) stress factors, and (9) individual biologic response.

The varying and sometimes prolonged interval between ingestion of elevated levels of fluorides and manifestation of the clinical signs of chronic fluoride toxicosis may in some cases complicate the clinical syndrome.

No single criterion should be relied upon in diagnosing and evaluating fluoride toxicosis. All clinical observations, necropsy findings, and chemical evidence must be carefully evaluated and correlated before a definite diagnosis and evaluation of fluoride toxicosis is made. The following factors are of particular diagnostic importance: (1) degree of dental fluorosis, (2) degree of osteofluorosis, (3) intermittent lameness, and (4) the amount of fluoride in the bone, urine, blood, and components of the ration.

Dental Fluorosis

Developing teeth are extremely sensitive to excessive fluoride. Fluorotic lesions in permanent dentition are one of the most obvious signs of

excessive fluoride ingestion if such ingestion occurs during the period of
tooth formation and mineralization [28,49,50].

Gross fluorotic lesions in the incisor enamel are generally described
as chalkiness (dull white, chalklike appearance), mottling (horizontal
white, chalklike striations or patches in the teeth), hypoplasia (defective
development), and hypocalcification (defective calcification). Teeth affected to a moderate, marked, or severe degree are subject to more rapid
attrition and in some cases to an erosion of the enamel from the dentin.

For the purpose of classifying various degrees of dental fluorosis
observed in research studies and endemic fluoride areas, the following
gradations have been developed (Fig. 2):

0. Normal: smooth, translucent, glossy white appearance of enamel; tooth
   normal shovel shape.

1. Questionable effect: slight deviation from normal; unable to determine
   exact cause; may have enamel flecks but no mottling.

2. Slight effect: slight mottling of enamel; best observed as horizontal
   striations with back lighting; may have slight staining but no increase
   in normal rate of attrition.

3. Moderate effect: definite mottling; large areas of chalky enamel or
   generalized mottling of entire tooth; teeth may show a slightly increased rate of attrition and may be stained.

4. Marked effect: definite mottling, hypoplasia, and hypocalcification;
   may have pitting of enamel; with use, tooth will have increased rate of
   attrition; enamel may be stained or discolored.

5. Severe effect: definite mottling, hypoplasia, and hypocalcification;
   with use, tooth will have excessively increased rate of attrition and
   may have erosion or pitting of enamel; tooth may be stained or discolored.

Dental fluorosis in animals is usually diagnosed by examining the incisor teeth. Cheek (premolar and molar) teeth are more difficult to examine in the live animal because of problems associated with proper restraint
of the animal being examined, poor illumination of the teeth, the presence
of the tongue and unswallowed food, and discoloration caused by vegetative
matter. The same criteria used in diagnosing and evaluating incisor lesions
are not used in diagnosing and evaluating cheek teeth for dental fluorosis

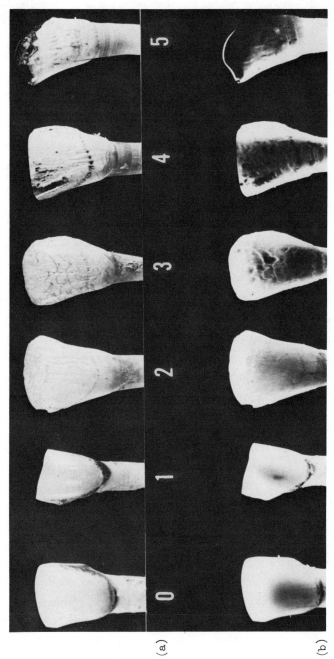

FIG. 2. Classification of representative incisor teeth from cattle is from 0 to 5 reading from left to right in (a) and (b): (a) is with front lighting, (b) with back lighting. (Reprinted with permission from Ref. 28.

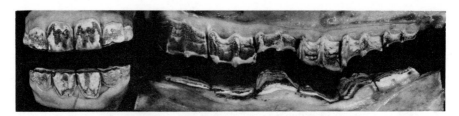

FIG. 3. Permanent equine incisor teeth and cheek teeth. Note pitting and discoloration of enamel and excessive abrasion of incisor teeth with excessive and irregular abrasion of cheek teeth.

[31,33]. Fluorosis of premolars and molars is estimated on the degree of selective abrasion and correlation with fluoride lesions in the incisor teeth (Fig. 3).

The degree of fluoride-induced dental lesions under controlled experimental conditions has been correlated with the amount of fluoride ingested, the age of the animal, the duration of excessive fluoride ingestion, the severity of osteofluorosis, and other factors influencing the biologic response to fluorides [28]. The dental lesions, therefore, are useful in clinically diagnosing chronic fluoride toxicosis (Fig. 4). To be most meaningful, however, the fluoride dental lesions should be evaluated with other tissue changes and signs induced by excessive fluoride ingestion. In other words, dental lesions should not be used as the sole criterion when diagnosing and evaluating the degree of chronic fluoride toxicosis [31,32].

Bone

The level of fluoride storage in bone can increase over a period of time without evidence of any demonstrable changes in bone structure and function. If the levels of fluoride ingestion are sufficiently higher than normal for an appreciable length of time, structural bone changes will become evident [24,25,28].

In livestock, the first clinically palpable bone lesions usually occur bilaterally on the medial surface of the proximal third of the metatarsal bones. Subsequently, palpable bone lesions occur on the mandible, metacarpals, and ribs. The severity of osteofluorotic lesions appears related in some degree to the stress and strain imposed on various bones and to the structure and function of the bones. This is exemplified by the difference in the osteofluorotic lesions of the ribs, mandible, and metaphyseal areas of the metatarsal and metacarpal bones as compared to the less severe lesions and lower fluoride content of the diaphyseal areas of the metatarsal and metacarpal bones [28]. Experiments with dairy heifers and cows showed an increase in bone alkaline phosphatase in response to increased dietary fluoride ingestion [51].

Grossly, bones that are severely affected by fluoride appear chalky white with a roughened irregular periosteal surface and are larger in diameter and heavier than normal (Fig. 5).

The type of bone changes depends on the levels and duration of fluoride ingestion, and one or more of the following conditions may occur: osteoporosis, osteosclerosis, hyperostosis, osteophytosis, or osteomalacia.

Although the precise mechanisms involved in osteofluorosis are not fully understood at this time, it appears that three different phases are involved with the changes found in bone that are associated with fluoride toxicosis. These three phases include (1) elevated levels of fluoride in bone without detectable changes in bone structure, (2) microscopic and radiographic changes in bone without detectable alteration of function, and (3) a sequence of progressive changes in bone structure that results in an alteration of its mechanical properties with resultant abnormal bone. Stimulation of abnormal osteoblastic activity apparently results in formation of an abnormal organic matrix with resultant irregular, disorderly, inadequate, and defective mineralization.

The osteofluorotic changes appear to occur in three stages: (1) an acceleration of the remodeling rate in existing bone; (2) a dissociation of the normal sequences of osteogenesis, and (3) the production of abnormal bone.

Some of the bone changes that have been associated with excessive fluoride ingestion are the following: There may be zones or areas of abnormal porosity due to excessive resorption or accelerated remodeling. The alteration of osteogenesis due to fluoride toxicosis often results in the production of abnormal osteones of various sizes and shapes with a number of osteocytes arranged in a tangled mass near the periphery of the affected osteone. Abnormal canaliculi are associated with these clumped cells. There may be a few cells in the remainder of the osteone. The osteocytes may or may not appear abnormal. Figure 6(a) is a microradiograph of a normal bone, and Fig. 6(b) shows the disorganized appearance of fluoride-damaged bone. The degree of progressive structural bone changes due to excessive fluoride ingestion and their types and severity or combinations

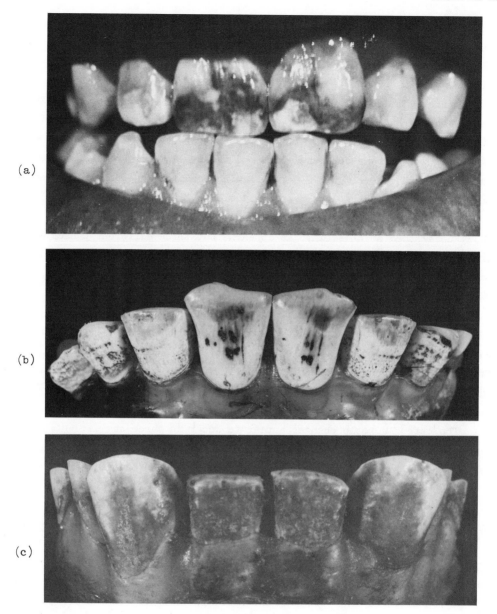

(a)

(b)

(c)

FIG. 4. Permanent incisor teeth with dental fluorosis: (a) human, (b) cattle, (c) sheep, (d) mule deer, (e) wapiti (elk), (f) bison (American buffalo).

(d)

(e)

(f)

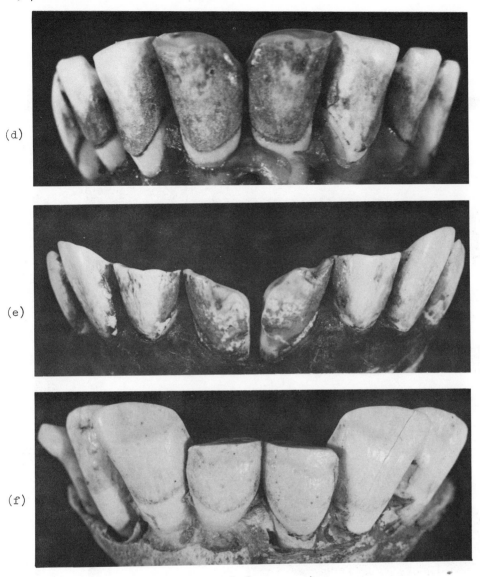

FIG. 4 (Continued)

are governed by the nine factors listed previously that influence the manifestations of fluoride toxicosis [24,25].

The amount of fluoride in different bones of the bovine skeleton varies
appreciably, with cancellous bones (such as those of the pelvis, head, ribs,

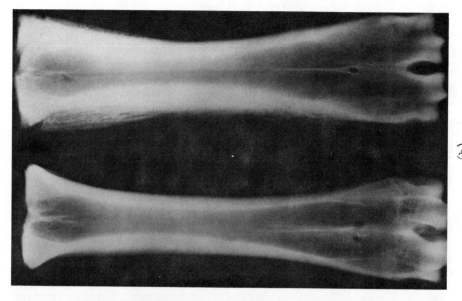

(b)

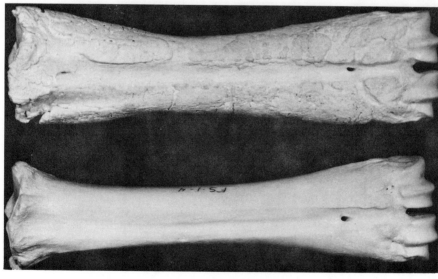

(a)

FIG. 5. Metatarsal bones from two cows of the same breed, size, and age. Left: normal, right: fluoride-induced osteofluorosis. Note normal-appearing articular surface. (a) Gross appearance, (b) radiographic appearance. (Reprinted with permission from Ref. 28.)

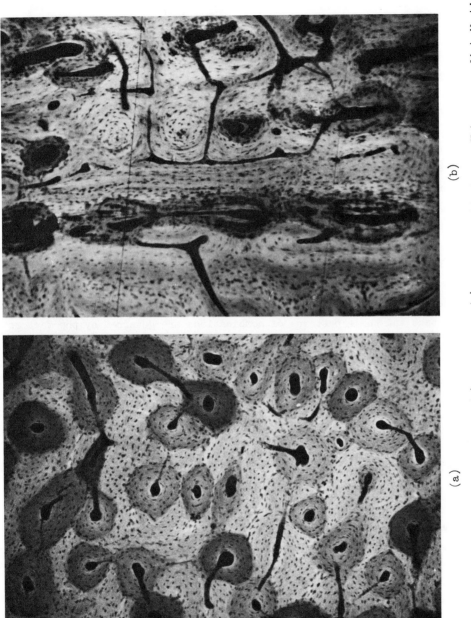

(b)

(a)

FIG. 6. Microradiographic appearance of (a) normal and (b) osteofluorotic bone. Note uneven distribution of variously sized, irregularly shaped osteocytes and osteones and interstitial changes in (b) (x 80).

and vertebrae) having higher fluoride contents than the more compact metacarpal and metatarsal bones. There is also a large variation in the fluoride
contents of different areas within some bones, such as the metacarpal or
metatarsal (the diaphyseal portion has a lower fluoride content than the
metaphyseal portion) [28]. It is extremely important, therefore, that
analysis of such bones be accompanied by a description of the method of
sampling and that the method of expressing these data (in terms of ash
weight or dry fat-free weight) be clearly indicated.

In experimental conditions where there is a constant and invariable
intake of fluoride, the amount of fluoride in the ration can be reasonably
estimated if the bone fluoride content and the period of exposure are known.
This cannot be assumed in field cases, which usually indicate varying amounts
of fluoride ingestion with differing degrees of dental lesions in range
cattle with similar bone fluoride concentrations [31,32,52]. Experiments
do indicate, however, that bone analysis is a good indication of total fluoride intake, but not necessarily of the concentration of fluoride in the
present rations [22,28].

The degree of progressive structural bone changes due to excessive fluoride intake and their patterns of combinations are governed by the factors
that influence the general degree and manifestation of fluoride toxicosis.
Some of the gross and histological changes induced by fluoride toxicosis
may resemble bone lesions and alterations that are associated with other
bone diseases. Therefore, the lesions observed must be carefully correlated with other lesions and signs in making a definitive diagnosis of
fluoride toxicosis [32,33].

Lameness and Stiffness

Stiffness and lameness are observed rather frequently in livestock.
Without supporting evidence, however, they are inconclusive measures of
fluoride toxicosis. In some severe cases, animals become progressively
worse and may eventually move around on their knees (Fig. 7). In most
cases, however, periods of stiffness and lameness are intermittent. The
complete cause and/or causes responsible for these locomotor difficulties
have not been determined, but they can deter the affected animals from
standing at the feeder or grazing. Subsequently, the reduced feed intake
may adversely reduce their levels of performance [34].

Crepitation, a sign of osteoarthritis, is not detectable in uncomplicated cases of fluoride toxicosis. Various degrees of osteoarthritis have

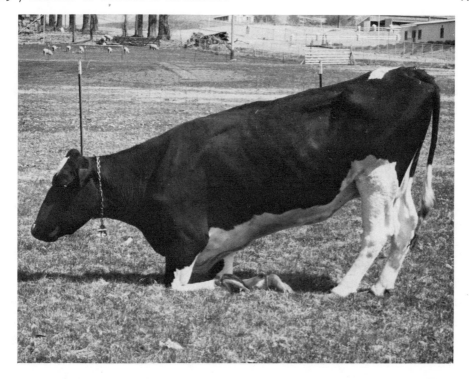

FIG. 7. Seven-year-old Holstein cow evidencing effects of severe fluoride toxicosis. Note posture because of extreme lameness. This cow had severe osteofluorosis.

been diagnosed in some field cases that were severely affected by fluorides. However, such arthritic changes and the signs of acute inflammatory arthritis, such as elevated body temperature, hot swollen joints, and suppressed ruminations, are not associated with the characteristic intermittent stiffness and lameness of advanced chronic fluoride toxicosis [48].

Osteoarthritic lesions are primarily intraarticular and may become secondarily periarticular.

Radiology

Radiographically in bones, porosis, sclerosis, hyperostosis, phytosis, malacia, or any combination of these conditions have been observed in animals that have ingested excessive levels of fluoride over long periods of time [15,24]. The radiographic findings vary, depending upon the interaction of factors influencing fluoride toxicosis.

Urine

A knowledge of the urinary fluoride concentration can be a useful diagnostic aid and to some extent can be correlated with dietary intake [29].
It is, however, affected by a number of important variables, including the
duration of fluoride ingestion, time of day the sampling is conducted, and
total urinary output. Because of variations in urinary output, results of
urinary fluoride analysis are usually expressed on a common specific gravity
basis, and are corrected to a specific gravity of 1.040.

Older animals often excrete more fluorides than do young animals raised
under the same conditions and ingesting the same amount of fluoride. This
occurs because bones of the older animals normally have a higher fluoride
content and so more fluoride is excreted.

Individual random samples of urine have little value for indicating
the fluoride intake of a herd of animals. Sufficient uncontaminated samples
should be taken at various intervals to ensure that they are representative
of the entire herd [29]. Urinary fluoride concentrations will remain high
for some time after the removal of animals from a high-fluoride ration [18,
36,53], and they are, therefore, not the best indicators of current exposure.

Under most conditions, specific gravity corrected values of less than
6 ppm F in the urine are considered normal.

Milk

The mammary gland is a minor source of fluoride excretion in animals
ingesting elevated amounts of fluoride. Even though the fluoride level in
milk rises slightly as the fluoride intake rises, not enough fluoride is
secreted in milk to constitute a health hazard under experimental conditions
[30].

Other Tissues

The ingestion of excessive amounts of fluoride by livestock will result
in increased concentrations of fluoride in blood, kidneys, and mineralizing
tissues. Recent advances in analytical methods have made it possible to
measure the plasma fluoride with sufficient accuracy to demonstrate a direct
correlation between fluoride intake and plasma fluoride concentration. This
does not appear to be a practical diagnostic aid, however.

Recovery from Fluoride Exposure

There have been only limited investigations of the response of animals
after they are removed from a diet containing excessive amounts of fluoride.
In these studies, a decline in the amount of skeletal fluoride has varied

from as low as 10% in 2 years to as much as 50% in a 4- to 5-year period.
Studies currently in progress have shown a loss in bone fluoride of 42% in
6 months and 66% in 24 months after Hereford cattle had accumulated 11,000
ppm fluoride in bone after a year's exposure and were removed to a low-fluoride ration. It appears that the percentage of fluoride loss varies inversely with the time it takes to reach a particular bone level. Animals
ingesting a high level of fluoride for a short time will be able to eliminate more fluoride during a subsequent recovery period than animals which
accumulate the same level over a longer period of time at a lower level of
intake.

Teeth that are formed after animals are removed from a high-fluoride
ration do not have dental fluorosis [31,32,49,50]. However, teeth which
have marked to severe fluoride lesions will continue to have an increased
rate of attrition in subsequent years [33].

Plasma fluoride concentrations drop to near normal a few days after
cattle are removed from a high-fluoride ration. Urinary fluoride concentrations decrease at a slower rate than plasma levels. There are periods
during which urinary fluoride concentrations do not reflect either current
intake or bone fluoride concentrations, and their use in diagnosis could be
very misleading unless properly interpreted.

The response of animals when moved from excessive to low levels of
fluoride intake thus depends on several factors. Each case should be indi-
vidually evaluated and the potential recovery rate considered. Caution
should be exercised in making a specific prognosis concerning subsequent
performance of animals after they have ingested damaging levels of fluoride.
When feed intake and performance are impaired as a result of molar abrasion,
there will be limited or questionable improvement after removal from a high-
fluoride ration [31-33]. However, if the described ration intake was due to
some metabolic effect, it will usually improve as the fluoride intake is
decreased.

OTHER EFFECTS

General Condition

Borderline cases of fluoride toxicosis may not be specific and thus
can be difficult to diagnose and evaluate. Certain signs and lesions due
to other causes may mimic some of the nonspecific signs and lesions of fluoride toxicosis [48] (see Table 2). The biological tolerances of various
animal species to fluoride are given in Table 2.

TABLE 2. Tolerance[a] of Animals for Fluoride (Concentration in Dry Matter in Ration)

Species	Breeding or Lactating Animals (ppm fluorine)[b]	Finishing Animals to Be Sold for Slaughter with Average Feeding Period (ppm fluorine)[b]
Dairy and beef heifers	30	100
Dairy cows	30	100
Beef cows	40	100
Steers	N.A.	100
Sheep	50	160
Horses	60	N.A.
Swine	70	N.D.
Turkeys	N.D.	100
Chickens	N.D.	150

[a]Tolerances based on sodium fluoride or other fluorides of similar toxicity.
[b]N.A.: not applicable; N.D.: not determined.

Appetite impairment resulting in general unthriftiness and loss of condition can be the result of excessive fluoride ingestion. Since many toxicities and deficiencies also result in impairment of feed intake, however, this criterion is not in itself a good diagnostic aid. Abnormal and excessive molar abrasion can also affect feed intake and utilization. A generalized unthriftiness characterized by dry hair and thick, nonpliable skin has been observed in animals with other unequivocal signs and lesions of fluoride toxicosis [28]. Reports of high incidences of diarrhea [54] have not been confirmed in controlled experimental studies or careful field investigations [28,30,38,45].

Diagnostic Aids

Signs and visible lesions sometimes are not definite enough to warrant an unequivocal diagnosis of fluoride toxicosis. Its subtle and insidious effects in some cases may interfere with normal performance and productivity. In such instances, or to substantiate a reasonably certain diagnosis, additional verification can be sought in several ways. When properly interpreted, urine analyses are useful diagnostic aids. Bone radiographs can supply valuable information. Biopsies or necropsies of properly selected cases can be used to obtain tissues for gross and histopathologic evaluations and chemical analyses for fluoride content. Correlation of signs, lesions, and chemical analyses of tissues with the ascertained fluoride contents of water and forage sources often can help substantiate suspected instances of fluoride toxicosis.

SUMMARY

Fluoride toxicosis in animals has become an important toxicologic problem in many parts of the world due to the expansion of certain types of industrial operations that emit excessive fluorides into the atmosphere in areas of animal habitat. Animals normally ingest low levels of fluoride with no adverse effects. Small amounts of fluoride may even have beneficial effects; but when excessive amounts are ingested for prolonged periods of time, adverse effects are induced.

Many sources may contribute to the total fluoride intake of animals. Various factors influence biologic responses of animals to excessive ingested fluorides. Signs and lesions of fluoride toxicosis in various species of animals are essentially similar. Fluoride standards and a comprehensive guide for use in diagnosing and evaluating fluoride toxicosis in animals are available. Prevention and control of fluoride toxicosis in animals can be achieved when the complexity of the disease is realized and the pathogenesis, symptomatology, and lesions are properly correlated, interpreted, and evaluated and when the source(s) of excessive fluorides are eliminated.

REFERENCES

1. H. Moissan, Le Fluor et ses Composés, Paris, 1900.

2. K. Roholm, Fluorine Intoxication. A Clinical-Hygienic Study with a Review of the Literature and Some Experimental Investigations (translated by W. E. Calvert), H. K. Lewis and Co., Ltd., London, 1937, pp. 1-364.

3. F. J. McClure, Water Fluoridation, in The Search and the Victory, National Institutes of Health, Public Health Service, Department of Health, Education and Welfare, Washington, D. C., 1970, pp. 29-35.

4. J. Velu, Le Darmous (ou Dermes) Fluorose Spontanée des Zones Phosphatées, Arch. Inst. Pasteur d'Algerie, 10, 41-118 (1932).

5. A.-P.-A. Rabuteau, Etude Experimentale sur les Effets Physiologiques des Fluorures et des Composés Metalliques en Général, Thèse, Paris, 1867.

6. C. Kuhns, Dtsch. Mschr. f. Zahnhlk., 6, 446 (1888).

7. E. Hupka and Götze, Zur Frage der Schädlichkeit des Fluors beim Rinde, Dtsch. Tierärztl. Wschr., 39, 203 (1931).

8. L. Slagsvold, Fluorforgiftning (German and English Summary), Norsk Vet. Tidsskr., 46, 2-16, 61-68 (1934).

9. Fluorides and Human Health, World Health Organization, Geneva, 1970.

10. J. L. Shupe, Fluorosis, International Encyclopedia of Veterinary Medicine, Vol. II, Sweet & Maxwell, London, 1966, pp. 1062-1068.

11. H. H. Messer, W. D. Armstrong, and L. Singer, Fertility Impairment in Mice on a Low Fluoride Intake, Science, 177, 893-894 (1972).

12. H. H. Messer, K. Wong, M. Wegner, L. Singer, and W. D. Armstrong, Effect of Reduced Fluoride Intake by Mice on Hematocrit Values, Nature New Biol., 240, 218-219 (1972).

13. K. Schwarz and D. B. Milne, Fluorine Requirement for Growth in the Rat, Bioinorg. Chem., 1, 331-338 (1972).

14. D. S. Bernstein and Phin Cohen, Use of Sodium Fluoride in the Treatment of Osteoporosis, J. Clin. Endocrinol., 27, 197-210 (1967).

15. N. C. Leone, C. A. Stevenson, T. F. Hilbish, and M. C. Sosman, A Roentgenographic Study of Human Population Exposed to High Fluoride Domestic Water: A 10-Year Study, Amer. J. Roentgen., 74, 874-885 (1955).

16. D. R. Taves, New Approach to the Treatment of Bone Disease with Fluoride, Fed. Proc., 29, 1185-1187 (1970).

17. Fluoridation Census, 1969, U.S. Department of Health, Education, and Welfare, Public Health Service, National Institutes of Health, Bethesda, 1970.

18. F. Blakemore, T. J. Bosworth, and H. H. Green, Industrial Fluorosis of Farm Animals in England, Attributable to the Manufacture of Bricks, the Calcining of Ironstone, and to the Enameling Process, J. Comp. Pathol., 58, 267-301 (1948).

19. J. L. Shupe, Fluorine Toxicosis and Industry, Amer. Ind. Hyg. Ass. J., 31, 240-247 (1970).

20. G. M. Merriman and C. S. Hobbs, Bovine Fluorosis from Soil and Water Sources, Tenn. Univ. Agric. Exp. Sta. Bull. No. 347, 1962, pp. 1-46.

21. J. W. Suttie, Fluoride Content of Commercial Dairy Concentrates and Alfalfa Forage, J. Agr. Food Chem., 17, 1350-1352 (1969).

22. J. L. Shupe, M. L. Miner, L. E. Harris, and D. A. Greenwood, Relative Effects of Feeding Hay Atmospherically Contaminated by Fluoride Residue, Normal Hay Plus Calcium Fluoride, and Normal Hay Plus Sodium Fluoride to Dairy Heifers, Amer. J. Vet. Res., 23, 777-787 (1962).

23. I. Zipkin, R. C. Likins, F. J. McClure, and A. C. Steere, Urinary Fluoride Levels Associated with the Use of Fluoridated Waters, Public Health Rep., 71, 767-772 (1956).

24. J. L. Shupe and E. W. Alther, The Effects of Fluorides on Livestock, with Particular Reference to Cattle, Handbook of Environmental Pharmacology, Vol. 20, Part 1 (O. Eichler, A. Farah, H. Herken, A. D. Welch, and F. A. Smith, eds.), Springer Verlag, New York, 1966, pp. 307-354.

25. L. C. Johnson, Histogenesis and Mechanisms in the Development of Osteofluorosis, Fluorine Chemistry (H. C. Hodge and F. A. Smith), Vol. IV (J. H. Simons, ed.), Academic, New York, 1965, pp. 424-441.

26. I. Schour and M. C. Smith, The Histologic Changes in the Enamel and Dentine of the Rat Incisor in Acute and Chronic Experimental Fluorosis. Arizona Agr. Exp. Sta. Tech. Bull. No. 52, University of Arizona, Tucson, 1934, pp. 69-91.

27. I. Zipkin, E. D. Eanes, and J. L. Shupe, Effect of Prolonged Exposure to Fluoride on the Ash, Fluoride, Citrate, and Crystallinity of Bovine Bone, Amer. J. Vet. Res., 25, 1591-1597 (1964).

28. J. L. Shupe, M. L. Miner, D. A. Greenwood, L. E. Harris, and G. E. Stoddard, The Effect of Fluorine on Dairy Cattle: II. Clinical and Pathologic Effects, Amer. J. Vet. Res., 24, 964-984 (1963).

29. J. L. Shupe, L. E. Harris, D. A. Greenwood, J. E. Butcher, and H. M. Nielsen, The Effect of Fluorine on Dairy Cattle: V. Fluorine in the Urine as an Estimate of Fluorine Intake, Amer. J. Vet. Res., 24, 300-306 (1963).

30. D. A. Greenwood, J. L. Shupe, G. E. Stoddard, L. E. Harris, H. M. Nielsen, and L. E. Olson, Fluorosis in Cattle, Utah Agr. Exp. Sta. Spec. Rep. 17, Utah State University, Logan, 1964, pp. 1-36.

31. J. L. Shupe, Diagnosis of Fluorosis in Cattle (Guest, Introductory Lecture: Fourth International World Congress for Diseases of Cattle), Publ. der IV. Internationalen Tagang der Weltgesellschaft für Buiatrik, Zurich, Switzerland, 1966, pp. 4-9, 1-18.

32. J. L. Shupe, Fluorosis: Bovine Medicine and Surgery, American Veterinary Publications, Wheaton, Ill., 1970, pp. 288-301.

33. J. L. Shupe and A. E. Olson, Clinical Aspects of Fluorosis in Horses, J. Amer. Vet. Med. Ass., 158 (2), 167-174 (1971).

34. G. E. Stoddard, G. Q. Bateman, L. E. Harris, J. L. Shupe, and D. A. Greenwood, Effects of Fluorine on Dairy Cattle: IV. Milk Production, J. Dairy Sci., 46, 720-726 (1963).

35. J. N. Agate, G. H. Bell, G. F. Boddie, R. G. Bowler, M. Buckell, E. A. Cheesman, T. H. J. Douglas, H. A. Druett, J. Garrad, D. Hunter, K. M. A. Perry, J. D. Richardson, and J. B. de V. Weir, Industrial Fluorosis: A Study of the Hazard to Man and Animals Near Fort William, Scotland, A Report to the Fluorosis Committee, Med. Res. Council Memo. No. 22, His Majesty's Stationery Office, London, 1949, pp. 1-131.

36. R. Allcroft, K. N. Burns, and C. N. Hebert, Fluorosis in Cattle. II. Development and Alleviation: Experimental Studies, Ministry of Agriculture, Fisheries and Food, Animal Disease, Surveys Report No. 2, Part II, Her Majesty's Stationery Office, London, 1965, pp. 1-58.

37. H. J. Schmidt, G. W. Newell, and W. E. Rand, The Controlled Feeding of Fluorine, as Sodium Fluoride, to Dairy Cattle, Amer. J. Vet. Res., 15, 232-239 (1954).

38. J. Suttie and P. H. Phillips, Studies of the Effects of Dietary Sodium Fluoride on Dairy Cows: V. A 3-Year Study on Mature Animals, J. Dairy Sci., 42, 1063-1069 (1959).

39. R. Allcroft and J. S. L. Jones, Fluoroacetamide Poisoning: I. Toxicity in Dairy Cattle: Clinical History and Preliminary Investigation, Vet. Rec., 84, 399-402 (1969).

40. R. Allcroft, F. J. Salt, R. A. Peters, and M. Shorthouse, Fluoroacetamide Poisoning: II. Toxicity in Dairy Cattle, Confirmation of Diagnosis, Vet. Rec., 84, 403-409 (1969).

41. Effects of Fluorides in Animals, National Academy of Sciences, National Research Council, Washington, D. C., 1974, pp. 1-70.

42. O. Krug, Eine Vergiftung von Milchkühen durch Kieselfluornatrium, Z. Fleisch- u. Milchhyg., 37, 38-39 (1927).

43. N. C. Leone, E. F. Geever, and N. C. Moran, Acute and Subacute Toxicity Studies of Sodium Fluoride in Animals, Public Health Rep., 71, 459-467 (1956).

44. J. S. Cass, Fluorides: A Critical Review: IV. Response of Livestock and Poultry to Absorption of Inorganic Fluorides, J. Occup. Med., 3, 471-477, 527-543 (1961).

45. K. N. Burns and R. Allcroft, Fluorosis in Cattle: 1. Occurrence and Effects in Industrial Areas of England and Wales 1954-57, Ministry of Agriculture, Fisheries and Food, Animal Disease Surveys Report No. 2, Part I, Her Majesty's Stationery Office, London, 1964, pp. 1-51.

46. C. S. Hobbs and G. M. Merriman, Fluorosis in Beef Cattle, Tenn. Agr. Exp. Sta. Bull. No. 351, University of Tennessee, Knoxville, 1962, pp. 1-183.

47. P. H. Phillips, E. B. Hart, and G. Bohstedt, Chronic Toxicosis in Dairy Cows Due to the Ingestion of Fluorine, Wisc. Agr. Exp. Sta. Res. Bull. No. 123, University of Wisconsin, Madison, 1934, pp. 1-30.

48. J. L. Shupe, Arthritis in Cattle, Can. Vet. J., 2 (10), 369-376 (1961).

49. W. A. B. Brown, P. V. Christofferson, M. Massler, and M. B. Weiss, Postnatal Tooth Development in Cattle, Amer. J. Vet. Res., 21, 7-34 (1960).

50. N. L. Garlick, The Teeth of the Ox in Clinical Diagnosis: IV. Dental Fluorosis, Amer. J. Vet. Res., 16, 38-44 (1955).

51. G. W. Miller and J. L. Shupe, Alkaline Bone Phosphatase Activity as Related to Fluoride Ingestion by Dairy Cattle, Amer. J. Vet. Res., 23 (92), 24-31 (1962).

52. F. N. Mortensen, L. G. Transtrum, W. P. Peterson, and W. S. Winters, Dental Changes as Related to Fluorine Content of Teeth and Bones of Cattle, J. Dairy Sci., 47, 186-191 (1964).

53. P. H. Phillips, J. W. Suttie, and E. J. Zebrowski, Effects of Dietary Sodium Fluoride on Dairy Cows: VII. Recovery from Fluoride Ingestion, J. Dairy Sci., 46, 513-516 (1963).

54. D. H. Udall and K. P. Keller, A Report of Fluorosis in Cattle in the Columbia River Valley, Cornell Vet., 42, 159-184 (1952).

TOXICITY OF BERYLLIUM AND OTHER
ELEMENTS IN MISSILE PROPELLANTS

Farrel R. Robinson[*]
Armed Forces Institute of Pathology
Washington, D. C.

"Beryllium disease" has been known since 1933. It became of prominence in the United States in the late 1940s, when it was associated with a disease of workers in the fluorescent lamp industry. Currently, beryllium is used experimentally as a missile propellant, in high-performance aerospace craft, and for other industrial purposes. Beryllium is an expensive metal and, in some of its forms, is quite toxic.

At one time beryllium-powered motors were used in the United States, but the effluent was trapped and not discharged into the general environment. Later small motors were fired in the western states without entrapment. When it was proposed that larger beryllium motors were to be employed, local governments brought political pressure and public opinion to bear, causing a cessation of firings within the continental limits of the United States. These motors were subsequently tested on remote Pacific islands.

Until recent years industrial exposures have been the topic of most importance. More recently, however, the emphasis has shifted away from purely industrial exposures to concern for general environmental contamination as the result of new uses of beryllium.

HISTORICAL BACKGROUND

Beryllium disease was first recognized in Germany in 1933, in the U.S.S.R. in 1936, and in the United States in the 1940s. It was initially thought that the toxicity of beryllium was related only to the acute disease,

[*]Present Affiliation: Purdue University School of Veterinary Medicine, West Lafayette, Indiana.

which was self-limiting if the patient was removed from the contaminated
environment. Dermatitis, conjunctivitis, and inflammation of various points
of the respiratory tract were observed with exposure to a high concentration
of beryllium.

The chronic disease was described much later. It often developed long
after the exposure ceased and was characterized by a granulomatous interstitial pneumonitis. Frequently, other tissues such as skin, liver, lymph
nodes, and muscle were also involved.

Some chronic cases of beryllium disease have not been diagnosed until
many years following the initial exposure. There are some cases in which
the initial exposure to beryllium is not known or documented. The mechanism
of the variable latency may depend on immunologic or hormonal factors, as
suggested by exacerbations of symptoms during pregnancy.

There are over 700 cases of beryllium disease in the beryllium case
registry [1]. Many of these arose as a result of the use of beryllium
phosphors in the fluorescent lamp industry in the 1940s [2,3]. The acute
disease was soon associated with these phosphors, and industrial precaution-
ary measures were taken to eliminate the possibility of human exposure to
beryllium-containing compounds. After 1950, many workers still became ill
as the result of exposures in extraction, metallurgical, or metal-working
operations [4]. The incidence of cases has declined rapidly since 1950,
probably because of improved industrial hygiene practices. However, there
are apparently enough acute and chronic cases of recent onset to establish
that the disease is of more than purely historical interest.

Not only do workers in industry develop beryllium disease, but there
are also those known as "neighborhood" cases. These are persons with evidence of close contact either with a beryllium worker or with a worker's
clothes or with a history of time spent close to one of the plants. Trace
levels of beryllium are also found in many environmental materials [5].

DIAGNOSIS OF THE DISEASE

The diagnosis of beryllium disease is often difficult and is based on
two sets of criteria, one epidemiologic and the other clinical. The epidemiologic criterion is a significant beryllium exposure, i.e., an exposure
to beryllium or its toxic compounds that has produced illness in others.
The clinical criteria include (1) diffuse densities on roentgenograms, with
or without symptoms; (2) patterns of respiratory insufficiency initially

characterized by reduction in lung volumes and/or diffusion capacity with later obstructive defect, depending on the degree of fibrosis; (3) interstitial pneumonitis, usually granulomatous, determined by examination of pulmonary biopsy or autopsy specimens; (4) systemic toxicity demonstrated by functional or pathologic abnormalities in other tissues; and (5) beryllium in tissues [6]. A diagnosis consists of the determination of significant exposure and the finding of at least the first two clinical criteria [6]. The demonstration of beryllium in pulmonary tissue is also contributory.

Beryllium may be absorbed by routes other than respiratory, but deposition in the pulmonary tract is the principal way in which its compounds are absorbed in man. Granulomas appear clinically and can be induced experimentally in tissues other than pulmonary. Beryllium can also be distributed from the lungs to other organs after absorption. The different forms of beryllium are not equally toxic, and the relative toxicity of various inhaled forms of beryllium has been demonstrated. Soluble forms are responsible for the acute disease, and there is general agreement that exposure to beryllium oxide, which is relatively insoluble, can result in chronic toxicity. Exposure to fumes and the dust of beryllium alloys has resulted in disease with metallurgical and metal-working operations [4]. Beryllium disease in the industrial setting is presumably related to beryllium or its oxides and not to other constituents of alloys. Beryl, an ore form of beryllium, has not been reported to cause disease in man; it is found in coal and other sources. This is one source of the inert beryllium in tissues that is a confusing factor in the interpretation of tissue analyses.

Experimental evidence indicates that beryl causes pulmonary tumors in rats [7], suggesting that the records of beryl mine workers should be reviewed for the possibility of disease conditions related to this ore.

EXPERIMENTAL STUDIES

Differences in toxicity between high-fired and low-fired beryllium oxides have been demonstrated [8]. The high-fired oxide (calcined at 1600° C) has crystals of 1500 Å, is poorly soluble in acid, and in animals is retained nearly completely in the lungs in a presumably relatively inert form. The low-fired oxide (calcined at 500° C) has 150 Å crystallites, is soluble in hydrochloric acid, and is much more readily translocated in the body. Pul-

monary tumors have been reported in rats exposed to the high-fired material,
although much less frequently than in those exposed to the low-fired oxide
[8]. The beryllium-powered motor burns at a very high temperature, resulting
in the production of oxides similar to the high-fired beryllium oxides.
Pulmonary tumors have also been produced in rats breathing beryllium sulfate
[9,10].

Pulmonary tumors have been induced in monkeys chronically exposed to
beryllium sulfate [11] and beryllium oxide [12]. In addition, osteosarcomas
have developed in rabbits given injections of beryllium compounds [13,14].
Although neoplasia in animals can be related to beryllium exposure, a causal
relationship of pulmonary neoplasia to inhaled beryllium in man has not yet
been established [12].

Pulmonary granulomas developed in two beagle dogs killed 30 months after
exposure to a rocket exhaust containing beryllium oxide and in two other
beagles killed 36 months after exposure to a mixture of beryllium oxide,
beryllium fluoride, and beryllium chloride [15]. Beryllium was demonstrated
in pulmonary granulomas in these dogs by means of the laser microprobe and
emission spectroscopy [15]. The ability to detect minute amounts of beryllium in tissue sections of necropsy and biopsy material is a significant
aid in the diagnosis of both the acute and chronic forms of beryllium disease [16]. Tissues of the latter two dogs were examined on the ultrastructural level and appeared to exhibit primarily the typical reaction of the
lung to a foreign body. There was a significant increase in septal collagen
with little evidence of an immunologic response [17].

Later studies with monkeys and dogs exposed to a different beryllium-
containing exhaust product revealed no evidence of beryllium-induced disease
2 years after exposure [18]. These studies are continuing in order to include examination 5 years or more after exposure.

Conventional spectrographic analysis of lung tissue removed at autopsy
from persons who have had no known industrial exposure to beryllium may
reveal concentrations of beryllium as high as 1.98 µg/100 g of tissue [19].
Experimental evidence indicates that the microemission spectrographic technique is best used in conjunction with conventional spectrography [20].
The latter provides data on the average beryllium content on the basis of
micrograms per 100 g of tissue, while the microemission spectrographic
technique allows the localization of the beryllium to microscopic areas if
the beryllium has been concentrated to at least 50 µg/g. This information

can then be correlated with clinical data and histopathologic lesions in support of a diagnosis of chronic berylliosis.

OTHER ELEMENTS

Boron compounds have been used as high-energy fuels in rocket motors, but they are not employed at the present time nor are they apparently being considered for immediate future use. The boron hydrides, particularly decaborane and pentaborane, were the compounds previously used and they were quite toxic [21,22]. These compounds were expensive and presented no distinct advantages over cheaper and simpler propulsion-system fuels. Signs of decaborane toxicity include central nervous system signs and symptoms, such as dizziness, weakness, headache, tremors, and involuntary contractions of muscles.

Four exhaust products from beryllium-motor firings were analyzed for beryllium and other elements [8]. While beryllium oxide was the chief component in all four samples, many other elements were also identified by emission spectroscopy: aluminum, copper, iron, magnesium, manganese, nickel, and silicon. Other elements identified in the water-soluble fraction were boron, chromium, lead, tin, sodium, titanium, zinc, and silver. Rats were exposed to these samples, and beryllium was the only element to which toxicity could be related [8].

One author, in studying tissues from 58 cases of possible chronic berylliosis, suspected the presence of excessive amounts of certain elements in tissues as the result of unknown environmental exposures. These elements were boron, strontium, barium, chromium, vanadium, copper, silver, and lead [23].

SUMMARY

At present there does not appear to be an extensive problem of general environmental contamination from beryllium compounds or other elements related to missile propellants. Various beryllium compounds have been and are continuing to be studied to define their toxic properties. Unless there is a change in national policy to permit beryllium-powered rocket motors to be fired within the continental United States, the most likely application of this information is in the field of industrial toxicology and general environmental contamination from industrial uses.

REFERENCES

1. H. L. Hardy, New Engl. J. Med., 273, 1188 (1963).

2. F. R. Dutra, Amer. J. Pathol., 24, 1137 (1948).

3. D. G. Freiman and H. L. Hardy, Human Pathol., 1, 25 (1970).

4. J. Lieben, J. Occup. Med., 11, 480 (1969).

5. W. R. Meehan and L. E. Smythe, Environ. Sci. Technol., 1, 839 (1967).

6. J. D. Stoeckle, H. L. Hardy, and A. L. Weber, Amer. J. Med., 46, 545 (1969).

7. W. D. Wagner, D. H. Groth, J. L. Holz, G. E. Madden, and H. E. Stokinger, Toxicol. Appl. Pharm., 15, 10 (1969).

8. H. C. Spencer, S. E. Sadek, J. C. Jones, R. H. Hook, J. A. Blumenshine, and S. B. McCollister, AMRL-TR-67-46, June 1967, Aerospace Medical Research Laboratories, Wright-Patterson AFB, Ohio.

9. A. L. Reeves and A. J. Vorwald, Cancer Res., 27, 446 (1967).

10. A. J. Vorwald and A. L. Reeves, Arch. Ind. Health, 19, 190 (1959).

11. A. J. Vorwald, in Use of Nonhuman Primates in Drug Evaluation, Symposium (H. Vagtborg, ed.), University of Texas Press, Austin, 1968.

12. A. J. Vorwald, A. L. Reeves, and E. C. J. Urban, in Beryllium: Its Industrial Hygiene Aspects (H. E. Stokinger, ed.), Academic, New York, 1966.

13. E. Tapp, Arch. Pathol., 88, 89 (1969).

14. E. Tapp, Arch. Pathol., 88, 521 (1969).

15. J. R. Prine, S. F. Brokeshoulder, D. E. McVean, and F. R. Robinson, Amer. J. Clin. Pathol., 45, 488 (1966).

16. S. F. Brokeshoulder, F. R. Robinson, A. A. Thomas, and J. Cholak, Amer. Ind. Hyg. Ass. J., 27, 496 (1966).

17. F. R. Robinson, F. Schaffner, and E. Trachtenberg, Arch. Environ. Health, 17, 193 (1968).

18. C. Conradi, P. H. Burri, Y. Kapanci, F. R. Robinson, and E. R. Weibel, Arch. Environ. Health, 23, 348 (1971).

19. J. Cholak, Arch. Ind. Health, 19, 123 (1959).

20. F. R. Robinson, S. F. Brokeshoulder, A. A. Thomas, and J. Cholak, Amer. J. Clin. Pathol., 49, 821 (1968).

21. L. L. Foster and W. N. Scott, SAM-TR-67-103, USAF School of Aerospace Medicine, Brooks Air Force Base, Texas, October 1967.

22. J. H. Merritt, Review 3-66, USAF School of Aerospace Medicine, Brooks Air Force Base, Texas, June 1966.

23. G. W. H. Schepers, Diseases Chest, 42, 600 (1962).

THE LESSER METALS

Robert P. Beliles
Litton Bionetics, Inc.
Kensington, Maryland

This chapter is devoted to metallic elements that are presumably less hazardous from a toxicologic point of view. The exposure to these metals in the industrial, medical, or environmental sense may be small. The scientific documentation of their effects is more voluminous than that of lead, mercury, and cadmium, which have been covered in other chapters. Not all of the elemental metals to be discussed in this chapter fit clearly into one of the above categories. For example, aluminum, included in this chapter, is the third most abundant element in the earth's crust. Iron is also included, but the frequency of accidental iron poisoning from overdoses is significant; also the average human daily intake is approximately 3000 times larger than that of mercury. In addition, this chapter deals with uranium, a relatively rare metal with respect to its concentration in the earth's crust or in the total body burden (based on a 70-kg man). Uranium has one of the smallest body burdens of the metallic elements. However, our knowledge of uranium with respect to its hazards and experimental toxicity is well documented.

The presence of a metal in the environment, through natural occurrence or contamination, where knowledge is sufficient, is reviewed. The industrial exposure and hazards, if known, are discussed with regard to each element. The use and exposure in cosmetics and drugs are also mentioned if the form is a frequent source of accidental poisoning.

The ethical and medicinal use of a metal, while not directly related to environmental toxicity, is also discussed. This use of metals is generally decreasing with the advent of more sophisticated organic materials, although lithium might be considered an exception to this general trend in

IA								VIII		IB	IIB					VIIA	Zero
1 H	IIA											IIIA	IVA	VA	VIA	1 H	2 He
3 Li	4 Be											5 B	6 C	7 N	8 O	9 F	10 Ne
11 Na	12 Mg	IIIB	IVB	VB	VIB	VIIB						13 Al	14 Si	15 P	16 S	17 Cl	18 Ar
19 K	20 Ca	21 Sc	22 Ti	23 V	24 Cr	25 Mn	26 Fe	27 Co	28 Ni	29 Cu	30 Zn	31 Ga	32 Ge	33 As	34 Se	35 Br	36 Kr
37 Rb	38 Sr	39 Y	40 Zr	41 Nb	42 Mo	43 Tc	44 Ru	45 Rh	46 Pd	47 Ag	48 Cd	49 In	50 Sn	51 Sb	52 Te	53 I	54 Xe
55 Cs	56 Ba	57 *La	72 Hf	73 Ta	74 W	75 Re	76 Os	77 Ir	78 Pt	79 Au	80 Hg	81 Tl	82 Pb	83 Bi	84 Po	85 At	86 Rn
87 Fr	88 Ra	89 #Ac															

*LANTHANIDE SERIES	58 Ce	59 Pr	60 Nd	61 Pm	62 Sm	63 Eu	64 Gd	65 Tb	66 Dy	67 Ho	68 Er	69 Tm	70 Yb	71 Lu
#ACTINIDE SERIES	90 Th	91 Pa	92 U	93 Np	94 Pu	95 Am	96 Cm	97 Bk	98 Cf	99 Es	100 Fm	101 Md	102 No	103 Lr

FIG. 1. Periodic table of the elements.

medicine. Furthermore, the medical experience often provides an insight into the type of toxicity one should expect following absorption or excessive exposure as well as an understanding of the distribution in the human body. The main emphasis is on the toxicity to man. Experimental data are presented to provide a basis for ascertaining the possible hazard.

In considering toxicity, one must rightly evaluate safety. The safety of man in an industrial setting has apparently received the most consideration. The concentrations in the work area to which man might be safely exposed have been suggested by the American Conference of Government Industrial Hygienists (ACGIH). These values, known as threshold limit values (TLV), based on an average 40-hr work week, are continually being revised; and those used in this chapter are related to the extent of our knowledge at the present time [1].

The discussion of elements included in this chapter is in relation to the periodic table (Fig. 1). This table may be of some help in organizing one's thoughts and providing an interesting basis for comparison in many instances.

THE ALKALINE METALS (GROUP IA)

This group of elements composed of lithium (Li), sodium (Na), potassium (K), rubidium (Rb), cesium (Cs), and francium (Fr) are all reactive chemically and never occur as free metals in nature. Sodium and potassium have great physiological importance. However, except in certain disease

states or after massive doses which might overwhelm the physiological homeostatic mechanism, they are of little toxicological significance. Francium
occurs only at trace levels in uranium ores and is a radioactive material
with a short half-life. Thus, only lithium, rubidium, and cesium are considered.

Lithium

The pure metal never occurs in nature; but salts, especially as silicates, are common. The concentration in the earth's crust is 30 ppm.
Lithium is used in alloys, as a catalytic agent, in heat exchangers for air
conditioning systems, and as a lubricant. Lithium hydride is used in manufacturing electronic tubes and ceramics and in chemical synthesis. Lithium
salts have been used as a sodium chloride substitute in low-sodium diets and
recently used medicinally in the treatment of manic depressive illness.

Lithium's similarity to sodium and potassium, two other members of
periodic table Group IA, accounts for many of its characteristic actions:
physiologic, pharmacologic, and toxicologic. However, lithium is not considered an essential element; and only recently has there been a suggestion
of a deficiency disease. Regional epidemiologic studies have indicated an
inverse correlation between atherosclerotic heart disease and levels of
lithium in water. The lithium content of water and vegetables varies from
region to region and is related to the hardness of water [2]. The presence
of lithium has been verified in many plant and animal tissues, and the daily
intake is estimated to be about 2 mg.

Lithium salts are almost completely absorbed from the gastrointestinal
tract and excreted in the urine. Lithium ion is more evenly distributed
throughout the body water than either sodium or potassium. The peak serum
concentration of lithium after oral ingestion occurs in about 30 min and
plateaus in 12-24 hr. Lithium ion crosses the cell boundary slowly. This
may account for the delay of 6-10 days in achieving full therapeutic response and the delay of excretion. The excretion is biphasic with an initial phase of 24 hr half-time followed by slower excretion of the remainder
of the dose in 10-14 days. In the glomeruli and proximal tubule lithium is
handled almost identically to sodium. Extracellular volume reduction by
sodium depletion will increase reabsorption of both Na^+ and Li^+. Thus, Li^+
reabsorption probably explains the severe lithium toxicity when it is used
as a taste substitute for NaCl in low-sodium diets and the lithium toxicity
induced after Na^+ depletion. The distal tubules do not reabsorb significant
amounts of lithium [3].

Neither the amounts of lithium normally ingested in food and water nor the occupational exposures to lithium salts (except for lithium hydride) result in toxicity. Inhalation of lithium hydride irritates the throat and lungs because of the formation of hydroxides and their caustic action on moist surfaces. Eye and skin irritation may also occur for the same reason [4]. The TLV for lithium hydride is 0.025 mg/m^3 [1].

The toxicity of lithium salts may occur as a consequence of therapy or as an accidental oral ingestion. These effects are related to the imperfect substitution of lithium for other cations (Na$^+$, K$^+$) that normally affect proper electrochemical gradients and maintain osmotic balance. Additional effects of lithium are caused when it affects cellular homeostatic balance.

The therapeutic use of lithium carbonate produces unusual sequelae of toxicity. These include neuromuscular changes (tremor, muscle hyperirritability, and ataxia), central nervous system changes (blackout spells, epileptic seizures, slurred speech, coma, psychosomatic retardation, and increased thirst), cardiovascular changes (cardiac arrhythmia, hypertension, and circulatory collapse), gastrointestinal changes (anorexia, nausea, and vomiting), and renal damage (albuminuria and glycosuria). These changes appear to be more frequent when the serum levels increase above 1.6 mequiv/l. Thyrotoxic reactions, including goiter formation, have also been suggested [5]. There is clinical evidence to suggest that some of the neurological effects may be irreversible [6]. Neither the mechanism of these changes nor the mechanism of beneficial effects of lithium is completely understood at this time. Incomplete ion substitution coupled with interference with cyclic AMP-mediated processes plus hormonal activity and secretion probably combine to bring on the sequelae of lithium toxicity.

Careful monitoring and control of serum lithium levels when used in therapy should be the rule. Several cases of serious lithium intoxication at constant levels of intake have resulted from loss of sodium due to vomiting or severe reduction of sodium intake due to food refusal. Diphenylhydantoin was used successfully to control convulsions which resulted [7]. Hemodialysis has also been used in the management of lithium intoxication [6].

While there has been some indication of adverse effects on fetuses following lithium treatment, none were observed in rats (4.05 mequiv/kg), rabbits (1.08 mequiv/kg), or primates (0.67 mequiv/kg). This dose to rats was sufficient to produce maternal toxicity and effects on the pups of treated, lactating dams [8]. In other studies with possibly higher serum lithium levels, cleft palate, eye defects, and auricular defects have been demonstrated in rats and mice [9].

Based on 118 children born to mothers receiving lithium treatment during the first trimester of pregnancy, it was concluded that the risk in women was not so high as suggested by the studies in rats and mice [10]. It must be assumed that excessive lithium serum levels may still present difficulties. Careful monitoring of lithium serum levels is required even in late pregnancy and after delivery because renal lithium clearance is higher during pregnancy than after [11]. Women on lithium treatment should avoid nursing as it has been shown that the serum concentration of the children is about one-third to one-half the concentration of their mothers' [12].

Rubidium

Rubidium is found in the earth's crust at a level of 120 ppm. Rubidium is produced as a by-product of potassium and molybdenum production. Its chief industrial use is in the manufacture of photoelectric cells.

Biologically, rubidium seems to be an acceptable substitute for potassium in many physiological processes. While rubidium will prevent the kidney and muscle lesions characteristic of potassium depletion, there is no evidence that rubidium itself is an essential element. It is widespread in nature at trace levels, and it is found in beef, grains, milk, fruits, and vegetables at significant levels [13].

The average daily intake is about 10 mg and the body burden is 1200 mg [14]. Rubidium is fairly well absorbed orally and resembles potassium in its pattern of distribution and excretion. The highest concentrations are in the heart and skeletal muscles, while bone contains almost none. The muscle acts as the primary storage site under conditions of excess. In the blood the largest amount is partitioned in the red blood cells. The urine is the major route of excretion.

Purified diets containing up to 200 ppm Rb were not toxic in rats. Levels of 1000 ppm decreased growth, reproductive performance, and survival time [13].

The recent use of lithium, another alkali metal, in the treatment of manic episodes in manic-depressive psychosis has revived interest in the possible therapeutic use of rubidium. The initial impression was that since rubidium and lithium have many antagonistic actions, rubidium might have useful pharmacologic properties. Historically, rubidium salts have been used in the treatment of cardiovascular disease, epilepsy, and other nervous system disorders and as a hypnotic. Parenteral administration of rubidium does induce behavioral changes (aggressiveness in experimental animals) [15]. However, oral administration of rubidium chloride produced gastrointestinal irritation at about 50 mg Rb/kg in dogs. Results from rat studies further suggest possible kidney and hematological changes [16]. In man a single oral administration of 0.5-1.0 g of rubidium produced plasma levels of 0.014-0.041 mequiv/l per 8.2 mequiv ingested. The half-life was long (50-60 days). In repeated dose studies no adverse effects were produced, but the maximum plasma rubidium levels were less than 0.40 mequiv/l. Results with regard to the potassium balance aspect of this study confirmed animal data suggesting that total body potassium is replaced by rubidium approximately mequiv for mequiv following excessive oral ingestion [17]. The desired pharmacologic antidepressant effect could not be substantiated in this study.

Cesium

Cesium occurs in nature as pollucite, a hydrous cesium-aluminum silicate. The concentration in the earth's crust is low (1 ppm). Its main industrial uses are as a catalyst in the polymerization of resin-forming materials and in photoelectric cells. It is useful in this respect because the range of sensitivity is approximately that of the human eye. Radioactive cesium is a constituent of nuclear fallout.

Ingested cesium salts are absorbed and cesium is bound within the cells of the soft tissues such as kidney and muscle. However, because of its scarcity in nature, the human body burden is less than 0.01 mg. It is in the red blood cells and may, in some circumstances, be able to replace potassium. The urine is the main route of excretion. Increased potassium levels facilitate cesium excretion. The radioactive material is found in milk.

No cases of industrial injury related to the chemical toxicity of cesium have been reported. It must be assumed that (indefinite) replacement of potassium by cesium would produce ill effects, probably neuromuscular in nature, as demonstrated in experimental animals [18].

A TLV for cesium hydroxide of 2 mg/m^3 has been proposed [1]. This is because of its basic and corrosive nature.

ALKALINE EARTH METALS

Beryllium (Be), magnesium (Mg), calcium (Ca), strontium (Sr), barium (Ba), and radium (Ra) compose Group IIA of the periodic table. Beryllium is discussed in Chapter 24. Calcium as an essential element plays numerous physiological roles; but because of its homeostatic regulation, harmful effects are rare and tend to occur only infrequently as in cases involving overloading of the regulating mechanisms. The harmful effects of radium emanate from its natural radioactivity. Its chemical toxicity, per se, has not been significantly studied and so will not be discussed. In biological systems all the elements of Group IIA are bone seekers and perhaps in other tissues concentrations are correlated with calcium content.

Magnesium

Magnesium is found at a concentration of 20,900 ppm in the earth's crust. The primary ores of magnesium are magnesite and dolomite. Magnesium may also be obtained from brinewells and salt deposits. It is used in alloys, particularly those requiring light weight. It is used in wire and ribbon for radios as well as for incendiary materials such as flares.

Magnesium is an essential nutrient. It is a co-factor of many enzymes and is contained in metalloenzymes; it is apparently associated with phosphate in these functions. Magnesium deficiency, per se, generally occurs in the face of some underlying disease such as chronic malabsorption syndrome, severe diarrhea, chronic renal failure, chronic alcoholism, and chronic malnutrition. The average daily requirement has been estimated at between 200 and 700 mg. The latter estimate is based on an interpretation of experimental data from rats that suggested magnesium intakes near the lower limit may have adverse effects on the arterial walls. This interpretation is not widely accepted at the present time [2]. Experimentally, magnesium deficiency has also been produced in man. Despite adequate intakes of calcium and potassium, hypocalcemia and hypokalemia were evident among the clinical chemistries, suggesting a strong interrelationship of magnesium to these ions. From this experimentally induced magnesium deficiency it was concluded that magnesium is essential to man for the proper mobilization of calcium from the bone and/or soft tissue and for the cellular retention of potassium. The signs of this artificially induced magnesium deficiency suggested neurological or gastrointestinal changes of varying degrees. These signs included tremors, hyporeflexia, apathy, weakness, anorexia, nausea, vomiting, electrocardiographic and electromyographic changes [19]. Experimental hypomagnesium has produced cardiomyopathy and myopathy of the skeletal muscles. Renal lesions have also been produced in experimental animals [20]. The deficiency is called "grass staggers" in cattle and "magnesium tetany" in calves.

Magnesium citrate, oxide, sulfate, hydroxide, and carbonate are widely taken as antacids or cathartics. The hydroxide (milk of magnesia) is one of the constituents of the universal antidote for poisoning. Topically, the sulfate is also used widely to relieve inflammation. Magnesium sulfate may be used as a parenterally administered central depressant. Its most frequent use for this purpose is in the treatment of seizures associated with eclampsia of pregnancy and acute nephritis.

The average city water contains about 6.5 ppm but varies considerably, increasing with the hardness of the water. Nuts, cereals, seafoods, and meats are high dietary sources of magnesium. The daily intake has been estimated at 500 mg, one of the highest of the materials considered in this chapter [21].

Magnesium salts are poorly absorbed from the gastrointestinal tract. In cases of overload this may be due in part to their dehydrating action. Magnesium is absorbed mainly in the small intestine. The colon also absorbs some. Calcium and magnesium are competitive with respect to their absorptive sites, and excess calcium may partially inhibit the absorption of magnesium.

The kidney is the principal organ responsible for regulating the magnesium content of the body. It allows for wide variations in dietary intake by increasing or reducing urinary secretion of magnesium in maintaining its normal serum concentration. Parathyroid hormone also plays an important role in the homeostatic regulation of magnesium and may influence renal tubular reabsorption [22]. It has been shown that parathyroid hormones make bone magnesium more available in magnesium-deficient rats and that this gland influences transport mechanisms in the intestine, liver, and kidneys [23].

Magnesium is excreted into the digestive tract by the bile, pancreatic and intestinal juices. A small amount of radiomagnesium given intravenously appears in the gastrointestinal tract. The serum levels are remarkably constant. There is an apparent obligatory urinary loss of magnesium which amounts to about 12 mg/day, and the urine is the major route of excretion

under normal conditions. Magnesium found in the stool is probably not absorbed. Magnesium is filtered by the glomeruli and reabsorbed by the renal
tubules. In the blood plasma about 65% is in the ionic form, while the
remainder is bound to protein. The ionic portion is that which appears in
the glomerular filtrate. Mercurial diuretics cause excretion of magnesium
as well as potassium, sodium, and calcium. Excretion also occurs in the
sweat and milk. Endocrine activity (particularly of the adrenal cortical
hormones, aldosterone and parathyroid hormone) has an effect on magnesium
levels, although these effects may be related to the interaction of calcium
and magnesium. Tissue distribution studies indicate that of the approximate
20 g body burden the majority is intracellular in the bone and muscle. Bone
concentration of magnesium decreases as calcium increases. Most of the remaining tissues have higher concentrations than blood, except for fat and
omentum. With age, the aorta tends to accumulate magnesium along with calcium, perhaps as a function of atherosclerotic disease [21].

Magnesium and alloys containing 85% of the metal are generally considered together in respect to their toxicologic properties. In industry,
their toxicity is regarded as low, although the fumes of magnesium oxide,
as with those of other metals, can cause metal fume fevers (see zinc). Some
investigators have reported that there is a high incidence of digestive disorders in magnesium plant workers, suggesting that a relationship may exist
between magnesium absorption and gastroduodenal ulcers. Slivers of magnesium penetrating the skin could cause damage from the evolution of hydrogen.
Generally speaking, magnesium compounds do not present a real hazard in
industry. The greatest danger in the handling of magnesium (in grinding)
is when small fragments of the metal are ignited and burn at very high
temperatures [24]. The threshold limit value for magnesium oxide fumes is
10 mg/m^3, and that for magnesite (magnesium carbonate) is that of a nuisance particle, 10 mg/m^3 [1]. Conjunctivitis, nasal catarrh, and coughing
up discolored sputum result from industrial particulate exposure to magnesium. With industrial exposure, increases of serum magnesium up to twice
the normal levels failed to produce ill effects, but were accompanied by
calcium increases.

Intoxication occurring after oral administration of magnesium salts is
rare, but may be present in the face of renal impairment. The results are
characterized by a sharp drop in blood pressure and respiratory paralysis
due to central nervous system depression [18].

Strontium

Strontianite ($SrCO_3$) is the basic mineral form of strontium. The element is found at a level of 450 ppm in the earth's crust. Industrial uses of strontium are limited to the manufacture of pyrotechnique devices, the processing of steel and paint, and the refining of sugar. Strontium bromide is often used for x-ray diagnostic work and as a therapeutic agent in reducing gastric hyperacidity.

The biological action or function of strontium resembles that of calcium, especially with regard to the bone. There is some evidence that strontium is essential for the growth of animals, especially for the calcification of bones and teeth. An apparent homeostatic regulating mechanism between strontium and calcium exists which favors the absorption of calcium and the preferential excretion of strontium.

Strontium is present in many foods. Spices, seafood, cereals, grains, roots, leafy vegetables, and legumes contain high concentrations. Unlike most water-borne elements, strontium is absorbed from the cooking water by vegetables. Water supplies contain variable amounts of strontium. Those in the United States have a mean value of 110 ppb strontium (range 2.2-1200 ppb). Strontium is not routinely measured in air but might be considered a natural pollutant from dust [25].

Daily intake of strontium from all sources has been estimated at approximately 2 mg. An ingestion of 1.99 mg of strontium by human volunteers over an 8-day period led to an almost complete recovery. The majority of the ingested strontium appeared in the feces and about 20% appeared in the urine. Considerable strontium can be excreted in the sweat; milk is a secondary route of excretion [13]. Approximately 99% of strontium in the body is in the bone or in the soft tissue; the largest concentrations are found in the aorta, larynx, trachea, and lower gastrointestinal tract. Strontium levels in the lung tend to increase with age, suggesting it is retained in the lungs after inhalation. The total body burden is about 140 mg. Adults and children from the Far East have more strontium in the bone than Americans. This is presumed to be the result of their low calcium intake. Strontium is found in high concentrations in newborn infants, indicating that it passes the placental barrier [25].

While the radiation hazard of ^{90}Sr from nuclear fallout is clear, there is no evidence associating stable strontium with any chronic disease. Increased salivation, nausea, diarrhea, and death due to respiratory paral-

ysis have been produced experimentally. Electrocardiographic changes may
occur after intravenous injection of massive doses, perhaps altering the
ionic balance as might occur following calcium overload.

Barium

Barite ($BaSO_4$) and witherite ($BaCO_3$) are the more common mineral forms
of barium. Barium is used in various alloys, in paints, soap, paper, and
rubber, and in the manufacture of ceramics and glass. Barium fluorosilicate
and carbonate have been used as insecticides. Barium sulfate, an insoluble
compound, is used as a radiopaque aid to x-ray diagnosis. This compound is
also used as a lubricating agent in drilling oil wells.

Barium is relatively abundant in nature (400 ppm in the earth's crust)
and is found in plants and animal tissue; some plants accumulate barium
from the soil. Studies suggest that barium may be an essential element inasmuch as rats and guinea pigs maintained on barium-free diets fail to grow
normally [13]. Brazil nuts have very high concentrations (3000-4000 ppm).
An average barium concentration in U.S. urban air of 0.09 $\mu g/m^3$ has been
reported [26]. Some water contains natural amounts of barium. An upper
limit of 0.01 mg/l has been established for barium in drinking water, but
maximum concentrations of 1.55 have been reported in community water supplies
[27]. The normal daily intake is 1.2-16 mg.

The soluble compounds of barium are absorbed after oral ingestion, and
small amounts are retained in the body to account for a body burden of approximately 20 mg. The muscle, lung, lower gastrointestinal tract, skin,
and fat contain relatively high concentrations when the soft tissues are
considered. The lung concentrations increase with age, probably from intake and retention related to atmospheric contamination. However, the
largest fraction of the body burden is in the skeleton [25].

Once absorbed, the soluble compounds are transported by the plasma.
The biological half-life is short (less than 24 hr). Feces are the major
excretion route of absorbed barium although some excretion is through the
kidney. The renal tubules reabsorb barium in the filtrate. The insoluble
forms of barium, particularly barium sulfate, are not toxic by the oral
route because of minimal absorption. One of the few complications of the
innumerable barium enemas performed each year has been the occasional formation of rectal barium granulomas [28].

The soluble barium compounds are highly toxic, in contrast to calcium
and strontium, the other members of this group in the periodic table.

Accidental poisoning from ingestion of soluble barium salts has resulted in gastroenteritis, muscular paralysis, decreased pulse rate, ventricular fibrillation, and extrasystoles. Potassium deficiency occurs in acute poisoning and the heroic measure, treatment with intravenous potassium, appears beneficial. The digitalis-like toxicity, muscle stimulation, and central nervous system effects have been confirmed by experimental investigation.

Accidental ingestions of barium chloride mixed with flour, mistaken for salt or barium carbonate, have resulted in serious cases of barium intoxication. Successful treatment of barium intoxication resulting from an attempted suicide by ingesting a commercial depilatory (12.8 g barium) has been reported. Paralysis of the respiratory muscles and hypokalemia resulting from the ingestion were reversed in 19 hr by giving respiratory assistance until acidosis was reversed, injecting intravenously 260 mequiv of potassium, and inducing diuresis by saline and furosemide [29].

Baritosis, a benign pneumoconiosis, is an occupational disease arising from the inhalation of barium sulfate, a (barite) dust, and barium carbonate. It is not incapacitating, but does produce radiological changes in the lungs. The radiological changes are reversible with cessation of exposure [18,30]. An acceptable average concentration (TLV) of 0.5 mg/m^3 for soluble barium compounds has been suggested for occupational exposures [1].

LANTHANONS (RARE EARTHS) AND SIMILAR ELEMENTS

On the conventional periodic table, IIIB is the next group of elements to consider. This group is composed of scandium, yttrium, lanthanum, and actinium. This group of elements might be regarded as the first group in the series of transition metals. However, the arrangement of the periodic table is somewhat irregular with regard to the lanthanide elements, atomic numbers 58-71. Therefore, because of their similar characteristics the lanthanons (rare earths) consisting of the elements with atomic numbers 57 through 71 will be considered along with yttrium and scandium. Actinium (atomic number 89), also of Group IIIB in the periodic table, is radioactive and its chemical toxicity has not been established. The rare earths or lanthanides compose approximately one-fifth of the known elements, and the use of the description "rare" is misleading in that some (yttrium, cerium, and neodymium) are more plentiful in the earth's crust than lead, as shown in Table 1. The rare earths are conventionally divided into two groups. The "light" group (or cerium group) is composed of lanthanum (La), cerium

TABLE 1. Rare Earths and Similar Elements

Name	Symbol	Atomic Number	Concentration in the Earth's Crust ($\% \times 10^{-5}$)
Scandium	Sc	21	50
Yttrium	Y	39	310
Lanthanum	La	57	50
Actinium	Ac	89	--[a]
Cerium	Ce	58	220
Praseodymium	Pr	59	35
Neodymium	Nd	60	120
Promethium	Pm	61	--[a]
Samarium	Sm	62	65
Europium	Eu	63	1.4
Gadolinium	Gd	64	63
Terbium	Tb	65	10
Dysprosium	Dy	66	50
Holmium	Ho	67	7
Erbium	Er	68	40
Thulium	Tm	69	5
Ytterbium	Yb	70	26
Lutetium	Lu	71	7

[a] Radioactive.

(Ce), praseodymium (Pr), neodymium (Nd), and promethium (Pm). The light
elements are separated by conventional crystallization procedures. Cerium
is the most widely distributed. Various special chemical methods are available for the separation of cerium. The "heavy" group (or yttrium group)
includes yttrium (Y), samarium (Sm), europium (Eu), gadolinium (Gd), terbium
(Tb), dysprosium (Dy), holmium (Ho), erbium (Er), thulium (Tm), ytterbium
(Yb), and lutetium (Lu). The heavy lanthanons, samarium through lutetium,
are separated by ion exchange. Natural mixtures of the heavy rare earths
are found together with yttrium oxide composing up to 80% [31]. Before
these separation techniques were available, the main use of these elements
was in mantles for gas lights. However, they are now used in control rods
for atomic reactors, in alloys with nickel and chrome, in microwave devices,
lasers, masers, and in television sets.

Neodymium and several other rare earths have been tried clinically as anticoagulants. Cerium oxalate has been used to remedy the vomiting during pregnancy, and other salts of this element have been used as central nervous system depressants, astringents, and antiseptics. Only samarium has been reported as a constituent of U.S. urban air. The level detected was 0.07 $\mu g/m^3$ [26].

Only small amounts of the stable rare earths are absorbed from the gastrointestinal tract. The percentage of oral absorption and retention of cerium is greater in neonates than in older mice [32]. Subcutaneous injection reveals slow excretion, mostly by the gastrointestinal route. Scandium after intravenous injection is concentrated in the liver and reticuloendothelial system; the bone concentration is low. Thulium is concentrated in the skeleton. Parenteral injection to rats of the elements lanthanum through samarium revealed an approximate 50% liver and 25% skeletal deposition. Excretion was via the bile with a 15-day half-life. Elements (65-71) terbium to lutetium have a skeletal retention of 50% or more with a longer biological half-life. Cerium (^{144}Ce) is deposited in the kidneys, spleen, cartilage, and adrenal cortex as are ^{180}Tb and ^{169}Yb. Promethium (^{147}Pm) and holmium (^{160}Ho) are taken up in the kidney and cartilage.

The oral toxicity of the rare earths is low due to poor gastrointestinal absorption. Based on scattered acute parenteral toxicity studies, these elements can be considered only slightly toxic. The signs of acute toxicity determined in rodents consisted of writhing, ataxia, labored respiration, and sedation. The maximum incidence of death occurred at 48 to 96 hr. There was a tendency for the females to be more sensitive than the males. Intravenous injection of various salts of the rare earths (lanthanum through samarium) caused splenic and hepatic degeneration in various rodents. The intravenous administration of neodymium and other rare earths for their anticoagulant effect, while apparently useful, produced undesirable side effects, primarily hemolysis resulting in hemoglobinuria [33,34]. Feeding up to 1% of the rare earths caused liver nuclear vacuolization in the case of gadolinium, terbium, thulium, and ytterbium. Incorporation of scandium in drinking water of mice at 5 ppm in the diet reduced growth, but no increase in tumors as compared to controls was observed. Ytterbium in the drinking water of mice at 5 ppm suppressed growth. Since all tumors of the yttrium-treated group were malignant, the authors felt that this was suggestive of carcinogenic properties, although the data were not conclusive [35].

Inhalation exposures in man, while infrequent, have caused sensitivity to heat, itching, and an increased awareness of odor and taste. Intratracheal administration or inhalation exposure of experimental animals to fluorides or oxides, or a combination thereof, resulted in transient pneumonitis, subacute bronchiolitis, and regional bronchiolar stricturing. The formation of granulomas, while rare, has been reported.

Skin damage by the rare earths is apparently not an important factor unless the skin is abraded. Applications to abraded skin cause epilation and scar formation. Intradermal injections produce granulomas in guinea pigs and man. The rare earths irritate the conjunctiva, but not the cornea. However, in rabbits when the cornea is denuded, scandium, yttrium, lanthanum, cerium, praseodymium, neodymium, samarium, and gadolinium cause permanent corneal opacity.

Lanthanum oxide fume and dust generated from arc light carbons used to produce intense white illuminations in the lithographic industry may be responsible for workers' frequent complaints of headache and nausea. Cerium is the most widely used of this group, and no records of human injury from industrial or medicinal use are reported [18]. A TLV for yttrium of 1 mg/m^3 has been set [1].

GROUP IVB (Ti, Zr, Hf)

Titanium, zirconium, and hafnium make up Group IVB in the periodic table. These members of the transition series of metals are relatively inert biologically, being neither essential nor markedly hazardous.

Titanium

Rutile (TiO_2) and ilmenite ($FeTiO_3$) are the primary ores of titanium. It is abundant in the earth's crust, at a level of 4400 ppm. Titanium is used as a deoxidizer, in permanent magnets, in corrosion-resistant alloys, in pigments, in welding rods, in electrodes and lamp filaments, and in surgical appliances. Titanium dioxide salve has been used in the treatment of burns. It is also used in some cosmetics.

Titanium is a contaminant of U.S. urban air. The average concentration was 0.04 $\mu g/m^3$ with values as high as 1.10 $\mu g/m^3$ recorded [36]. Titanium is found in North American rivers at levels of 2-107 $\mu g/l$. The mean concentration in municipal U.S. drinking water is 2.1 $\mu g/l$. Titanium has been detected in some foods: butter, corn oil, shrimp, lettuce, pepper, and other condiments. The daily intake is about 0.3 mg. Part of the food content may be due to contamination during processing. Oral absorption of titanium is limited; only about 3% of that ingested is absorbed. The majority of that absorbed is excreted in the urine.

The estimated body burden of titanium is about 15 mg. Most of it is in the lungs, probably as a result of inhalation exposure. Inhaled titanium tends to remain in the lungs for long periods. It has been estimated that about one-third of the inhaled titanium is retained in the lungs. There is some geographic variation in lung burden, dependent on air concentration. For example, concentrations of 430, 1300, and 91 in ppm of ash have been reported for the United States, Delhi, and Hong Kong, respectively. Titanium is not constantly present in newborns [37].

Slight fibrosis ("titanicosis") of lung tissue has been reported following inhalation exposure to titanium dioxide, but the injury was not disabling. Otherwise, titanium dioxide has been considered physiologically inert by all routes (ingestion, inhalation, dermal, and subcutaneous) [38]. The metal and other salts are also relatively nontoxic, except for titanic acid which, as might be expected, will produce irritation [18]. The TLV of 10 mg/m^3 established for titanium dioxide is based on the nuisance value of the particulate [1].

Incorporation of titanium at 5 ppm into the drinking water of mice for their lifetime produced no effects on growth, survival, longevity, or tumor incidence [39]. However, 5 ppm of titanium as titanate in the drinking water for three generations resulted in reduction of rats surviving to the third generation, reduction of the male/female ratio, and an increase in runts in all generations [40]. Intramuscular injection of titanocene caused a variety of neoplasms at the site of injection and in other organs of mice and rats. However, similar results were not obtained with titanium dioxide [41].

Zirconium

Zircon ($ZrSiO_4$) is the primary ore of zirconium. It is common for zirconium and hafnium to occur together. This is to be expected because of their chemical similarities. The concentration of zirconium in the earth's crust is 170 ppm. It is used in the nuclear industry as a shielding material, in metal alloys, as a catalyst in organic reactions in the manufacture of water-repellent textiles, in dyes, pigments on ceramics, and in abrasives and cigarette lighter flints. The metallurgical difficulties probably prevent even wider application. Zirconium oxychloride has been

used as an antiperspirant. Zirconium carbonate and oxide are used for dermatitis. Intravenous injection of zirconium has been advocated for prophylactic use to prevent skeletal deposition of certain radioelements, especially plutonium.

The daily oral intake in man has been estimated at 1-6 mg. Lamb, pork,
eggs, dairy products, and grains have the highest concentration. Plant
uptake of zirconium from soil and fertilizer has been demonstrated. Zirconium has been detected in rivers at 0.1 ppb. Because the common salts
are insoluble, the water concentrations are of small and doubtful significance in urban water supplies.

With the relatively large average body burden of 250 mg, fat, gall
bladder, aorta, liver, red blood cells, diaphragm, lung, kidney, muscle,
brain, pancreas, stomach, spleen, and testes have mean concentrations over
1 μg Zr per gram of tissue (wet weight). Zirconium is excreted by the intestine, probably in the bile. Zirconium levels are negligible in the
urine. Milk is a secondary route of excretion. Significant amounts of
zirconium are found in fetuses. While metabolic studies are lacking, it
must be assumed from tissue concentrations that significant amounts of
zirconium may be absorbed orally. It has been suggested that some homeostatic mechanism exists in respect to zirconium [42].

Inhalation exposure of $ZrOCl_2$ (water soluble) revealed the highest
concentration of zirconium in the lungs and pulmonary lymph nodes. Deposition and retention in the bone (femur) was greater than in the liver. Inhalation exposure of $ZnCl_4$ (6 mg Zr/m^3) for 60 days produced slight decreases
in hemoglobin and red blood count in dogs and increased mortality in rats
and guinea pigs. Zirconium oxide at 75 mg/m^3 caused no effect [43].

Granulomatous lesions, probably of allergic epithelioid origin have
been observed following the use of deodorant sticks and poison ivy lotions
containing zirconium. Rabbits developed pulmonary granulomata following
zirconium lactate inhalation exposure [44,45].

The TLV for zirconium compounds (as Zr) is 5 mg/m^3 [1]. This is based
on animal experiments and human experience. No evidence of industrial
diseases related to zirconium exposure has been documented [46].

The oral toxicity of zirconium compounds is low. The addition of 5
ppm of zirconium as the sulfate to the drinking water of mice for their
lifetime did not increase the incidence of tumors or the zirconium tissue
levels as compared to the controls [47]. The addition of 5 ppm of Zr to

the drinking water of rats for their lifetime produced only a slight increase in the frequency of glycosuria [48].

It has been suggested that since zirconium is incapable of forming a bond with organic carbon, its replacement of certain other toxic metals in selected manufacturing processes, such as chrome tannage, would be advantageous in respect to overall safety [49].

Hafnium

Hafnium is found in most minerals containing zirconium and its concentration in the earth's crust is about 25 ppm. Because of their similarity and difficulty in separation, it must be assumed that all zirconium contains 0.5-2% hafnium. Hafnium has been used in radio tubes, television tubes, incandescent lights, and x-ray tube cathodes.

There are no reports of human toxicity. In animals, the principal toxic effect is the production of nonhealing ulcers following dermal application (hafnyl chloride) to abraded skin. In a 90-day feeding study 1% produced slight liver changes [50]. A TLV of 0.5 mg/m^3 has been established for hafnium [1].

GROUP VB (V, Nb, Ta)

Group VB of the periodic table is comprised of vanadium, niobium, and tantalum. These transition metals are somewhat more interesting than the previous group. The lightest of the group, vanadium, has biological activity suggestive of usefulness, if not essentiality. The industrial use of vanadium is expanding and its potential for hazard may not be fully evident. It is interesting to observe that vanadium is the last of the lightest metals in any of the transitional series triads to be without marked biologic effect. The next heavier element of this triad, niobium, basically is toxic. The heaviest of this triad, tantalum, is apparently of little potential hazard.

Vanadium

Vanadium occurs in several ores. Carnolite and patronite are of commercial importance. The concentration in the earth's crust is 110 ppm. Vanadium can also be obtained as a by-product of petroleum refinement. Vanadium pentoxide is used as a catalyst in the production of various materials, of which sulfuric acid may be the most important. Ammonium metavanadate is also used as a catalyst. In addition, vanadium compounds are used in the hardening of steel, the manufacture of pigments, in photography,

and as insecticides. Various salts of vanadium have been used medicinally
as antiseptics, spirochetocides, and as antituberculosis and anti-anemic
agents, as well as a general tonic. These uses are without proven efficacy.

There has been some suggestion that vanadium is useful (if not essential) in various biological systems. In mammals, it may accelerate bone
mineralization and has an anticaries effect. Vanadium also has been shown
to inhibit cholesterol synthesis thus decreasing plasma phospholipid and
cholesterol concentrations and reducing aortic cholesterol accumulations.
Vanadium counteracts the stimulation of cholesterol synthesis induced by
manganese [13]. However, the essentiality of vanadium in man has not been
established [2].

Vanadium is a ubiquitous element. It is common in many foods; significant amounts are found in milk, seafoods, cereals, and vegetables. Vanadium
has a natural affinity for fats and oils; food oils have high concentrations.
Municipal water supplies may contain on the average about 1-6 ppb. Urban
air contains some vanadium, perhaps due to the use of petroleum products or
from refineries [51]. The average U.S. urban air concentration was 0.05
$\mu g/m^3$, but values as high as 2.2 $\mu g/m^3$ have been reported [36]. The average
daily intake is between 1 and 4 mg. The average body burden of vanadium has
been estimated at about 30 mg. The largest single compartment is the fat.
Bone and teeth stores contribute to the body burden. It has been postulated
that some homeostatic mechanism maintains the normal levels of vanadium in
the face of excessive intake, since the element in most forms is moderately
absorbed.

The principal route of excretion for excess vanadium is the urine, although under normal conditions none may be present in the urine. Parenteral
administration increases levels in the liver and kidney, spleen and testes,
but these increased amounts may be only transient. Some of the injected
vanadium may be excreted in the feces. The lung tissue may contain some
vanadium, depending on the exposure by that route [18,51].

The hazard of excessive vanadium is largely confined to the respiratory
tract and then only after inhalation exposure. Threshold limit values of
0.5 mg V/m^3 for vanadium pentoxide dust and 0.05 (ceiling) mg/m^3 of the fume
have been established [1]. Exposure effects are chiefly irritation of the
eyes, throat, and respiratory tract. Eczematous lesions of the skin and
discoloration (greenish-black) of the tongue may occur. Chronic exposure
may lead to fibrosis and emphysema. Edema of the lungs was the cause of

death in rabbits exposed to 200 mg/m^3 V_2O_5, confirming the possibility of severe pulmonary effects in animals.

Large doses of vitamin C or calcium ethylenediaminetetraacetate (EDTA) have been recommended for treatment of vanadium toxicity. Urinary values in excess of 30 µg V/l are indicative of excessive exposure [52].

An epidemiological investigation has indicated clear correlation between urban air levels of vanadium in Britain and the incidences of severe respiratory disease, bronchitis, and pneumonia [53]. The best correlation was among males. It has been suggested that inhibition by vanadium of alveolar macrophages, a means of defense against respiratory insults, may be an underlying mechanism in the apparent increase in vanadium-related pulmonary disease [54]. It has been postulated that vanadium air pollution is related to heart disease and may act with cadmium to produce these adverse effects [55].

The oral toxicity of vanadium compounds is minimal, and amounts of 4.5 mg or more per day have been given to man without effects. Higher doses produced only gastrointestinal distress and the green tongue. Renal toxicity was suggested by injection of pentavalent vanadium salts in rats and rabbits [51]. Incorporation of 5 ppm of vanadyl sulfate into the drinking water of rats over their lifetime produced only lower serum cholesterol values when the treated and control groups were compared [48].

Niobium

Niobium (columbium) is found with tantalum in the primary ore of tantalite and columbite. It is used in the manufacture of high-temperature steel alloys, corrosion-resistant chromium-steel alloys, and electronic equipment. It has a low thermal neutron cross section and has growing use in nuclear energy and chemistry.

Niobium is ubiquitous in nature, occurring at a level of 24 ppm in the earth's crust. Most grains, meats, and dairy products contain significant amounts of niobium. Fats and oils tend to have the largest amounts, whether of vegetable or animal origin. Total daily intake of niobium is estimated at 0.6 mg.

A little less than half the daily intake is absorbed; this is excreted in the urine. In the body, niobium is carried mainly in the red blood cells. The total body burden is approximately 100 mg. The red blood cells, liver, kidney, fat, hair, lungs, and pancreas contain the highest concentrations; but niobium is found in most other organs. The "normal" concentrations in the red cells, serum, and urine are about 5, 0.7, and 0.25 µg/g, respectively. Niobium is present in the newborn and in milk [56]. Inhalation studies in rats have shown that the largest amounts are retained in the lungs with secondary deposition in the bones. The biological half-life was 120 days after aerosol exposure [57].

Incorporation of niobium (sodium niobate) in the drinking water of mice at 5 ppm caused liver degeneration [47]. At the same levels in rats the growth rate in the male was increased, and glycosuria was more frequently observed than in the controls [48].

Intravenous administration of 30 mg/kg niobium as potassium niobate to dogs and rats produced severe nephrotoxic effects. Tubular epithelial damage was predominant in the convoluted tubule. In contrast, uranium in moderate doses injured only the distal portion of the proximal tubule, decreasing the tubular secretion of para-aminohippurate (PAH), but not the reabsorption of glucose. Niobium damages both the proximal and distal sections of the tubules and abolishes the renal response to the antidiuretic hormone (ADH). After treatment with both uranium and niobium, the secretion of PAH and reabsorption of glucose are decreased. Mercurials injure the proximal portion of the proximal tubule, having no effect on PAH secretion, but reducing glucose reabsorption. The mercury-poisoned kidney may remain responsive to ADH [58]. Niobium pentachloride produces moderate transient irritation of the eye and severe dermal irritation in experimental animals [59].

No cases of occupational disease from niobium are known. It has been suggested that the safety levels of niobium exposure should be about the same as for tantalum [60].

Tantalum

The concentration of tantalum in the earth's crust is less than 1 ppm. It is found with niobium in tantalite or columbite. Tantalum is used in electronics, in cutting alloys, in chemical manufacturing as a catalyst, and for acid-resistant materials. Tantalum is used as a supporting gauze in the repair of hernias, as a dressing for burns, in prosthetic appliances, and in local radiation for bladder cancer after neutron activation.

Oral salts of tantalum are poorly absorbed. After intramuscular injection the liver, bone, and kidney contain significant amounts [61].

A few animal experiments have suggested that after inhalation, tantalum may produce some pulmonary effects, benign and nonfibrotic in nature [34].

No adverse effects have been reported as a result of industrial exposure. Implantation of tantalum has not shown any adverse tissue reaction either in man or experimental animals [18]. The TLV of tantalum is 5 mg/m^3 [1].

GROUP VIB (Cr, Mo, W)

Chromium, molybdenum, and tungsten comprise the Group VIB triad. Chromium is also used in explosives, ceramics, and photography. The medicinal uses of chromium are limited to external application of chromium activity.

Chromium, in some form, also has clearly demonstrable toxic effects and is an industrial hazard. Molybdenum will be discussed in another chapter. Some similarity, principally lack of marked toxicity, exists between tungsten, the heaviest of the triad, and tantalum, which occupies the same position in Group VB of the periodic table.

Chromium

Chromium is found in nature at levels of 100 ppm in the earth's crust. Chromite (FeOCr$_2$O$_3$) is the most important chrome ore. Chromium plating is one of the major uses of this metal. Steel fabrication, paint, pigment manufacturing, and leather tanning constitute other major uses of chromium. Chromium is also used in explosives, ceramics, and photography. The medicinal uses of chromium are limited to external application of chromium trioxide as a caustic and intravenous sodium radiochromate to evaluate the life span of red cells.

Chromium exists in several valence states. Only the trivalent and hexavalent are biologically significant. Trivalent chromium is essential in animals. It plays a role in glucose and lipid metabolism. Chromium deficiency mimics diabetes mellitus and produces aortic plaques in rats. Trivalent chromium is thought to form a complex between sulfhydryl groups on the A-chain of insulin and to potentiate insulin activity. In addition, it bonds to plasma albumin and interacts with manganese in glucose metabolism. Chromium supplementation improves or normalizes glucose tolerance in diabetics, older people, and malnourished children. It has been suggested that chromium deficiency may be a basic factor in atherosclerosis. The hexavalent material is the cause of most of the adverse effects of chromium. While conversion from the trivalent (chromic) to the hexavalent (chromates) and other states is important chemically, the inner conversion from chromic to chromate apparently does not occur biologically. However, the conversion from hexavalent to trivalent does take place in the body [62,63].

The average concentration in U.S. urban air is 0.01 $\mu g/m^3$; however, levels as high as 0.35 $\mu g/m^3$ have been detected. While community air quality standards have not been set for chromium compounds in the United States, the U.S.S.R. has adopted a standard of 15 $\mu g/m^3$ for chromates and 80 $\mu g/m^3$ for average 24-hr exposures to trivalent chromium [64]. Chromium is a consistent contaminant of street dust found at a level of 0.11 lb/mile. This source (street dust) contributes to air pollution by reflotation of the particles into the atmosphere and therefore to water pollution by runoff into the streams [65]. The concentration in natural water supplies is low. However, U.S. municipal water supplies have been reported as showing concentrations up to 0.79 mg/ml, despite a mandatory tolerance level of 0.05 mg/l [27]. Hexavalent chromium is more toxic to fish under most test conditions than lead. In addition, chromium appears to be toxic to algae at levels of less than 10 ppm [66]. The major environmental exposure to chromium occurs as a consequence of its presence in food. Brown sugar and animal fats, especially butter, are chromium rich. The daily intake of chromium has been estimated at 60 μg (30-100 μg) of which about 10 μg is due to the concentration of the material in the water. However, its absorption is limited to approximately 1% [67].

The total chromium body burden of man has been estimated at less than 6 mg. Oral administration of trivalent chromium results in little chromium absorption. Absorption is slightly better following administration of hexavalent compounds. Once absorbed, trivalent chromium is bound to the plasma proteins. Under normal conditions the body contains stores of chromium in the skin, lungs, muscle, and fat. The bone contains chromium, but this is not due to selective deposition. The caudate nucleus has high concentrations. Skin reduces the hexavalent chromium to the trivalent form. In the blood little hexavalent chromium can be detected. The reticuloendothelial system, liver, spleen, testes, and bone marrow have an affinity for chromite, possibly as the result of phagocytosis of colloid particles formed at higher tissue concentrations. On the other hand, chromates are bound largely to the red blood cells. Subcellular distribution studies have indicated that the nuclear fraction contains almost one-half the intercellular chromium [62].

Perhaps the suggested homeostatic mechanism for trivalent chromium involving hepatic or intestinal transport systems rejects excessive accumulation and prevents undue hazard from chronic oral intake. Furthermore, ascorbic acid plays an important role in accelerating the conversion of the hexavalent chromium to the trivalent. Ascorbic acid will reduce the

dermal toxicity of chromate if given orally within an hour or two of exposure, and will reduce the gastrointestinal injury from hexavalent chromium
[68]. Water-soluble chromates disappear from the lungs into the circulatory
system after intratracheal application, while the trivalent chromic chloride
remains largely in the lungs. Urinary excretion accounts for about 80% of
injected chromium. However, elimination via the intestine may play a role
in chromium excretion. Milk is another secondary route of excretion [62].
Normal urinary and blood ranges are 1.5-11.0 µg/l and 1.0-5.5 µg/100 g.

Chromium is transported across the placenta and concentrated in the
fetus. The tissue concentrations decline rapidly with age, except for the
lung concentration, which tends to increase. The decline of chromium levels
with age does not take place in rats. Wide geographic variations in tissue
concentration, presumably on account of dietary intake and atmospheric concentration, have been reported [69].

Chromium is one of the most common causes of skin allergy. The presence of chromium in cement is responsible for the high incidence of allergy
in the building industry. Its use in primer paints, in auto rust coating,
and in alloys and electrodes are further sources of trouble. Even house-
wives may develop dermatitis, perhaps related to chromium in detergents
and bleaching agents. The photosensitivity caused by chromates has been
suggested as a reason for geographic variation for frequency of eczema [70].
Occupational exposure to hexavalent chromium compounds (Cr^{6+}) causes dermatitis, penetrating ulcers on the hands and forearms, perforation of the
nasal septum and inflammation of the larynx and liver. The dermatitis is
probably due to an allergenic response, although hexavalent chromium-sensi-
tive persons respond to large amounts of the trivalent ion [71]. The ulcers
resulting from chromium exposure are believed due to chromate ion and not
related to sensitization. Chromic acid and, to a lesser extent, chromate
are presumably the causative agents in perforation of the nasal septum [18].

Chrome ulceration due to penetration of the skin through cuts and abra-
sions is frequently reported. Unchecked, the ulcer penetrates deeply into
the soft tissue and may reach the underlying bone. If irritated, ulceration
of the nasal septum may occur. Neoplastic changes are not associated with
this lesion. The chelating agent, $CaNa_2$ (EDTA), in a 10% ointment reduces
the frequency of dermal and nasal septum ulcers when used prophylactically
or after irritating exposure. Inhalation of dust or mist containing hexavalent chromium is irritating to the mucous membrane. In a few cases,

presumably because of sensitization, asthmatic attacks occurred with repeated exposure.

Epidemiological studies suggest that chromate is probably a carcinogen,
with the lung as the principal site (bronchogenic carcinoma). The skin lesions, as a rule, are not metaplastic. A recent review of respiratory cancer in chromate workers again confirmed the occupational hazard of this
metal. Latent periods appear to be from 10-15 years. The risk for respiratory cancer among chromate plant workers was estimated at 20 times the
rate in the control population. In this report, experimental studies were
considered, and they suggested that calcium chromate may be the specific
carcinogenic agent [72]. The TLV for chromic acid and chromates (as CrO_3)
is 0.1 mg/m^3; that for soluble chromic and chromate salts (as Cr) is 0.5
mg/m^3. The TLV for tert-butyl chromate (as CrO_3) is 0.1 mg/m^3, and exposure
of the skin is to be considered of special consequence. In view of the
carcinogenic potential the TLV for the chromates and insoluble salts will be
0.1 mg/m^3 [1].

The possibility of nonoccupational lung cancer has been suggested [73].
The hexavalent form is generally considered the most harmful causative agent.
However, some investigators have produced cancer in experimental animals
with injections of either the trivalent or hexavalent form [74]. Incorporation of hexavalent chromium (chromate) into the drinking water of mice at
5 ppm over their lifetime reduced their growth in the first 6 months of the
study and produced a slightly higher incidence of malignant tumors than the
controls, although this difference was not remarkable [35]. Trivalent chromium (chromium acetate) given to rats under similar conditions produced no
effect [47].

Chromic acid used for cauterization has been reported in rare instances
as causing fatal nephritis. Ingestion of potassium chromate generally causes
vomiting because of its irritant property. However, in several cases symptoms referable to central nervous system and hepatic disturbances have been
observed [18].

Tungsten

The concentration of tungsten in the earth's crust is 70 ppm. Wolf-
ramite [(Fe, Mn)WO_4] and scheelite ($CaWO_4$) are the chief ores. Tungsten is
used in making high-speed tool steel and in other alloys. In addition, it
is used in filaments for x-ray tubes, radio tubes, and light bulbs, in pigments, and in waterproofing textiles.

Tungsten is not a normal complement of animal tissues. It is absorbed to some extent from the gastrointestinal tract and retained largely in the bone, although smaller amounts have been assayed in the spleen, liver, and kidney. The oral toxicity of tungsten compounds varies depending on the salt. The signs of toxicity by oral and parenteral administration are nervous prostration, diarrhea, coma, and death due to respiratory paralysis. Oral toxicity is apparently not a significant problem in man.

Some controversy exists over the effects of tungsten by inhalation. It is difficult to ascertain whether tungsten or cobalt is the causative agent in the pneumoconiosis of the tungsten carbide tool industry. Animal experiments suggest that the effects on the lungs are due not so much to tungsten itself as to other components, especially cobalt [18]. The TLV of insoluble tungsten compounds is 5 mg W/m^3, while that of the soluble compounds is lower, 1 mg W/m^3 [1].

Experimentally, tungsten has interactions with two other elements. The addition of soluble tungsten to the diet reduced the mortality and liver lesions characteristic of high levels of selenium intake. Increased tungsten intake also decreased molybdenum deposition in the livers of rats and reduced intestinal xanthine oxidase. Sufficient amounts of tungsten caused molybdenum deficiency in chicks [18].

GROUP VIIB (Mn, Tc, Re)

Only manganese (Mn), the lightest element of the triad, is of biological significance. Technetium (Tc) is radioactive and was the first artificially produced element. This element will not be considered in this section. Rhenium (Re) is a rarity in nature and very little is known of its biological activity, either useful or hazardous.

Manganese

Manganese is abundant in the earth's crust (1000 ppm). The principal ore of manganese is pyrolusite (MnO_2). Manganese or its compounds are used in making steel alloys, as oxidizing agents, and in the manufacture of dry cell batteries, electrical coils, ceramics, matches, glass, and dyes, in fertilizers and welding rods, and as animal food additives. The primary uses in medicine are as antiseptics and germicides. Potassium permanganate ($KMnO_4$) is applied dermally for these effects and for its slight astringent action. This is virtually the only manganese compound of medicinal use at the present time. Manganese chloride was administered intravenously for

schizophrenia, but was abandoned due to lack of effect and the danger of
flocculation.

Manganese is an essential element and is present in all living organisms. Manganese deficiency has not been recognized in man, probably because
of its ubiquitous nature in foodstuffs. It has been assumed that 2-3 mg/day
is adequate to meet the necessary requirements. It is a co-factor in a
number of enzymatic reactions, particularly those involved in phosphorylation, cholesterol, and fatty acid synthesis [2].

Manganese is present in most water supplies and in urban air. The
average concentration in U.S. urban air is 0.10 $\mu g/m^3$, but concentrations
as high as 9.98 have been measured [36]. Iron and steel manufacturing and
burning of diesel fuel are the major sources of manganese air pollution.
Possible use of organic manganese compounds as antiknock gasoline additives
may prove to be another source of atmospheric contamination. The use of
manganese in some fertilizers contributes to further air and water pollution.
The ability of manganese dioxide to catalyze the conversion of sulfur dioxide to sulfur trioxide and ultimately to sulfuric acid may be an important
secondary action played by high levels of manganese in adverse effects of
air pollution on health [64]. Nevertheless, the principal portion of the
daily intake (2-5 mg) is derived from food. Vegetables, the germinal portions of grains, fruits, nuts, tea, and some spices are rich in manganese.

The body burden has been estimated at 20 mg. The liver, kidney, intestine, and pancreas contain the highest concentrations. No significant
changes in tissue concentrations occur with age, except that tissues which
are normally low in concentration in adults tend to contain higher amounts
in the newborn. The lungs do not accumulate manganese with age despite
significant concentrations in urban air. The turnover of manganese is
rapid. Injected radiomanganese quickly disappears from the bloodstream;
it is concentrated in the mitochondria of the liver and pancreas. Administration of stable manganese in any valence state promotes rapid excretion
of radiomanganese. Serum manganese, normally about 2.5 $\mu g/l$, increases
after acute coronary occlusion and is claimed to be a more accurate index
of myocardial infarction than glutamic oxalacetic transaminase [75].

Studies have suggested that the major route of excretion is the gastrointestinal tract via the bile, and the excretion of manganese may be regulated by a homeostatic system maintaining relatively constant tissue levels.
This system apparently involves the liver, auxiliary gastrointestinal mechanisms for excreting excess manganese and perhaps the adrenal cortex [76-79].

In experimental animals, it is relatively clear that the excretion of manganese into the bile is accomplished by an active transport mechanism [80]. The consideration of the toxicity and environmental concentrations of manganese is complicated, inasmuch as only total manganese usually is measured; but eight valence states exist, and both cationic forms (Mn^{2+}) or anionic forms (MnO_4^-) may be present. In most cases the cations are more toxic than anions and Mn^{2+} is more toxic than Mn^{3+} [64]. This homeostatic regulating mechanism, plus the tendency for extremely large doses of manganese salts to cause gastrointestinal irritation, accounts for the lack of systemic toxicity following oral administration or dermal application. Experimental chronic oral intake of manganese in animals (rabbits, pigs, cattle) at levels of 1000 to 5000 ppm has reduced the accumulation and utilization of iron. Cereals rich in manganese contain only slightly more than 100 ppm. Thus, it is difficult to see how the effects reported in animals could apply to man [81]. A desirable level of 0.05 mg/l for manganese has been set for drinking water. The maximum concentration found in a survey of 969 communities was 1.32 mg/l, well above the limit. The limit was, in fact, exceeded in 211 of the total 2595 samples obtained [27].

Industrial toxicity through inhalation exposure, generally to manganese dioxide in mining or manufacturing, is of two types. The first is the result of acute short-term exposure and is a manganese pneumonitis. Men working in plants with high concentrations of manganese dust show an incidence of respiratory disease 30 times greater than normal. Pathological changes include epithelial necrosis followed by mononuclear proliferation. While the reproducibility of this type of manganese-related disease is difficult, manganese given to guinea pigs by intratracheal intubation along with an infective agent produces more response in the lung tissue than the agent as manganese dioxide dust only [82]. Several instances of manganic pneumonia allegedly caused by manganese air pollution have been reported. However, other studies have not been able to correlate low concentrations of Mn in the urban air with respiratory disease [63].

The second and more serious type of disease resulting from the chronic inhalation exposure to manganese dioxide, generally over a period of more than 2 years, involves the central nervous system. However, some cases have occurred after a few months' exposure to high concentrations of 30 mg/m^3 [83]. This occupational disease appears most frequently in mining operations. In iron-deficiency anemia the oral absorption of manganese is increased, and it may be that variations in manganese transport related to iron deficiency account for individual susceptibility [84]. Those who develop chronic manganese poisoning (manganism) exhibit a psychiatric disorder characterized by irritability, difficulty in walking, speech disturbances, and compulsive behavior that may include running, fighting, and singing. If the condition persists, a mask-like face, retropulsion or propulsion, and a Parkinson-like syndrome develop [85]. The outstanding feature of manganese encephalopathy has been classified as severe selective damage to the subthalmic nucleus and pallidum [86]. These symptoms and the pathological lesions, degenerative changes in the basal ganglia, make the analogy to Parkinson's disease feasible. In addition to the central nervous system changes, liver cirrhosis is frequently observed.

A TLV for occupational exposure to manganese and its compounds of 5 mg Mn/m^3 has been established. The TLV for methylcyclopentadienyl manganese tricarbonyl, a gasoline additive, is 0.2 mg Mn/m^3 (0.1 ppm). With this material skin contact should be held to a minimum, and consideration is being given to lowering the TLV to 0.1 mg/m^3 [1]. The U.S.S.R. has established a maximum allowable concentration (MAC) of 0.3 mg/m^3 for MnO_2 [87]. This difference in national standards is frequently seen for materials acting on the central nervous system (CNS).

Victims of chronic manganese poisoning tend to recover slowly, even when removed from the excessive exposure. Metal-sequestering agents have not produced remarkable recovery. L-Dopa, which is used in the treatment of Parkinson's disease, has been more consistently effective in the treatment of chronic manganese poisoning than in Parkinson's disease [88].

The syndrome of chronic nervous system effects has not been successfully duplicated in any experimental animals except monkeys, and then only by inhalation or intraperitoneal injection. After intraperitoneal administration of manganese to squirrel monkeys, dopamine and serotonin levels markedly decreased in the caudate nucleus, regardless of whether behavioral effects were present. Manganese levels were increased in the basal ganglia and cerebellum. Histopathological examination of animals did not reveal any morphological changes [89]. Exposure of rats to manganese dioxide at a concentration of 47 mg Mn/m^3 for 5 hr/day, 5 days a week for 100 days, while increasing the brain manganese concentration more than fourfold, produced no hematological, behavioral, or histological effects [90].

On the more positive side, intramuscular injection of manganese dust alone did not produce any sarcomas in rats at the site of injection. How-

ever, the frequency of such tumors following injection of nickel subsulfide
was reduced by injection of manganese dust along with the nickel [91].

Rhenium

Rhenium is scant in the earth's crust (0.001 ppm). Rhenium is obtained
as a by-product of molybdenum or copper processing. It is used in the electrical industry for electronic tubes and in marine engine magnetos because
of its resistance to salt corrosion. Also, it is used as a heater element.

Rhenium is excreted primarily in the urine. It tends to accumulate in
the thyroid. The basis of this accumulation is not binding, as is iodine.
No toxic effects have been reported [18].

GROUP VIII (Fe, Co, Ni, Ru, Rh, Pd, Os, Ir, Pt)

Group VIII in the periodic table is considered in two parts. Iron (Fe),
cobalt (Co), and nickel (Ni) are considered separately; and the remainder will
be considered together as the platinum group metals. The lightest two metals
of the group, iron and cobalt, superficially share the biological ability to
prevent anemia, although the mechanism of action is quite different. Nickel
has no established role in metabolism but, at least with regard to some compounds, is most hazardous when long-term atmospheric exposure is encountered.

Iron

Iron is widespread in nature, occurring at a level of 50,000 ppm in the
earth's crust. The principal ores of iron are oxides. The industrial uses
of iron are numerous, mainly in the fabrication of steel. Iron carbonate is
used as a trace mineral and is added to food. Ferbam, ferric dimethyldi-
thiocarbamate, is an iron-containing fungicide. It has a relatively high
threshold limit value of 10 mg/m^3 [1]. When it is heated, ferbam decomposes
and emits highly toxic fumes.

Iron has been used therapeutically since at least 1500 B.C. Its medicinal uses have included treatment of acne, alopecia, hemorrhoids, gout, pulmonary diseases, excessive lacrimation, weakness, edema, and fever, to name
a few. The primary therapeutic use of iron salts today is in the treatment
of iron-deficiency anemia and is available in nonprescription forms. Parenteral dosage forms, generally iron carbohydrate complexes, are available for
treating iron deficiency that does not respond to oral treatment and for
physiological anemia due to rapid growth (for example, anemia of baby pigs).

Iron is an essential element; its major function in the animal body is the formation of hemoglobin. In addition, enzymes also contain iron; these include cytochrome and xanthine oxidase [92].

Urban air and water may contain significant amounts of iron from industrial or geological sources. The average concentration in the U.S. urban air was 1.58 $\mu g/m^3$; however, concentrations as high as 22 $\mu g/m^3$ have been recorded [36]. Iron is widely distributed in food, animal tissues tending to contain considerably more than plants. The average daily intake is about 500 mg, the highest of any metal under normal conditions. Every tissue of the body contains iron. Under normal conditions the body burden is about 4 g. Hemoglobin is the major iron compound in the body and is highly concentrated in the erythrocytes. Sixty-seven percent of the total body iron is contained in hemoglobin. Twenty-seven percent is stored as ferritin, mainly in the liver, or as hemosiderin, in cases of excess intake.

The oral absorption of iron is complicated, and the intestinal mucosa is the principal site for limiting the absorption of iron. Under normal circumstances the iron from food is not well absorbed in nonanemic persons. In this homeostatic mechanism, the divalent iron is absorbed into the gastrointestinal mucosa and converted to the trivalent form, where it is attached to ferritin. The ferritin passes into the bloodstream and is then converted to transferrin where the iron remains in the trivalent form or is transported to the liver or spleen for storage as ferritin or hemosiderin. The absorption of iron from the gastrointestinal tract may be dependent upon hepatic and pancreatic secretions. However, the adequacy of iron stores in the body seems to be the major controlling factor in the absorption of iron by the gastrointestinal tract [93]. Dietary factors such as ascorbic acid, carbohydrate, and alcohol may also influence iron absorption. Extrinsic factors may cause soluble complexes of ferric iron to form, depending on the pH of the duodenal contents, increasing absorption [94]. Certain organic iron compounds such as ferrocene may permit the absorption of iron unregulated by the normal homeostatic mechanisms.

Iron crosses the placenta and concentrates in the fetus. However, this concentration of the iron may serve a valuable physiological purpose, inasmuch as it prevents anemia caused by rapid growth in the absence of sufficient supplies of iron in the mother's milk.

When iron intake increases beyond the physiological requirements, most is excreted in the feces; but small amounts may accumulate. Some iron may

be excreted via the bile. In cases of overload, iron is excreted by loss
of epithelial cells of the gastrointestinal tract that limit iron intake.
Women tend to be more anemic than men. Menstrual bleeding accounts for increased iron loss and is the reason why under conditions of limited iron
intake, anemia may develop [92]. Inhalation exposure of rats to labeled
iron oxide revealed that exposure was accompanied by renal excretion of
iron for about 1 week; thereafter, excretion was largely by the feces. The
iron deposited in the upper respiratory tract was largely cleared in 24 hr,
while the alveolar clearance required considerably longer, about 60 days.
This is comparable to alveolar clearance in dogs [95].

Long-term inhalation exposure to iron, particularly iron oxide, has
resulted in mottling of the lungs (siderosis). This is considered a benign
pneumoconiosis and does not ordinarily cause a significant physiological
impairment [34]. However, hematite miners in certain areas have from 50 to
70% higher death rates attributable to lung cancer. It has been suggested
that at least part of the increased incidence may be due to radioactivity
in the mine fields surveyed [96]. An industrial threshold of 10 mg/m^3 has
been suggested to prevent the development of x-ray changes in the lungs on
the basis of long-term exposure. This concentration of iron oxides is not
irritating to the mucous membranes. A community air quality level for iron
oxide of 100 μg/m^3 over a 30-day period with a 24-hr maximum of 250 μg/m^3
has been recommended. However, these recommendations are based on annoyance
factors such as reduced visibility and soiling, not health effects [97].
The current TLV for occupational exposure with regard to iron oxide fumes
is 10 mg/m^3. A lower value of 5 mg/m^3 has been proposed. The TLV for soluble iron salts is 1 mg Fe/m^3, that for ironpentacarbonyl is 0.08 mg/m^3
(0.01 ppm). The TLV for ferrovanadium dust is 1 mg/m^3 [1].

Chronic excessive oral intake of iron may lead to hemosiderosis or
hemochromatosis. Hemosiderosis refers to a condition in which there is
generalized increased iron content in the body tissues, particularly in the
liver and reticuloendothelial system, but affecting other organs as well.
Hemochromatosis, on the other hand, indicates demonstrable histological
hemosiderosis and diffused fibrotic changes of the affected organ.

Excessive dietary iron intake appears to be the cause of abnormal iron
accumulation in the notable condition known as "Bantu siderosis" occurring
in South Africa. Bantu siderosis is more frequent in men than in women.
The disease is probably brought about by the use of iron pots in food preparation and the brewing of beer in iron containers. This type of disease

is marked by iron accumulations in the Kupffer cells of the liver and in
the reticuloendothelial cells of the spleen and bone marrow. In addition,
a glucose test indicates that 20% of the patients with hemochromatosis have
abnormal glucose metabolism. Increase in heart disease may also accompany
hemochromatosis. It has been reported that high dietary iron intake from
other sources, for example red wine, may also play a role in the etiology
of hemochromatosis in some areas of the world. It is possible that high
alcohol content is a factor in these iron overload diseases, perhaps related to alcoholic cirrhosis [98]. Numerous investigators have attempted
to produce hemochromatosis in experimental animals either by parenteral or
oral administration of iron in large doses over a protracted period. Although it is possible to induce hemosiderosis in the liver and other viscera,
fibrosis has not been clearly demonstrated. In experimental animals the
production of hemosiderosis, accompanied by cellular injury and fibrosis,
apparently requires a choline-deficient diet. Administration of folic acid
to rats receiving a choline-deficient diet has prevented cellular necrosis
and fibrosis [93].

An unusual disorder (Kaschin-Beck disease) has been reported in Asia.
This has been ascribed, perhaps in error, to the consumption of drinking
water with excessive iron content and resulted in an arthritic-type disease.
An upper desirable limit of 0.3 mg Fe/l has been established for drinking
water. In a survey of 969 U.S. community water supplies, the maximum concentration measured was 26 mg Fe/l, approximately 100 times the desirable
limit. Of 2595 samples taken, 223 exceeded the desirable level [27].

The compulsory or excessive fortification of foods, especially bread,
has led to objections. These are based on the possibility of iron toxicity
due to vitamin E deficiency. This vitamin (E) has been shown to reduce the
toxicity of iron. In addition, the possibility of hazardous excessive
dietary iron in males, especially in the face of high alcohol intake, has
been postulated.

Acute poisoning from accidental ingestion of ferrous sulfate tablets
occurs more frequently in children than in adults. About 2000 such cases
occur annually. Only acute intoxications from aspirin, other unknown medications, and phenobarbital occur more frequently than acute iron poisoning
[99]. In children, prior to the advent of deferoxamine, the death rate was
higher from this form of intoxication than from acetylsalicylic acid [100].

The primary acute toxicity from oral iron preparations is due largely
to the irritation of the gastrointestinal tract; vomiting may be the first

sign; there may be some gastrointestinal bleeding, lethargy, restlessness, and gray cyanosis. This may be followed by a short period of recovery which takes place from several hours to 1 or 2 days after the poisoning. This is followed by a third phase of acute iron toxicity in which signs of pneumonitis and convulsions may occur. Gastrointestinal bleeding generally continues throughout this entire period; and some neurological manifestations, including coma, are predominant during this phase. Signs of hepatic toxicity, such as jaundice, may be observed. Most deaths occur during this time. In those patients surviving 3 or 4 days, recovery is generally rapid. Later sequelae occur rarely, but pyloric constriction and gastric fibrosis have been observed 6 weeks after the acute phase of iron poisoning. Marked leucocytosis may occur.

Acute iron poisoning in rabbits produces prolongation of coagulation time and prothrombin time, increased thrombocyte count, and qualitative changes in fibrin formation. Serum glutamic oxalacetic and glutamic pyruvic transaminase are increased. The severity of the clinical course seems to be proportional to the increase in the serum iron concentration. It has been hypothesized that the severe gastrointestinal necrosis facilitates direct access of the iron into the bloodstream, circumventing the mucosal block. Electron microscope examinations have found livers of rabbits experimentally poisoned with large intravenous doses of iron to have degenerative mitochondria accompanying the marked hepatic degeneration. Fatty degeneration of the myocardium and masses of granular material in the kidneys have been reported [93].

Iron poisoning has been treated with dimercaprol (British antilewisite [BAL]), diethylenetriaminepentaacetate (DTPA), and ethylenediaminetetraacetate (EDTA). However, these agents have been completely supplanted by deferoxamine.

Cobalt

Cobalt is a relatively rare metal produced primarily as a by-product of other metals, chiefly copper. Its concentration in the earth's crust is 23 ppm. It is used in high-temperature alloys and in permanent magnets. Its salts are useful in paint driers, as catalysts, and in the production of numerous pigments. Cobalt salts have been used in the treatment of cyanide poisoning and to correct anemias.

Cobalt is an essential element in that 1 µg of vitamin B12 contains 0.0434 µg of cobalt. Vitamin B12 is essential in the prevention of per-

nicious anemia. This form, vitamin B12, is the only way in which man is
known to utilize cobalt. Deficiency diseases of cattle and sheep caused by
insufficient natural levels of cobalt are characterized by anemia and loss
of weight or retarded growth. However, ruminants can convert cobalt into
vitamin B12. This is accomplished by ruminal microflora [2].

Average urban air concentration has been reported to be less than
0.0005 $\mu g/m^3$. However, a maximum concentration of 0.060 was reported [36].
Foods containing relatively high concentrations (>1 $\mu g/g$) of cobalt include
fish, cocoa, bran, and mollusks.

Cobalt salts are generally well absorbed after oral ingestion, probably
in the jejunum. Despite this fact, increased daily intake above an average
of about 0.3 mg does not result in significant accumulation. The majority,
about 80% of the ingested cobalt, is excreted in the urine. Of the remaining,
about 15% is excreted in the feces by an entero-hepatic pathway, while the
milk and sweat are other secondary routes of excretion. Significant species
differences have been observed in the excretion of radiocobalt. In rats and
cattle, 80% is eliminated in the feces [101]. The muscle contains the
largest total fraction, but the fat has the highest concentration. The liver,
heart, and hair have significantly higher concentrations than other organs,
but the concentration in these organs is relatively low. The total body
burden has been estimated at about 1 mg. The normal levels in human urine
and blood are about 98 $\mu g/l$ and 0.18 $\mu g/l$, respectively. The blood level
is largely in association with the red cells.

Polycythemia is the characteristic response of most mammals, including
man, to ingestion of excessive amounts of cobalt. This response is due in
part to the creation of intracellular hypoxia. Toxicity resulting from
overzealous therapeutic administration has been reported to produce vomiting,
diarrhea, and a sensation of warmth. Intravenous administration leads to
flushing of the face, increased blood pressure, slowed respiration, giddiness,
tinnitus, and deafness due to nerve damage [18].

High levels of chronic oral administration may result in the production
of goiter. Epidemiological studies suggest that the incidence of goiter is
higher in regions containing increased levels of cobalt in the water and
soil [102]. The goitrogenic effect has been elicited by the oral administration of 3-4 mg/kg to children in the course of sickle-cell anemia therapy
[18].

Cardiomyopathy has been caused by excessive intake of cobalt, particularly in beer with cobalt added to enhance its foaming qualities. The onset

of the poisoning occurred about 1 month after cobalt was added in concentrations of 1 ppm. Why such a low concentration should produce this effect in the absence of any similar change when cobalt is used therapeutically is unknown. The signs and symptoms were those of **congestive** heart failure. Autopsy findings revealed a 10-fold increase in the cardiac levels of cobalt. Alcohol may have served to potentiate the effect of the cobalt [103].

Since coffee has been implicated in cardiac pathology, it is interesting to note that the average content of seven brands was 0.93 µg/g. Instant coffee powder had the highest concentration. Tea contained significantly less cobalt than did coffee [104].

Hyperglycemia due to alpha cell pancreatic damage has been reported after injection into rats. Inhibition of glucose oxidation has also been reported [105]. Reduction of blood pressure has been observed in rats after injection and has led to some experimental use in man [101].

Industrial exposure to cobalt salts leads to respiratory effects, although there is some question as to whether cobalt is the sole agent responsible for these effects. Most industrial exposure comes from the cemented carbide industry, where 1-2 mg/m^3 have produced pulmonary effects. Sensitization may be an important part of this effect. Experimental studies in animals, however, confirm the lung-irritant effect of the metal as used in this industry, but not with other cobalt compounds. Skin and eye lesions similar to allergic dermatitis have also been reported. Skin tests show positive sensitization to cobalt but not to other material used in the cemented carbide industry. Gastric disturbances occurring shortly after daily exposure to cobalt acetate progressing to epigastric pain, pain in the limbs, hematuria and occult blood in the stool have been reported. Recovery was complete in 3 weeks [18,106]. Subcutaneous injections of cobalt salts have produced sarcomas in rodents, but this observation does not suggest an environmental hazard [41], because many materials induce tumors when administered by this route to experimental rodents. A safe occupational exposure level of 0.1 mg/m^3 has been set in the United States for cobalt dust and metal fume [1].

Nickel

In its principal ores nickel is found in combination with iron or copper. Nickel occurs in the earth's crust at a level of 80 ppm. The main uses of nickel are in electronics, coins, steel alloys, batteries, food processing (Ni-Cu Monel), and stainless steel. Nickel is also used as a catalyst in the hydrogenation of fats and oils.

No functional action has been described for nickel in the intact animals, although in vitro it will activate enzymes. Nickel is a constituent
of urban air, possibly as a result of fossil fuel combustion, with incinerators contributing to the nickel content in the atmosphere. The average
concentration in U.S. urban air was 0.034 $\mu g/m^3$, although concentrations
as high as 0.46 $\mu g/m^3$ occurred [36]. Nickel is not a normal constituent of
water. While some nickel is found as a contaminant from food processing
(gelatin and baking powder), relatively large amounts occur naturally in
vegetables, legumes, and grains. The average daily intake is about 0.45 mg.

The average body burden has been estimated at < 10 mg, but wide geographic variations occur. Nickel is present in the lung, liver, kidney, and
intestine of most stillborn infants. The concentration in the lung increases
with age. In rats the bones accumulate a major portion of increased intake.
Excretion is largely in the feces, probably through bile. A mechanism for
limiting intestinal absorption has been suggested. Many nickel salts have
astringent and irritant properties which limit their absorption [107].

Dietary nickel acetate at levels of 100 to 1000 ppm as nickel depressed
growth, red cell indexes, tissue cytochrome oxidase, and alkaline phosphatase activities in rats. Nickel accumulated in the heart, liver, testes,
and to the greatest extent in the kidneys [108]. The administration of 5
ppm nickel in the drinking water of rats for three generations caused a
reduction in the size of the litters in successive generations and a drastic
reduction in the number of males by the third generation [40]. However, the
exposure of 5 ppm nickel in the drinking water of rats for their lifetime
was not toxic. No accumulation of nickel in the tissues was observed.
Nickel, under these conditions, was not tumorgenic or carcinogenic; growth
was, in fact, enhanced and survival and longevity were unaffected [109].

Dermatitis (nickel itch) is the most frequent effect of exposure to
nickel. This occurs from direct contact with metals containing nickel such
as coins and costume jewelry. It has been estimated that of all eczema, 5%
is caused by nickel or nickel compounds. The dermatitis is a sensitization
reaction and contact in some cases may produce paroxysmal asthmatic attacks
and pulmonary eosinophilia [110]. Except for nickel carbonyl, perhaps,
nickel salts are not absorbed through the skin in sufficient amounts to
cause intoxication [111].

Nickel carbonyl [$Ni(CO)_4$] is the most toxic of nickel compounds. It
is recognized as a carcinogen in man, and a TLV for occupational exposure
of 1 ppb (0.007 mg/m^3) has been established [1]. It has been estimated as
lethal in man at atmospheric exposures of 30 ppm for 30 min [111]. This

material is formed by nickel or its compounds in the presence of carbon
monoxide. The initial symptoms of toxicity consist of headache and vomiting.
These are relieved by fresh air. Delayed symptoms occurring in 12-36 hours
consist of dyspnea, cyanosis, leukocytosis, and increased body temperature.
Delirium and other central nervous system signs usually appear. Acute chemical pneumonitis results. Death may occur between the 4th and 11th day.

Chronic exposure to nickel carbonyl has been implicated epidemiologically
as an occupational carcinogen affecting the lungs and nose. These findings
have been confirmed by inhalation exposure in experimental animals. It has
been pointed out that cigarette smoke contains significant amounts of nickel
carbonyl [112].

While dietary nickel is excreted largely in the feces, inhalation of
nickel carbonyl results in the appearance of significant increases in urinary nickel, both with regard to concentration and relative to that in the
stools. The increase of nickel in the urine has been used clinically to
confirm exposure and levels above 0.5 mg/l are considered serious. Diethyl-
dithiocarbamate trihydrate (Dithiocarb), a metal binding agent, has been
used successfully to treat acute poisoning [111].

There are no studies in man which confirm the systemic toxicity at
reasonable exposure levels of nickel or its compounds, except $Ni(CO)_4$. Oral
doses of nickel sulfate (0.1-0.5 mg/kg) for 161 days have induced myocardial
and liver damage. High doses of the soluble salts induce giddiness and
nausea. Nickel dust and the oxide by inhalation have induced malignant
pulmonary neoplasia in guniea pigs and rats.

The increase of serum nickel in humans after myocardial infarction is
of unknown significance [113]. A TLV for nickel metal and its soluble salts
of 1 mg Ni/m^3 has been set [1].

Platinum-Group Metals

These metals may be grouped together because of their similar chemical
properties. They are found together in sparsely distributed deposits. The
concentration of each of these elements in the earth's crust has been indicated in Table 2. These rare metals are also obtained as a by-product of
refining other metals, chiefly nickel and copper. Ruthenium (Ru), rhodium
(Rh), and palladium (Pa) are the lighter triad, while osmium (Os), iridium
(Ir), and platinum (Pt) encompass the heavier.

The main use of ruthenium is as a hardener in platinum and palladium
alloys used in jewelry and electrical contacts. Rhodium is used in the

TABLE 2. Platinum-Group Metals

Name	Symbol	Atomic Number	Concentration in the Earth's Crust ($\% \times 10^{-7}$)
Ruthenium	Ru	44	18
Rhodium	Rh	45	1
Palladium	Pd	46	50
Osmium	Os	76	50
Iridium	Ir	77	10
Platinum	Pt	78	200

manufacture of rhodium-platinum alloys, in electroplating, electronic components, and movie projectors, and in reflectors for searchlights. Medicinal uses are not made of the reported slight chemotherapeutic activity against certain mouse viruses [18]. The industrial uses of palladium include alloys (especially those used in the communication industry), as a catalyst, for decoration and jewelry, dental alloys, and in cigarette lighters. Palladium in colloidal form has been given medicinally for tuberculosis, gout, and obesity. These uses were without significant benefits. This metal, along with platinum, is utilized in the catalytic converters on automobiles to reduce air pollution. Osmium is used in the hard points of fountain pens and engraving tools. It is used in staining tissues for electron microscopy and in fingerprinting. Formerly, it was employed in the manufacture of electrical lights. Iridium is used to harden platinum jewelry and as an alloy with osmium for hard points of fountain pens and engraving tools. Platinum is widely used as a catalyst in the chemical industry and in electronics. It is alloyed with other metals and used in jewelry.

Osmium metals and most of its salts are of little toxicological significance. Osmium tetroxide, produced by heating the metal, is toxic. Its action is mainly on the eyes. Lacrimation and halo vision occur, probably due to effects on the cornea. Irritation of the respiratory tract and headache may occur. One fatal case due to pulmonary irritation has been reported. Some renal toxicity has been ascribed to osmium tetroxide exposure [114].

No reports implicating iridium as an industrially hazardous agent have appeared [34].

Platinosis is an industrial disease caused generally by platinum's complex salts, mainly chloroplatinate. Cutaneous and respiratory allergic manifestations occur in platinum-refining workers. These reactions may occur by platinum salts combining with protein to form a complex antigen in which platinum salts act as a haptene. Thus, the substance is capable of both sensitizing and releasing histamine at first contact. Scratch tests are only positive from the time the workers begin to show symptoms. Thus, the signs may arise on exposure; but workers have been known to use platinum salts for long periods of time before developing untoward reactions [115, 116]. In cancer chemotherapy cis-diammenedichloroplatinum has been used. Nephrotoxicity, gastrointestinal side effects, hyperuremia, and erythro-suppression occurred [117].

The TLV of the soluble salts of platinum is very low at 0.002 mg Pt/m^3. Osmium tetraoxide, the only compound of that element apparently considered an industrial hazard, has a TLV of 0.002 mg/m^3 (0.0002 ppm). The TLV of the soluble salts of rhodium is 0.001 mg/m^3, while that for the metal fume and dust is 0.1 mg Rh/m^3 [1].

Intratracheal injections of radioruthenium chloride are retained in the lungs, suggesting that there might be pulmonary retention after inhalation. Toxicological information is limited to references in the literature indicating that fumes may be injurious to eyes and lungs [18].

Rhodium trichloride produced death in rats and rabbits within 48 hr after intravenous administration at doses near the LD$_{50}$ (approximately 200 mg/kg). Histological evaluation revealed no changes; however, it was suggested that death was attributable to central nervous system effects [118].

When administered orally, palladium is excreted in the feces. Intravenous administration results in rapid and almost complete excretion in the urine. Palladium chloride is not readily absorbed from subcutaneous injection. No adverse effects have been reported from industrial palladium exposure. Subcutaneous injection of palladium chloride in rabbits leads to gray-brown discoloration at the site of injection. Intravenous administration in lethal doses causes loss of appetite, hemolysis, renal deposits, and bone marrow injury. Colloid palladium [Pd(OH$_2$)] reportedly increases body temperature, produces discoloration and necrosis at the site of injection, decreases body weight, and causes slight hemolysis [18,34]. While dermatitis and sensitization are generally accepted as a hazard of platinum exposure, at least one case of palladium sensitization and dermatitis has been reported [119]. In a single study, incorporation of rhodium (rhodium chloride) or palladium (palladous chloride) into the drinking water of mice at a concentration of 5 ppm over the lifetime of the animals produced a minimally significant increase in malignant tumors. Most of these tumors were classified as of the lymphoma-leukemia type [35].

THE NOBLE METALS (GROUP IB)

The metals of Group IB, copper (Cu), silver (Ag), and gold (Au), are chemically inactive; all are found to some extent as free metals in nature. Mercury is the only other common metal which occurs as a free metal. All elements of this group have intrinsic value and have been used in monetary systems. Copper, an essential element and the most abundant of the group, is discussed in Chapters 22, 27, and 29.

Silver

Silver occurs in many ores. The primary silver ore is argentite (Ag_2S). Silver is also obtained as a by-product in the purification of copper, lead, and other metals. The concentration in the earth's crust is 0.1 ppm. Silver is employed in electrical applications because of its excellent properties of conduction. Jewelry, coins, and eating utensils are some of the principal uses of the metal. Silver halides are used in photography; silver nitrate is used for making indelible inks and for medicinal purposes. The application of silver nitrate for prophylaxis of ophthalmia neonatorium was a legal requirement in some states. Other medicinal uses of silver salts have been as caustics, germicides, antiseptics, and astringents [120].

Silver does not occur regularly in animal or human tissue. The average human body burden is less than 1 mg [14]. The chief effect of excessive absorption of silver is local or generalized impregnation of the tissues and is referred to as argyria. It can be absorbed from the gastrointestinal tract and lungs. Some ingested silver is retained in the cells of the gastrointestinal tract, while the majority is excreted. Urinary excretion has not been reported even after intravenous injection. Intravenous injection produces accumulation in the spleen, liver, bone marrow, lungs, muscle, and skin.

Industrial argyria, a chronic occupational disease, has two forms: local and generalized. The local form involves the production of gray-blue patches on the skin or manifestation in the conjunctiva of the eye. In generalized argyria the skin shows widespread pigmentation, often spreading from the face to most uncovered parts of the body. In some cases the skin may become bluish-black with a metallic luster. The eyes may be affected to such a point that the lens and vision are disturbed. The respiratory tract may also be affected in severe cases [18]. The ACGIH has assigned a TLV of 0.01 mg/m^3 to metallic silver and its soluble compounds [1].

Silver oxide is used as a catalyst in the purification of water and in glass to produce a yellow color. An upper mandatory level for drinking water is 0.05 mg/l. The maximum concentration found in 969 community water supplies was 0.03 mg/l [27]. The administration of $AgNO_3$ to rats in their drinking water showed increases of silver in the basement membranes and phagocytic cells. When treatment was discontinued for up to 4 weeks, silver deposition was continued in these areas, possibly because of relocation from the cells of the gastrointestinal tract. The glomerular basement membrane was one of the first sites of deposition. The deposition occurred later in the basement membrane of the urinary bladder. Organ deposition may be related to fluid movement across the basement membrane. A level of 24 mM $AgNO_3$ (~ 2.6 mg Ag/ml) produced deterioration of general appearance, listlessness, and death. It was suggested that vitamin E deficiency may increase toxicity [121].

Orally, large amounts of silver nitrate cause severe gastrointestinal irritation due to its caustic action. Lesions of the kidneys and lungs and the possibility of arteriosclerosis have been attributed to both industrial and medicinal exposures. Large doses of colloidal silver administered intravenously to experimental animals produced death due to pulmonary edema and congestion. Hemolysis and resulting bone marrow hyperplasia have been reported. Pulmonary changes (chronic bronchitis) have also been reported after medicinal administration of silver in this form [18,120].

Gold

Gold is rather widely distributed in small quantities in the earth's crust (0.005 ppm), but the major economically usable deposits occur as the free metal in quartz veins or alluvial gravel. It may be naturally alloyed as sylvanite $(AuAg)Te_2$. Gold is used in jewelry, for other ornamental uses, and for special industrial purposes where its properties of electrical and heat conductivity, malleability, and ductility outweigh its expense. While gold and its salts have been used for a wide variety of medicinal purposes, their present uses are limited to the treatment of rheumatoid arthritis and rare skin diseases such as discoid lumps. Sea water contains 3 to 4 mg per ton; and small amounts, 0.03 to 1 mg%, have been reported in many foods.

Gold salts are poorly absorbed from the gastrointestinal tract. The normal body burden is estimated at less than 1 mg. The majority of the information available concerning the distribution of gold salts originates from its therapeutic use or through experimental studies. Gold seems to have a long biological half-life, and detectable blood levels can be demonstrated for 10 months after the cessation of treatment. Most of the retained gold salts are found in the kidney; less is present in the liver and other organs, including the spleen. Colloidal gold may be collected by the reticuloendothelial system and larger amounts are found in the liver. After injection of most soluble salts, gold is excreted via the urine, while the feces account for the major portion of insoluble compounds [120].

The toxicity of gold and its salts seems to be associated largely with its therapeutic use rather than its industrial use. Dermatitis is the most frequently reported toxic reaction, sometimes accompanied by stomatitis. The skin lesions tend to disappear after the cessation of therapy. Dermatitis resulting from gold jewelry and dental fillings has been reported, and the patient was positive to skin tests with sodium aurothiomalate [122].

Nephritis with albuminuria, encephalitis, gastrointestinal damage, hepatitis, and blood dyscrasia, including leukopenia, agranulocytosis, thrombopenia, or aplastic anemia, have been reported with less frequency [123,124]. A 2-year, double-blind study using gold sodium thiomalate in the treatment of arthritis produced some improvement in the disease; but skin rashes, albuminuria, hematuria, pruritis, and stomatitis necessitated alterations in original treatment plan in 9 of 13 patients [125]. The gold-induced nephropathy has been postulated to involve a tissue immune response [126]. In rats, larger doses produce proximal tubular necrosis, whereas smaller doses elicit a slowly progressive renal disease involving the glomerular membrane [127].

GROUP IIB METALS

Group IIB is composed of zinc (Zn), cadmium (Cd), and mercury (Hg). Cadmium and mercury, which have been established as serious environmental hazards, are discussed in Chapters 12-14 and 26-28. Zinc interacts with cadmium, being antagonistic to many of the toxic effects of the latter. Zinc is furthermore unique in this group, inasmuch as it is an essential element.

Zinc

The principal ore of zinc is sphalerite (largely ZnS). Zinc is present in the earth's crust at a level of 50 ppm. The main uses of zinc are in the manufacture of galvanized iron, bronze, paint (white), rubber, glazes, enamel, glass, paper, and as a wood preservative ($ZnCl_2$, fungicidal action). Therapeutically, zinc compounds are used as topical astringents, dermal products, antiseptics, and emetics. The total exposure to zinc is increased through the widespread use of zinc undecylenate (preparations for athletes' foot) and zinc pyridinethione in antidandruff shampoos. Zinc is also contained in medicinal preparations of insulin and in zinc bacitracin.

Zinc has a ubiquitous distribution and is an essential trace element. It is necessary for normal growth and develepment in mammals and birds. Zinc is present in a number of metalloenzymes, including carbonic anhydrase, carboxypeptidase, alcohol dehydrogenase, glutamic dehydrogenase, lactic dehydrogenase, and alkaline phosphatase [128]. Both in natural and contaminated states it is generally accompanied by cadmium. The zinc/cadmium ratio plays a vital role in the effect zinc has on living organisms. Disease states related to zinc deficiency in the diet include growth failure, sexual infantilism in teenage individuals, anorexia, hyposmia, hypogensia, and impaired wound healing as signs and symptoms. The zinc deficiency may be worsened by the presence of phytate (inosital hexaphosphate) which binds zinc in the presence of calcium, thus decreasing the biological availability of zinc. Requirements of as much as 54.5 mg of zinc daily have been suggested for lactating women if the bioavailability is low [2].

Zinc is found in U.S. urban air at an average concentration of 0.67 $\mu g/m^3$ with concentrations as high as 58.0 $\mu g/m^3$ having been reported [36]. Zinc is present in natural water supplies, but the content in water may be increased by its flow through galvanized, copper, or plastic pipes. An upper desirable limit in community water supplies of 5 mg/l has been established. The maximum concentration in 969 communities was 13 mg/l. Of 2595 samples, only eight exceeded the desirable level [27].

Meat, eggs, milk products, and shellfish are zinc-rich foods. The average American intake has been estimated at about 12 mg/day, mainly from foods; only a small fraction of the ingested zinc is absorbed. As previously mentioned, the presence of phytate in food reduced absorption. On the other hand, vitamin D increases absorption. In addition, a homeostatic mechanism, perhaps involving the control of absorption as well as excretion, operates to regulate zinc balance [129].

Of the approximate 2-g body burden in man, most is found in skeletal muscle and bone. However, the prostate, liver, and kidney contain high concentrations. As one might expect because of the essentiality of zinc, it is found in newborns. After birth, the zinc body burden declines, then rises to a peak at about 45 years of age and declines thereafter [130].

The feces are the primary route of zinc excretion. A large percentage of absorbed zinc is eliminated by way of pancreatic juices. Urine, milk, and sweat are secondary vehicles for zinc excretion. The body pool of zinc is apparently not freely changeable and this, plus the essential nature of the metal, may account for a long ($\sim$300 days) biological half-life.

While a few instances of acute oral zinc intoxication have been described due to acid food intake from galvanized iron containers, it has been suggested that the gastroenteritis is similar to that resulting from cadmium salts. This seems plausible, inasmuch as galvanized pails contain 1.0% or more cadmium. Vomiting occurs after ingestion of zinc at 2-g oral dose of zinc sulfate, while 45 g of zinc sulfate is reported to be lethal [129]. In rats, zinc salts in the diet at 2500 ppm Zn has no effect. Higher levels (5000-10,000 ppm) reduce growth and produce anemia. Pregnant rats were not affected at 2000 ppm in the diet, but 4000 ppm caused fetal death and resorption [13].

Ingestion of 12 g (150 mg/kg) of metallic zinc by a 16-year-old boy produced lethargy and elevated amylase several days after ingestion. Dimercaprol was used as therapy and the whole blood zinc concentration fell from 8.1 to 0.8 mg/kg/l in 7 days. The normal range of whole blood zinc is 4.6-6.7 [131].

With regard to industrial exposure, the inhalation of freshly formed fumes of zinc oxide resulting in metal fume fever presents the most significant effect. Only the freshly formed material is potent, presumably because of flocculation in the air, thereby preventing deep penetration into the lungs. After the initial response resulting in "chills," repeated exposures often cause no reaction. Workers have noted that this effect appears most frequently on Mondays or after holidays. The primary symptom, fever, has been reproduced in rabbits; and it is postulated that the increased body temperature is due to the action of the fumes on endogenous pyrogen in the leucocytes. All evidence affirms that metal fume fever is an allergic-like reaction. Even in the most severe cases recovery is usually complete in 24-48 hr. There is no evidence that chronic effects have resulted from zinc oxide inhalation [132]. While zinc oxide fumes are the most common cause of metal fume fever, inhalation of other metal oxides may induce this reaction.

Dermal toxicity following exposure to $ZnCl_2$ has resulted from consistently handling these salts, and inhalation of mists or fumes may give rise to irritation of the gastrointestinal or respiratory tract. A gray cyanosis, dermatosis, and ulceration of the nasal passages have resulted from the inhalation of this caustic material.

The ocular hazard of zinc salts varies with the salt. Zinc chloride, while used as an astringent in eye drops at 0.2 to 0.5%, may cause damage at higher concentrations. Zinc sulfate in concentrations as high as 20% has been applied to the cornea for therapeutic purposes [18,120].

The TLV for zinc oxide fume is 5 mg/m^3, while that for zinc chloride fume is 1 mg/m^3. A TLV for zinc stearate of 10 mg/m^3 has been proposed on the basis of the particulate nuisance [1].

Testicular tumors have been produced by direct intratesticular injection into rats and chickens. This effect is probably related to the zinc concentration, normally in the gonads, and may be hormonally dependent. Other routes have not produced carcinogenic effects by zinc salts [112].

The antagonistic action between cadmium and zinc in the rat with respect to increased growth, prevention of dermal lesions, interaction with copper metabolism, and maintenance of circulation and body temperature by adequate intake of the latter has been demonstrated. Therefore, it is suggested that, in a sense, cadmium can be considered as an antimetabolite of zinc [133].

THE BORON FAMILY (GROUP IIIA)

The elements of this group, boron (B), aluminum (Al), gallium (Ga), indium (In), and thallium (Tl), present a series of contrasts. Most thallium compounds are poisonous, while aluminum is virtually innocuous. Aluminum is the most abundant metal, composing about 7% of the earth's crust, while indium is only found at about 1×10^{-5}%. While boron is actually not a metal, it will be discussed.

Boron

Boron is, strictly speaking, a nonmetal; however, it is in the Group IIIA of the periodic table and is of some toxicologic concern. Its concentration in the earth's crust is 16 ppm. Borax ($Na_2B_4O_7$) is the most important mineral. Borax is used in soldering and welding to remove oxide film, for softening water, in soaps, and in glass, pottery, and enamels.

Boric acid is useful medicinally as a mild antiseptic, especially as an eyewash. While boric acid has been used in the past to preserve food, this application has been declared unacceptable by the Food Agriculture Organization/World Health Organization (FAO/WHO) Expert Committee on Food Additives [2]. The borane hydrides, particularly decaborane and pentaborane, have various industrial uses. The former is used in vulcanizing rubber, and both were once used as high-energy fuels in rocket motors.

Boron occurs regularly in natural water supplies. An upper mandatory limit of 5.0 mg/l has been set for drinking water; frequently concentrations greater than 1.0 mg/l, the desirable upper limit, have been found in U.S. community water supplies [27]. Boron is essential to plants, but its necessity in animal diets has not been adequately demonstrated. An excess of soil boron may reduce plant growth. The average daily human intake has been estimated at 3 mg [2].

Boron as sodium borate or boric acid in the food (mostly in fruit and vegetables) is almost completely absorbed. However, it is also rapidly eliminated in the urine. The body burden is estimated at less than 10 mg. Treatment of large burned areas with boric acid results in systemic absorption. Large amounts of absorbed boron may accumulate in the brain [13].

Death has been reported due to dermal application of boric acid for burns and cuts. Central nervous system depression and gastrointestinal irritation are the most severe symptoms. Infants appear to be more susceptible to the toxic effects than adults. Skin irritation has occurred in infants following dermal application. Two cases of chronic borax intoxication in infants have been reported following the use of a borax and honey mixture for dry mouth. Recurrent generalized convulsions occurred in both infants. This symptom has been associated with boric acid poisoning. The child with the highest estimated intake (10 g/week for 12 weeks) had severe anemia, suggesting bone marrow depression. The estimated intake of the other child was 2 g/week for 5 weeks [134].

Chronic oral administration (2 years) of both borax and boric acid to rats and dogs produced no adverse effects at the 350 ppm boron level. Testicular degeneration was produced in males of both species at levels of 1170 ppm of boron by both borax and boric acid. Red cell indexes were also reduced in both species at higher levels (≥ 1170 ppm) of the test materials [135].

Industrial poisoning has not been reported from exposure to boron salts except for the boranes. The boranes, diborane, decaborane, and pentaborane, are highly toxic. Pentaborane is the most hazardous. Diborane is an irritant to the lungs and kidneys. Decaborane and pentaborane are central nervous system poisons; however, the liver and kidneys may also be damaged if the exposure is severe [18]. The toxicity of decaborane, which can produce effects after penetration through the skin, may be due to degradation products which act by reducing pyridoxal phosphate [136].

TLV values for industrial exposure to various boron compounds have been set: boron oxide 10 mg/m^3, boron tribromide 10 mg/m^3, boron trifluoride 3 mg/m^3 (ceiling), diborane 0.1 mg/m^3, pentaborane 0.01 mg/m^3, and decaborane 0.3 mg/m^3 [1].

Aluminum

Aluminum is the third most plentiful element and the most abundant metal in the earth's crust (81,300 ppm). Its principal ore is bauxite. Aluminum is widely used as a building material and for other applications where light weight and corrosion resistance are important. It also has industrial uses as an abrasive and catalyst. Medicinally, various soluble salts of aluminum have efficacy as astringents, styptics, and antiseptics. The insoluble salts serve as antacids and as antidiarrheal agents. Inhalation of aluminum hydroxide has been utilized as a prophylactic and curative agent for silicosis.

Practically no absorption of ingested aluminum or its compounds occurs, despite a daily intake of 10-100 mg. Many aluminum salts are converted to the phosphate salt in the gastrointestinal tract and excreted in the feces as such. Milk is a secondary route of excretion. Parenteral injection of aluminum salts results in excretion in both the feces and urine. Administration of aluminum by this route may cause slightly increased concentrations in the liver and spleen. Because of the widespread distribution, there is some aluminum in the body. Most soft tissues contain between 0.2 and 0.6 ppm [13]. The human body burden is 50-150 mg. The body burden is apparently not increased by heavy intake, much less at normal daily intake levels [18].

Only massive oral doses of aluminum are toxic, inducing gastrointestinal irritation and producing rickets by interfering with phosphate absorption. The use of aluminum in cooking utensils and cans produces no significant absorption or toxic effect [13].

Shaver's disease is the only suggested human manifestation of aluminum-induced industrial disease. It results from bauxite fume and the use of abrasive wheels containing aluminum. Exposure to the fume may produce weakness, fatigue, and respiratory distress. Chest x-ray may reveal extensive fibrosis with large blebs. Spontaneous pneumothorax is a frequent complication. Aluminum may not play a solitary role in the disease because silica is also frequently inhaled. In addition, fibrosis has been noted after such aluminum dust inhalation. Similar changes can be reproduced by intratracheal injection to experimental animals [18,137]. With regard to safe industrial exposure, the TLV is 10 mg/m^3 for alundum (A_2O_3) [1]. Powdered aluminum used in pyrotechnique devices and paints will ignite, and precautions against fire should be taken.

Gallium

Gallium is obtained as a by-product of copper, zinc, lead, or aluminum. It occurs at low levels in the earth's crust (5 ppm). It is used in high-temperature thermometers, as a substitute for mercury in arc lamps, in the manufacture of alloys and as a seal for glass and vacuum equipment. The metal is a liquid at temperatures greater than 29.9° C. Radioactive gallium has been given for diagnostic purposes to localize bone lesions.

Gallium is not readily absorbed by the oral route and occurs in bone at concentrations less than 1 ppm. Increased intake produces slightly higher levels in the liver, spleen, and kidney, as well as bone. The urine is the major route of excretion.

There are no reported adverse effects of gallium following industrial exposure. Therapeutic use of radiogallium has produced some consequences, chiefly dermal and gastrointestinal in nature. The bone marrow depression reported may be due largely to the radioactivity. In animals gallium acts as a neuromuscular poison and causes renal damage. Photophobia, blindness, and paralysis have been reported in rats. Renal damage ranging from cloudy swelling to necrosis has been reported. Aplastic changes in the bone marrow have been observed in dogs [18].

The incorporation of gallium into the drinking water for the lifetime of mice at a level of 5 ppm depressed growth slightly, and the survival of the females was less than that of the controls. No carcinogenic potential was suggested by the results of this study [35].

Indium

Indium is produced as a by-product in the manufacture of other metals, chiefly zinc, but also tin and lead. The concentration of indium in the earth's crust is low (less than 1 ppm). The industrial applications are in electroplating of nontarnishing silver and copper plate, corrosion-resistant alloys, glass manufacture, in nuclear energy processes, and in the manufacture of containers for foodstuffs.

Indium is poorly absorbed from the gastrointestinal tract. It is excreted in the urine and feces. Its tissue distribution is relatively uniform. The kidney, liver, bone, and spleen have relatively high concentrations. Intratracheal injections produce similar concentrations, but the accumulations in the tracheobronchial lymph nodes are increased.

While absorption from indium-plated silver in utensils may occur, this is without known toxic effect [18]. No industrial injury has been reported from the use of indium, although a TLV for indium and its compounds of 0.1 mg/m^3 has been set [1].

The knowledge of indium toxicity is based largely on results of animal experiments. Intravenous injection of indium chloride or hydrated indium oxide is followed by hind leg paralysis and inactivity. The liver and kidneys are adversely affected [138]. When administered to pregnant hamsters, malformations of limb buds in the fetuses were observed [139]. The incorporation of indium into the drinking water of mice for their lifetime at a level of 5 ppm produced only a slight suppression of growth. Neither longevity nor tumor frequency was adversely affected as compared to controls [35].

Thallium

The concentration of thallium in the earth's crust is less than 1 ppm. It is obtained as a by-product of iron, cadmium, and zinc; and it is used as a catalyst and in certain alloys, optical lenses, jewelry, low-temperature thermometers, dyes and pigments, and scintillation counters. It has been used as a depilatory. Thallium compounds, chiefly thallous sulfate, have been employed as rodenticides and insecticides.

Thallium is not a normal constituent of animal tissues. It is absorbed through the skin, gastrointestinal tract, and from parenteral sites, and can be identified in the urine within a few hours. The highest concentrations after poisoning are in the kidney and urine. The intestines, thyroids, testes, pancreas, skin, bone, and spleen have lesser amounts. The brain and liver concentrations are still lower. Thallium is excreted slowly. Following the initial exposure, large amounts are eliminated in the urine during the first 24 hr. After that period the feces may be an important route of excretion.

There have been many cases of poisoning from the medicinal use of thallium, and accidental poisoning occurs from thallium rodenticides. Acute thallium poisoning is characterized by gastrointestinal irritation, acute ascending paralysis, and psychic disturbances. In man, fatty infiltration and necrosis of the liver, nephritis, gastroenteritis, pulmonary edema, degenerative changes in the adrenals, degeneration of peripheral and central nervous system, alopecia, and, in some cases, death have been reported as a result of long-term systemic thallium intake. These cases usually are caused by the contamination of food or the use of thallium as a depilatory [18].

Acute toxicity studies in rats have indicated that thallium is quite toxic (oral LD_{50} approximately 30 mg/kg). The estimated lethal dose in humans is 8-12 mg/kg. Rat studies also indicate that thallium oxide, while relatively insoluble, is uniquely more toxic orally than by the intravenous or intraperitoneal route [140].

The signs of subacute or chronic thallium poisoning in rats were hair loss and hind leg paralysis occurring with some delay after the initiation of dosing. Renal lesions were observed at gross necropsy. Histological changes revealed damage of the proximal and distal renal tubules. The central nervous system changes were most severe in the mesencephalon, where necrosis was observed. Perivascular cuffing was also reported in several other brain areas. Electron microscopic examination indicated that the mitochondria in the kidney may have been the first organelle affected. Liver mitochondria also revealed degenerative changes. The livers of newborn rats whose dams had been treated throughout pregnancy showed these changes. Similar mitochondrial changes were observed in the intestine, brain, seminal vesicle, and pancreas. It has been suggested that thallium may combine with the sulfhydryl groups in the mitochondria and interfere with oxidative phosphorylation [141].

Occupational thallium poisoning is normally the result of moderate long-term exposure. The signs of this intoxication progress slowly and consist of polyneuritis followed by loss of hair. Urine thallium levels greater than 300 µg/l are considered suggestive of overexposure [142]. Industrial poisoning is a special risk in the manufacture of fused halides for the production of lenses and windows. Loss of vision, plus the other signs of thallium poisoning, has been related to industrial exposures [18]. A TLV of 0.1 mg/m^3 as Tl has been set for soluble thallium compounds [1]. It should be noted that absorption of thallium does occur through the skin, and good industrial hygiene practices should involve reduced topical exposure.

THE CARBON FAMILY (GROUP IVA)

Carbon (C) and silicon (Si) are the most abundant elements, carbon being a common constituent of living materials and silicon the chief inorganic element. Neither is a metal. Lead, which is of great environmental significance, is considered in Chapters 4-11, 26, and 28. Germanium, a metalloid, and tin are considered in this section.

Germanium

Germanium occurs in some mineral ores (1 ppm in the earth's crust) but is produced in the United States primarily as a by-product of zinc and can be obtained in the processing of coal. It is a semiconductor and has applications in electronics, in fine lenses, in certain aluminum alloys, and as a catalyst. However, only small amounts are actually used industrially; for example, only 7.5 tons were produced in the world in 1964.

One would expect significant amounts of germanium to be in the urban atmosphere as a result of its relatively high (1.6-7.5%) content in coal. Germanium is present in most foods. Raw clams, tuna, baked beans, and tomato juice have significant amounts. The average daily intake has been estimated at 1500 μg, but wide variations may occur.

Sodium germanite is rapidly absorbed from the gastrointestinal tract (96% in 8 hr). Germanium is transported at low serum levels unbound to plasma proteins. Some is also found in the red blood cells. Levels of 0.65 and 0.29 mg/ml have been reported as normal values for red blood cells and serum, respectively. In dogs 90% of radiogermanium oxide is excreted in the urine in 72 hr. The normal range of human urine concentration may be 0.40 to 2.16 μg/ml; milk and feces are secondary routes of excretion. The human body burden is minimal. In mice, continuous feeding of germanium causes accumulation in the spleen; however, the same apparently does not hold true for the rat [143]. Inhalation exposure of rats to germanium and germanium oxide revealed rapid removal from the lung tissue [18].

The toxicity of germanium and its compounds is low. The most widely studied is germanium oxide. The acute effects reported in animals are hypothermia, listlessness, diarrhea, respiratory and cardiac depression, edema, and hemorrhage in the lungs and gastrointestinal tract. The gaseous hydride, like other metal hydrides, is more toxic and causes hemolysis.

Germanium (sodium germanate) at 5 ppm in the drinking water of rats and mice for their lifetime produced increased germanium tissue levels. The incidence of some types of spontaneous tumors among treated groups was lower than in the control group [47]. Chronic administration to rats in food at 1000 ppm or in water at 100 ppm of germanium oxide caused growth inhibition and mortality. The survivors appeared to develop a tolerance. The cause of mortality was not apparent.

Exposure to germanium is not considered a serious industrial hazard, nor has it been implicated in any chronic diseases of man [18,143]. Occupational problems may arise if the dust of germanium oxide comes into contact with the eye and with the normal moisture forms germanic acid. In addition, inhalation exposure to metallic germanium, the dioxide, the tetrachloride, or the chloride causes pulmonary problems. The maximum allowable concentration established by the U.S.S.R. is 2 mg/m^3 for germanium and its oxides [144].

Tin

Tin occurs in the earth's crust at a level of 3 ppm. Cassiterite (SnO_2) is the most important ore of tin. It is used in the manufacture of tinplate and in food packaging, solder, bronze, and brass. Stannous and stannic chlorides are used in dyeing textiles. Organic, mainly trialkyl, tin compounds have been used as fungicides, bactericides, and slimicides, as well as in plastics as stabilizers. Stannous fluoride is used in toothpaste because of the anticavity effect of fluoride.

In ultraclean environments and by using a highly purified amino acid diet which retarded growth, some data suggestive of an essential role for tin in rats have been reported. Under these conditions, 2 mg Sn/kg (stannic sulfate) increased growth 59% [145]. However, evidence suggestive of an essential role in other species and in plants is lacking. The difficulties in the accurate determination of tin because of the high volatility of many tin compounds may tend to obscure the establishment of biological necessity. This difficulty also has led to unusual variations in reported Sn levels in tissues and foodstuffs and makes more difficult metabolic studies of tin.

The average concentration of tin in U.S. urban air was 0.02 $\mu g/m^3$ with detected values running as high as 0.5 $\mu g/m^3$ [36]. The daily intake of tin, mostly from foods as a result of processing, has been estimated at 3.5 to 17 mg. Diets of all canned foodstuffs (vegetables, fish, etc.) could raise this as high as 38 mg.

Of the 30-mg body burden in man the highest concentrations are found in the lungs and gastrointestinal tract. Newborns contain little tin; and the lungs tend to accumulate small amounts with age, probably due to atmo-

spheric contamination [146]. Only a small percentage of the inorganic tin
salts ingested are absorbed. Stannous (Sn^{2+}) salts may be somewhat better
absorbed than stannic (Sn^{4+}) salts. The use of radiolabeled tin in rats
has not revealed a significant difference in tissue distribution related
to the valence of the tin. Bone tin levels were increased. The increases
in liver and kidney were less marked. Following intravenous injection, 30%
of the tin was excreted in the urine, regardless of valence. Eleven percent
of the Sn^{2+} was recovered from the bile, but none of the Sn^{4+}. No significant amounts of radiolabeled tin were found in the brain after either oral
or intravenous administration [147].

Organic tin salts, particularly the lower alkyl tin compounds tend to
be absorbed more easily than inorganic tin. The highest tin concentrations
were found in the liver, blood, and skeletal muscle. Smaller amounts were
in the kidneys, spleen, heart, and brain when administration of the compound
ceased. Retention of tin in these tissues was not prolonged. Tetraethyl
tin and presumably other organic tin compounds are converted in vivo to the
more toxic triethyl tin [148].

Massive oral or intravenous doses of inorganic tin salts produce neurological, renal, and hepatic toxicity [146]. Oral intake by human volunteers
of tin in fruit juices at 1370 ppm (≥ 4.38 mg Sn/kg) produced only nausea
and diarrhea, probably due to local irritation of the gastrointestinal tract.
At 730 ppm (< 3.58 mg Sn/kg) there were no toxic effects [149]. In rats,
tin at a level of 0.3% (3000 ppm) in the diet for 13 weeks as stannous
chloride or other soluble salts produced depressed weight gain and red cell
indexes, induced slight liver changes, and caused bile duct epithelium proliferation. Increasing the iron intake was reported to lessen the anemia
[150]. Stannous tin at 5 ppm in the drinking water of rats and mice over
their lifetime did not produce any significant change in tumor incidence.
Some accumulation of tin in the tissue was noted [47].

Organic tin compounds tend to be considerably more toxic than inorganic
tin salts. An outbreak of almost epidemic nature took place in France due
to the oral ingestion of organic tin compounds used for skin disorders.
One hundred deaths resulted from this incident [148]. Excessive industrial
exposure to triethyl tin produced headaches, visual defects, and electro-
encephalogram (EEG) changes which were very slowly reversed [151]. Experimentally, triethyl tin produces depression and cerebral edema. The resulting
hyperglycemia may be related to the centrally mediated depletion of catecholamines from the adrenals [152]. Acute burns or subacute dermal irritation

has been reported among workers as a result of tributyl tin [34]. Triphenyl tin is a potent immunosuppressant [153]. Organic tin compounds used as plastic stabilizers produced fetal death when administered orally to pregnant rats [154]. Organic tin compounds, especially alkyl tins, have a hemolytic effect. This effect is reduced by sulfhydryl compounds [155]. Inhibition in the hydrolysis of adenosine triphosphate or uncoupling of oxidative phosphorylation taking place in the mitochondria has been suggested as the cellular mechanism of tin toxicity [156].

Tin inhalation in the form of dust or fumes over a considerable time span leads to benign pneumoconiosis. Tin hydride (SnH_4) is more toxic to mice and guinea pigs than is arsine; however, its effects appear mainly in the central nervous system and no hemolysis is produced [18].

A TLV for organic tin compounds of 0.1 mg Sn/m^3 has been established. Absorption through the skin should be taken into consideration during exposure. The TLV for inorganic tin compounds (except SnH_4 and SnO_2) is 2 mg Sn/m^3, while the TLV of tin oxide is 10 mg/m^3 and is considered a nuisance particulate [1]. A permissible limit of 250 ppm for tin in canned food has been applied [2], and this would seem adequate for inorganic compounds.

THE NITROGEN FAMILY (VA)

Group VA is composed of the gas nitrogen (N), phosphorus (P), arsenic (As), antimony (Sb), and bismuth (Bi). Progressing down the group in respect to atomic weight there is a transition from the nonmetal phosphorus to bismuth, which has many metallic chemical properties. Arsenic has been considered in Chapters 16, 17, and 26-29; thus, only antimony and bismuth are considered in this section.

Antimony

Antimony occurs in the earth's crust at less than 1 ppm. The primary ore of antimony is stibnite (Sb_2S_3). The important uses of this metal are with lead alloys, in storage battery grids, and in type alloys, pewter, bearing alloys, rubber, matches, ceramics, enamels, paints, lacquers, and textiles.

Antimony or its compounds were used medicinally as early as 4000 B.C. Its popularity in medicine has undergone several cycles of use and disuse. At the present time employment in this manner is declining with the advent of newer parasiticides. The therapeutic activity involves reaction with the sulfhydryl groups in enzymes and a selective toxicity due to concentration in the parasite. Both trivalent and pentavalent organic compounds have been administered parenterally for parasiticidal effect; however, based on the hypothesis for the mechanisms of effect, the trivalent forms would be expected to have greater efficacy. The probable in vitro conversion from the pentavalent to the trivalent forms may well account for the clinical effectiveness of the former. The trivalent compounds have been given orally as emetics and expectorants, but this procedure has been largely abandoned because of toxicity. The mechanism of emetic activity includes both a local and a central component [120].

Antimony is a common pollutant in urban air, occurring at an average concentration of 0.001 $\mu g/m^3$ and a maximum of 0.160 $\mu g/m^3$ [36]. Antimony may be present in food, resulting from the use of rubber, solders, and tinfoil for packaging. Leaching of antimony from cheap enameled vessels has caused some food contamination. Tartar emetic (antimony potassium tartrate) has been used as an insecticide.

The average body burden of antimony is about 90 mg [14]. Most of the information on the distribution and fate of antimony compounds is derived from investigational results on therapeutic compounds. Antimony compounds are slowly absorbed from the gastrointestinal tract and tend to produce vomiting. The distribution of antimony following intravenous or intramuscular administration is variable and cannot be fully accounted for solely on the basis of valence. The trivalent forms generally concentrate in red blood cells, while the pentavalent compounds are in the plasma. Trivalent forms accumulate in the liver and are slowly excreted, principally in the feces. In experimental animals significantly high concentrations are found in the thyroid after administration of trivalent compounds. The pentavalent forms tend to concentrate in the liver and spleen and are excreted in the urine. It is noteworthy that repeated dosages of labeled antimony tartar emetic were not accumulated in the body.

Acute poisoning has resulted from accidental or suicidal ingestion of antimonials. The symptoms are similar to those of arsenical poisoning and consist of vomiting, watery diarrhea, collapse, irregular respiration, and lowered temperature. Vomiting increases the chance of recovery. In fatal cases death occurs only a few hours after ingestion [18,120]. Chronic incorporation of potassium antimony tartrate (5 ppm) into the drinking water of rats caused a higher mortality rate and lower serum glucose and cholesterol levels. The incidence of tumors was not increased; but there was evidence of antimony accumulation in the soft tissue, contrary to what has

been reported by other investigators [48]. Accumulation in the tissue of
mice treated in a similar way has also been reported. In mice the life span
of females was slightly shortened [47]. Injection of antimony dextran gly-
coside into pregnant rats causes no adverse effects and antimony was not
detected in the fetuses [156].

Toxicity data have also been derived in connection with therapeutic
use of antimonials. Cardiac effects, in a few cases auricular fibrillation
due to a direct effect on the heart; liver toxicity, characterized by jaundice and fatty degeneration; pulmonary congestion and edema; papular skin
eruptions; and deaths have been reported [157].

Occupational poisoning by antimony is often difficult to establish
since the antimony used in industry may contain some arsenic. The toxicity
of antimony and arsenic are similar. The signs ascribed to industrial antimony poisoning include upper respiratory tract irritation, pneumonitis,
dizziness, diarrhea, vomiting, and dermatitis. An acceptable concentration
for occupational exposure of 0.5 mg/m^3 as Sb has been suggested for antimony
and its compounds [1].

Antimony miners have developed disabling, but benign, forms of silicosis. Some investigators have suggested a relationship between antimony and
pulmonary carcinogenesis on the basis of possible antimony-containing abnormal enzyme systems. However, no positive evidence has been produced that
diseased lung tissue contains excess amounts of antimony. Antimony and
antimony compounds may generate stibine (antimony hydride) under reducing
conditions. This has occurred during storage battery charging. Although
arsine is usually suspected in cases of industrially induced hemolytic anemia, stibine may be involved more frequently than is suspected. The lethal
exposure of stibine for mice is about 100 ppm for 1.6 hr, while that of arsine is 100 ppm for 3 hr. Stibine, like arsine, usually causes rapid destruction of red blood cells, hemoglobinuria, and anuria. Subjective signs
include headache, vomiting, nausea, and lumbar and epigastric pain [18].
An acceptable average occupational exposure for stibine is 0.5 mg/m^3 (0.1
ppm) [1].

Bismuth

Bismuth is obtained as a by-product of tin, lead, and copper ores.
The concentration in the earth's crust is less than 1 ppm. It is used in
the manufacture of type alloys, silvering of mirrors, low-melting solders
(sometimes in canning), and heat-sensitive devices such as automatic fire

extinguishers.   Bismuth telluride is used in the electronics industry as a
semiconductor.

Trivalent insoluble bismuth salts are used medicinally to control diarrhea and other gastrointestinal distress.   Some of these preparations are
available without prescription.   Various bismuth salts have been used ex-
ternally for their astringent and slight antiseptic properties.   Further
self-exposure comes from the use of insoluble bismuth salts in cosmetics.
Bismuth salts have also been used as radiocontrast agents.   Injections of
soluble and insoluble salts, suspended in oil to maintain adequate blood
levels, were used to treat syphilis.   Bismuth sodium thioglycollate, a
water-soluble salt, was injected intramuscularly for malaria (Plasmodium
vivax).   Bismuth glycoly arsanilate is one of the few pentavalent salts
that have been used medicinally.   This material was formerly used for treatment of amebiasis.   Exposure to various bismuth salts for medicinal use has
decreased with the advent of newer therapeutic agents.

Bismuth is one of the contaminants measured in U.S. urban air.   The
average concentration was <0.0005 $\mu g/m^3$, while the maximum concentration
reported was 0.064 $\mu g/m^3$ [36].

Most bismuth compounds that one is exposed to are insoluble and poorly
absorbed whether taken orally or applied to the skin, even if the skin is
abraded or burned.   Thus, most of the information on their distribution in
the body is related to therapeutic use.   Once the bismuth is absorbed from
the site, tissue binding appears minimal.   A diffusible equilibrium between
tissues, blood, and urine is established.   Tissue distribution, omitting
injection depots, reveals the kidney as the site of the highest concentration.   The liver concentration is considerably lower at therapeutic levels,
but with massive doses in experimental animals (dogs) the kidney/liver
ratio is decreased.   Passage of bismuth into the amniotic fluid and into
the fetus has been demonstrated.   The urine is the major route of excretion.
Traces of bismuth can be found in the milk and saliva.   The total elimination
of bismuth after injection is slow, depending on mobilization from the injection site [18].

Except for strong acidic salts such as bismuth trinitrate or violently
reactive compounds such as bismuth tripentafluoride, the bismuth compounds
do not present a hazard by dermal application, inhalation, or ingestion.
The dermal application of most bismuth compounds shows no systemic toxicity.
Oral administration of bismuth subnitrate produces poisoning through the
formation of nitrites.   Intravenous injections of bismuth salts are avoided

because of toxicity; the soluble salts have a tendency to flocculate. Intramuscular injections tend to be painful, and when sufficient doses are
employed, some necrosis is evident at the site of injection. In experimental animals renal and hepatic toxicity have been observed following the
achievement of sufficient systemic bismuth levels. The symptoms of chronic
bismuth toxicity in man consist of decreased appetite, weakness, rheumatic
pain, diarrhea, fever, metal line on the gums, foul breath, gingivitis, and
dermatitis. Jaundice and conjunctival hemorrhage are rare, but have been
reported. When nephritis does occur in man, albuminuria is used as a signal
to discontinue administration [120]. The renal effects include diuresis and
are similar to the effects of mercury. Microscopically, lipid-carbohydrate-
protein inclusions containing no bismuth are formed in the renal proximal
convoluted tubular cell shortly after treatment with bismuth. They are
apparently irreversible [158]. Bismuth poisoning may be treated with dimercaprol (British antilewisite). Industrial exposure resulting in poisoning is rare.

Bismuth telluride is the only compound for which a safe occupational
exposure level has been adopted. The TLV for this compound is 10 mg/m^3 [1].

THE OXYGEN FAMILY (VIA)

Of Group VIA elements composed of oxygen (O), sulfur (S), selenium
(Se), tellurium (Te), and polonium (Po), only tellurium will be discussed.
Polonium is a radioactive element and may be hazardous on the basis of its
α-particle emission following inhalation. Selenium and tellurium have certain metalloid characteristics, while oxygen and sulfur do not. Selenium
has been discussed in another section.

Tellurium

Tellurium is found in various sulfide ores along with selenium and is
produced as a by-product of metal refineries. The concentration of tellurium in the earth's crust is 0.002 ppm. Its industrial uses include applications in the refining of copper and in the manufacture of rubber. Tellurium vapor is used in "daylight lamps." It is used in various alloys as
a catalyst and is a semiconductor. Potassium tellurate has been used to
reduce sweating.

Condiments, dairy products, nuts, and fish are high in content. Food
packaging contains some tellurium; higher concentrations are found in aluminum cans than tin cans. Some plants, such as garlic, accumulate tellurium

from the soil. Tellurium found in food is probably in the form of tellurites.

The use of neutron activation analysis reveals much higher concentrations of tellurium in human organs than had been previously suggested. Of the 600 mg of average body burden in man, the majority is in the bone. This is a relatively high body burden for a nonessential element. It is, for example, about six times that of copper. The liver, brain, and kidney have high concentrations among the soft tissue. Soluble tellurites (tetravalent), absorbed into the body after oral administration, are reduced to tellurides, partly methylated, and then exhaled as dimethyl telluride. The latter is responsible for the garlic odor in persons exposed to tellurium compounds. The normal levels of serum and urine are similar. Normal ranges are 0.50-1.60 μg/ml and 0.26-1.09 μg/ml, respectively. At the usual level of intake, excretion and consumption are in balance. The urine is the principal route of excretion. Sweat and milk are secondary routes of excretion. Some data suggest that tellurium accumulates, probably as tellurite, in the bone and liver [159].

Tellurates and tellurium are of low toxicity, but tellurites are generally more toxic. Acute inhalation exposure results in decreased sweating, nausea, metallic taste, and sleeplessness. The typical garlic breath is a reasonable indicator of exposure to tellurium by the dermal, inhalation, or oral route. Serious cases of tellurium intoxication from industrial exposure have not been reported [160]. The TLV for tellurium is 0.1 mg/m^3 and is largely based on worker experience. It may not be low enough to prevent garlic breath when repeated exposures are involved. A TLV of 0.2 mg/m^3 (0.02 ppm) has been set for tellurium hexafluoride [1].

One of the few serious recorded cases of human tellurium toxicity resulted from accidental poisoning by injection of tellurium into the ureters during retrograde pyelography. Two of the three victims died. Stupor, cyanosis, vomiting, garlic breath, and loss of consciousness were observed in these unlikely incidents [161].

In rats, chronic exposure at high doses of tellurium dioxide has produced decreased growth and necrosis of the liver and kidney [18,162,163]. Sodium tellurite at 2 ppm or potassium tellurate at 2 ppm of tellurium in drinking water of mice for their lifetime produced no effects in the tellurate group. The females of the tellurite (tetravalent) group did not live as long [164].

In rats, 500 ppm in the diet of pregnant females induced hydrocephalus in the offspring. This was the only abnormality reported. Abortions were produced at 3600 ppm. Tellurium passes the rat placenta and is found in the fetal brain [165].

Dimercaprol (BAL) treatment for tellurium intoxication increases the renal damage. Ascorbic acid decreases the characteristic garlic odor but may also adversely affect the kidneys in the presence of increased amounts of tellurium [166].

ACTINIDE ELEMENTS

Of this series, only uranium will be discussed in detail. The members of this series are radioactive. Those with atomic number from 93 on have been made under artificial conditions. Thorium, however, because of its unfortunate history is probably worth some comment. Thorium is found in nature, $1.2 \times 10^{-3}\%$ in the earth's crust. It is present in monazite sand (2.5-28%), the source of the rare earths. Its hazardous effect is associated with its radioactivity. Unfortunately, thoratrast, a radiological contrasting agent containing thorium, caused cancer, probably as a result of radiation from amounts of thorium dioxide retained primarily in the liver, spleen, and bone marrow.

Uranium

The chief raw material of uranium is pitchblende or carnotite ore. Uranium occurs at only 2 ppm in the earth's crust. This element is largely limited to use as a nuclear fuel. While uranium is a radioactive element, it also has chemical toxicity and this may possibly present a hazard unrelated to radioactivity. Emission of an alpha particle, it should be noted, does not constitute an external radiation hazard, although internal effects, especially insofar as inhalation is concerned, are significant. The normal body burden of uranium is relatively small, 0.02 mg [14]. The uranyl ion is rapidly absorbed from the gastrointestinal tract. About 60% is carried as a soluble bicarbonate complex, while the remainder is bound to plasma protein. Sixty percent is excreted in the urine within 24 hr. About 25% may be fixed in the bone [167].

The soluble uranium compounds (uranyl ion) and those which solubilize in the body by the formation of a bicarbonate complex produce systemic toxicity in the form of acute renal damage. The classic impairment of renal function by uranium may result in death. However, if exposure is not too severe, the renal tubular epithelium is regenerated; and recovery occurs. Renal toxicity with the classic signs of impairment, including albuminuria, elevated blood urea nitrogen, and loss of weight, is brought about by filtration of the bicarbonate complex through the glomerulus, resorption by the proximal tubule, and liberation of uranyl ion with subsequent damage to the proximal tubular cells [168,169].

Uranium tetrafluoride and uranyl fluoride can produce a typical toxicity because of hydrolysis to HF. Skin contact (burned skin) with uranyl nitrate has resulted in nephritis [170].

Following inhalation of the insoluble salts, retention by the lungs is prolonged. Inhalation exposure of rats, dogs, and monkeys to uranium dioxide dust at a concentration of 5 mg U/m^3 for up to 5 years produced accumulation in the lungs and tracheobronchial lymph nodes which accounted for 90% of the body burden. No evidence of toxicity was observed at that time despite the unusually long duration of the experimental investigation [171]. Observations on the dogs and monkeys from the above study for a period of up to and over 6 years after exposure revealed retention in the tracheobronchial lymph nodes and lungs. Fibrosis was dose dependent and more marked in the primates. Frank neoplasms were found in four and foci of atypical epithelial proliferation were evident in six of 13 dogs surviving up to 75 months. The estimated dose to lungs of alpha radiation was 600-700 rads. No other adverse effects were observed [172].

The TLV for (natural) uranium compounds, regardless of their solubility, is 0.2 mg U/m^3 [1]. On the other hand, in the U.S.S.R. the soluble uranium compounds have an MAC of 0.015 mg/m^3 and that of the insoluble compounds is 0.075 mg/m^3 [173].

REFERENCES

1. American Conference Government Industrial Hygienists, J. Occup. Med., 16, 39 (1974).

2. World Health Organization, Trace Elements in Human Nutrition. WHO Technical Report Series No. 532, Geneva, 1973.

3. I. Singer and D. Rotenbenberg, New Engl. J. Med., 289, 254 (1973).

4. American Industrial Hygiene Association, Lithium Hydride, Hygienic Guide, 1964.

5. J. M. Davis and W. E. Fann, Ann. Rev. Pharmacol., II, 285 (1971).

6. B. V. Hartitzsch, N. A. Hoenich, R. J. Leigh, R. Wilkerson, T. H. Frost, A. Weddel, and G. A. Posen, Brit. Med. J., 4, 757 (1972).

7. G. K. Spring, Dis. Nervous System, <u>35</u>, 351 (1974).

8. E. J. Gralla and H. M. McIlhenny, Toxicol. Appl. Pharmacol., <u>21</u>, 428 (1972).

9. T. L. Wright, L. H. Hoffman, and J. Davies, Teratol., <u>4</u>, 151 (1971).

10. M. Schou, M. D. Goldfield, M. R. Weinstein, and A. Villeneurve, Brit. Med. J., <u>2</u>, 135 (1973).

11. M. Schou, A. Amdisen, and O. R. Steenstrup, Brit. Med. J., <u>2</u>, 137 (1973).

12. M. Schou and A. Amdisen, Brit. Med. J., <u>2</u>, 138 (1973).

13. W. J. Underwood, Trace Elements in Human and Animal Nutrition, 3rd Ed., Academic Press, New York, 1971.

14. H. A. Schroeder, J. Chronic Dis., <u>18</u>, 217 (1965).

15. B. S. Eichelman, Jr., Psychopharmacol. Bull., <u>10</u>, 27 (1974).

16. J. M. Stolk, Psychopharmacol. Bull., <u>10</u>, 32 (1974).

17. R. R. Fieve, H. Meltzer, D. L. Dunner, M. Levitt, J. Mendlewicz, and A. Thomas, Amer. J. Psychiatry, <u>130</u>, 55 (1973).

18. E. Browning, Toxicity of Industrial Metals, 2nd Ed., Butterworths, London, 1969.

19. M. E. Shils, Ann. N. Y. Acad. Sci., <u>162</u>, 847 (1969).

20. H. A. Heggtveit, Ann. N. Y. Acad. Sci., <u>162</u>, 758 (1969).

21. H. A. Schroeder, A. P. Nason, and I. H. Tipton, J. Chronic Dis., <u>21</u>, 815 (1969).

22. F. W. Heaton, Ann. N. Y. Acad. Sci., <u>162</u>, 775 (1969).

23. L. P. Eliel, W. O. Smith, R. Chanes, and J. Hawrylko, Ann. N. Y. Acad. Sci., <u>162</u>, 810 (1969).

24. D. C. Trainor, in International Labour Office Encyclopaedia of Occupational Health and Safety, Vol. II, McGraw-Hill, New York, 1972, pp. 809-811.

25. H. A. Schroeder, I. H. Tipton, and A. P. Nason, J. Chronic Dis., <u>25</u>, 491 (1972).

26. R. E. Lee, S. S. Goranson, R. E. Enrione, and G. B. Morgan, The National Air Surveillance Cascade Impactor Network Part II: Size Distribution Measurements of Trace Metal Components, presented at American Chemical Society, 163rd meeting, Boston, 1972.

27. U.S. Public Health Service: Community Water Supply Study, Analysis of National Survey Findings, U.S. Department of Health, Education, and Welfare, Washington, D.C., 1970.

28. S. Weitzner and D. H. Law, Amer. J. Digest, Dis., <u>17</u>, 17 (1972).

29. D. B. Gould, M. R. Sorrell, and A. D. Lupariello, Arch. Intern. Med., <u>132</u>, 891 (1973).

30. American Industrial Hygiene Association, Barium and Its Inorganic Compounds, Hygienic Guide, 1962.

31. T. A. Roscina, in International Labour Office Encyclopaedia of Occupational Health and Safety, Vol. II, McGraw-Hill, New York, 1972, pp. 1202-1203.

32. N. Matsusaka, J. Inaba, R. Ichikawa, M. Ikeda, and Y. Ohkudo, in Radiation Biology of the Fetal and Juvenile Mammal (M. R. Sikov and D. D. Mahlum, eds.), U.S. Atomic Energy Commission, Washington, D.C., 1969, pp. 217-226.

33. T. J. Haley, J. Pharm. Sci., $\underline{54}$, 663 (1965).

34. H. E. Stokinger, in Industrial Hygiene and Toxicology (D. W. Fasset and D. D. Irish, eds.), Vol. II, Interscience, New York, 1963, pp. 987-1194.

35. H. A. Schroeder and M. Mitchener, J. Nutr., $\underline{101}$, 1431 (1971).

36. G. B. Morgan, G. Ozolins, and E. C. Tabor, Science, $\underline{170}$, 289 (1970).

37. H. A. Schroeder, J. J. Balassa, and I. H. Tipton, J. Chronic Dis., $\underline{16}$, 55 (1963).

38. American Industrial Hygiene Association, Titanium, Hygienic Guide, 1973.

39. H. A. Schroeder, J. J. Balassa, and W. H. Vinton, J. Nutr., $\underline{83}$, 239 (1964).

40. H. A. Schroeder and M. Mitchener, Arch. Environ. Health, $\underline{23}$, 102 (1971).

41. A. Furst and R. T. Haro, Prog. Exp. Tumor Res., $\underline{12}$, 102 (1969).

42. H. A. Schroeder and J. J. Balassa, J. Chronic Dis., $\underline{19}$, 85 (1966).

43. C. J. Spiegl, M. C. Calkins, J. J. DeVoldre, J. K. Scott, L. T. Steadman, and H. E. Stokinger, Inhalation Toxicity of Zirconium Compound I Short Term Studies, University of Rochester Atomic Energy Report No. UR 460, 1956.

44. W. L. Epstein and J. R. Allen, J. Amer. Med. Ass., $\underline{190}$, 940 (1964).

45. J. T. Prior, G. P. Cronk, and D. B. Zielger, Arch. Environ. Health, $\underline{11}$, 297 (1960).

46. American Industrial Hygiene Association, Zirconium, Hygienic Guide, 1958.

47. M. Kanisawa and H. A. Schroeder, Cancer Res., $\underline{29}$, 892 (1969).

48. H. A. Schroeder, M. Mitchener, and A. P. Nason, J. Nutr., $\underline{100}$, 59 (1970).

49. W. B. Blumenthal, Amer. Ind. Hyg. Ass. J., $\underline{34}$, 128 (1973).

50. T. J. Haley, R. N. Komesu, and H. C. Upham, Toxicol. Appl. Pharmacol., $\underline{4}$, 238 (1962).

51. H. A. Schroeder, J. J. Balassa, and I. H. Tipton, J. Chronic Dis., $\underline{16}$, 1047 (1963).

52. American Industrial Hygiene Association, Vanadium Pentoxide, Hygienic Guide, 1957.

53. P. Stocks, Brit. J. Cancer, $\underline{14}$, 397 (1960).

54. M. D. Waters, D. E. Gardner, and D. L. Coffin, Toxicol. Appl. Pharmacol., $\underline{28}$, 253 (1974).

55. R. J. Hickey, E. P. Schoff, and R. C. Clelland, Arch. Environ. Health, $\underline{15}$, 728 (1967).

56. H. A. Schroeder and J. J. Balassa, J. Chronic Dis., $\underline{18}$, 229 (1965).

57. R. G. Thomas, R. L. Thomas, and J. K. Scott, Amer. Ind. Hyg. Ass. J., $\underline{28}$, 1 (1967).

58. L. C. K. Wong and W. L. Downs, Toxicol. Appl. Pharmacol., 9, 561 (1966).

59. W. L. Downs, J. K. Scott, F. S. C. Caruso, and L. C. H. Wong, Amer. Ind. Hyg. Ass. J., 26, 237 (1965).

60. J. L. Egorov, in International Labour Office Encyclopaedia of Occupational Health and Safety, Vol. II, McGraw-Hill, New York, 1972, pp. 935-936.

61. P. W. Durbin, Health Phys., 2, 223 (1960).

62. W. Mertz, Physiol. Rev., 49, 163 (1969).

63. H. A. Schroeder, A. P. Nason, and I. H. Tipton, J. Chronic Dis., 23, 123 (1970).

64. R. G. Smith, in Metallic Contaminants and Human Health (D. H. K. Lee, ed.), Academic, New York, 1972, pp. 139-157.

65. P. R. Harrison, Adv. Exp. Med. Biol., 40, 173 (1973).

66. R. Hartung, Adv. Exp. Med. Biol., 40, 161 (1973).

67. H. A. Schroeder, J. J. Balassa, and I. H. Tipton, J. Chronic Dis., 15, 941 (1962).

68. R. A. Shakman, Arch. Environ. Health, 28, 105 (1974).

69. L. B. Tepper, in Metallic Contaminants and Human Health (D. H. K. Lee, ed.), Academic, New York, 1972, pp. 229-241.

70. E. Feverman, Dermatologica, 143, 292 (1971).

71. S. Fregert and H. Rorsman, Arch. Dermatol., 90, 4 (1964).

72. P. E. Enterline, J. Occup. Med., 16, 523 (1974).

73. W. C. Hueper, Clin. Pharmacol. Ther., 3, 766 (1962).

74. W. C. Hueper and W. W. Payne, Arch. Environ. Health, 5, 445 (1962).

75. H. A. Schroeder, J. J. Balassa, and I. H. Tipton, J. Chronic Dis., 19, 545 (1966).

76. A. A. Britton and G. C. Cotzias, Amer. J. Physiol., 211, 203 (1966).

77. E. R. Hughes, S. T. Miller, and G. C. Cotzias, Amer. J. Physiol., 211, 207 (1966).

78. P. S. Papavasiliou, S. T. Miller, and G. C. Cotzias, Amer. J. Physiol., 211, 211 (1966).

79. A. J. Bertinchamps, S. T. Miller, and G. C. Cotzias, Amer. J. Physiol., 211, 217 (1966).

80. C. D. Klaassen, Toxicol. Appl. Pharmacol., 29, 458 (1974).

81. G. K. Davins, in Toxicants Occurring Normally in Foods, Food Protection Committee, National Academy of Science, Publ. No. 1354, Washington, D. C., 1967, pp. 229-235.

82. S. H. Zaidi, R. K. Dogra, R. Shanker, and S. V. Chandra, Environ. Res., 6, 287 (1973).

83. American Industrial Hygiene Association, Manganese and Its Inorganic Compounds, Hygienic Guide, 1963.

84. I. Mena, K. Horivchi, K. Burke, and G. C. Cotzias, Neurology, 19, 1000 (1969).

85. I. Mena, O. Marin, S. Fuenzalidia, and G. C. Cotzias, Neurology, 17, 128 (1967).

86. W. Pentschew, F. F. Ebner, and R. M. Kovatch, J. Neuropathol. Exp. Neurol., 22, 488 (1963).

87. C. Marti-Feced, in International Labour Office Encyclopaedia of Occupational Health and Safety, Vol. II, McGraw-Hill, New York, 1972, pp. 819-821.

88. G. C. Cotzias, P. S. Papavasiliou, J. Ginos, A. Stechk, and S. Duby, Ann. Rev. Med., 22, 305 (1971).

89. N. H. Neff, R. E. Barrett, and E. Costa, Experientia, 25, 1140 (1969).

90. M. T. Martone, M.S. Thesis, University of Rochester, Rochester, N.Y., 1964.

91. F. W. Sunderman, Jr., T. J. Lau, and L. J. Cralley, Cancer Res., 34, 92 (1974).

92. R. W. Beal, Drugs, 2, 190 (1971).

93. V. F. Fairbanks, J. L. Fahey, and E. Beutler, in Clinical Disorders of Iron Metabolism, 2nd Ed., Grune and Stratton, New York 1971.

94. M. J. Murray, Clin. Toxicol., 4, 545 (1971).

95. L. J. Casarett and B. Epstein, Amer. Ind. Hyg. Ass. J., 27, 533 (1966).

96. J. T. Boyd, R. Doll, J. S. Faulds, and J. Leiper, Brit. J. Ind. Med., 27, 97 (1970).

97. American Industrial Hygiene Association, Iron Oxide, Community Air Quality Guide, 1968.

98. R. Al-Rushid, Clin. Toxicol., 4, 571 (1971).

99. J. Greengard and J. T. McEnery, GP, 37, 88 (1968).

100. T. R. C. Sisson, Quart. Rev. Pediatr., 15, 47 (1960).

101. H. A. Schroeder, A. P. Nason, and I. H. Tipton, J. Chronic Dis., 20, 869 (1967).

102. J. H. Wills, in Toxicants Occurring Naturally in Foods, Foods Protection Committee, National Academy of Science, Publ. No. 1354, Washington, D. C., 1967, pp. 3-17.

103. Y. Morin and P. Daniel, J. Can. Med. Ass., 97, 926 (1967).

104. C. Horwitz and S. E. Van der Linden, S. Afr. Med. J., 48, 230 (1974).

105. G. E. Isom and J. L. Way, Toxicol. Appl. Pharmacol., 27, 131 (1974).

106. American Industrial Hygiene Association, Cobalt, Hygienic Guide, 1966.

107. H. A. Schroeder, J. J. Balassa, and I. H. Tipton, J. Chronic Dis., 15, 51 (1962).

108. P. D. Whanger, Toxicol. Appl. Pharmacol., 25, 323 (1973).

109. H. A. Schroeder, M. Mitchener, and A. P. Nason, J. Nutr., 104, 239 (1974).

110. F. W. Sunderman, Jr., in Laboratory Diagnosis of Diseases Caused by Toxic Agents (Sunderman and Sunderman, eds.), Warren and Green, St. Louis, 1970, pp. 389-395.

111. American Industrial Hygiene Association, Nickel Carbonyl, Hygienic Guide, 1968.

112. F. W. Sunderman, Jr., Food Cosmet. Toxicol., $\underline{9}$, 105 (1971).

113. American Industrial Hygiene Association, Nickel, Hygienic Guide, 1966.

114. American Industrial Hygiene Association, Osmium and Its Compounds, Hygienic Guide, 1968.

115. G. M. Levene, Brit. J. Dermatol., $\underline{85}$, 590 (1971).

116. J. L. Parrot, R. Herbert, A. Saindelle, and F. Ruff, Arch. Environ. Health, $\underline{19}$, 685 (1969).

117. A. H. Rossef, R. E. Slayton, and C. P. Porlia, Cancer, $\underline{30}$, 145 (1972).

118. R. R. Landolt, H. W. Berk, and H. T. Russell, Toxicol. Appl. Pharmacol., $\underline{21}$, 589 (1972).

119. D. Munro-Ashman and T. H. Hughes, Trans. A. Rep. St. John's Hospital Derm. Soc. (London), $\underline{55}$, 196 (1969).

120. T. Sollmann, Manual of Pharmacology, W. B. Saunders Company, Philadelphia, 1957, pp. 1191-1354.

121. F. Walker, Brit. J. Exp. Pathol., $\underline{52}$, 589 (1971).

122. M. L. Elgart and R. S. Higdon, Arch. Dermatol., $\underline{103}$, 649 (1971).

123. R. H. Freyberg, in Arthritic and Allied Conditions, 7th Ed., Lea and Febiger, Philadelphia, 1966.

124. P. W. Dale and M. B. Patterson, Electroenceph. Clin. Neurophysiol., $\underline{23}$, 493 (1967).

125. J. W. Sigler, G. B. Bluhm, H. Duncan, J. T. Sharp, D. C. Ensign, and W. R. McCrum, Ann. Intern. Med., $\underline{80}$, 21 (1974).

126. A. Katz and A. H. Little, Arch. Pathol., $\underline{96}$, 133 (1973).

127. A. H. Nagi, F. Alexander, and A. Z. Barabas, J. Exp. Mol. Pathol., $\underline{15}$, 354 (1971).

128. B. L. Vallee, Physiol. Rev., $\underline{39}$, 443 (1959).

129. J. A. Halsted, J. C. Smith, and M. I. Irwin, J. Nutr., $\underline{104}$, 345 (1974).

130. H. A. Schroeder, A. P. Nason, I. H. Tipton, and J. J. Balassa, J. Chronic Dis., $\underline{20}$, 179 (1967).

131. J. V. Murphy, J. Amer. Med. Ass., $\underline{212}$, 2119 (1970).

132. American Industrial Hygiene Association, Zinc Oxide, Hygienic Guide, 1969.

133. H. G. Petering, M. A. Johnson, and K. L. Stemmer, Arch. Environ. Health, $\underline{23}$, 93 (1971).

134. A. S. Gordon, J. S. Prichard, and M. H. Freedman, Can. Med. Ass. J., $\underline{108}$, 719 (1973).

135. R. J. Weir and R. S. Fisher, Toxicol. Appl. Pharmacol., $\underline{23}$, 351 (1972).

136. L. L. Naeger and K. C. Leibman, Toxicol. Appl. Pharmacol., $\underline{23}$, 517 (1972).

137. American Industrial Hygiene Association, Aluminum and Aluminum Oxide, Hygienic Guide, 1963.

138. F. P. Castronovo and H. H. Wagner, Brit. J. Exp. Pathol., 52, 543 (1971).

139. V. H. Ferm, Adv. Teratol., 6, 51 (1972).

140. W. L. Downs, J. K. Scott, L. T. Steadman, and E. A. Maynard, Amer. Ind. Hyg. Ass. J., 21, 399 (1960).

141. M. M. Herman and K. G. Bensch, Toxicol. Appl. Pharmacol., 10, 199 (1967).

142. J. Glomme, in International Labour Office Encyclopaedia of Occupational Health and Safety, Vol. II, McGraw-Hill, New York, 1972, pp. 1402-1403.

143. H. A. Schroeder and J. J. Balassa, J. Chronic Dis., 20, 211 (1967).

144. O. J. Mogilevskaja, in International Labour Office Encyclopaedia of Occupational Health and Safety, Vol. I, McGraw-Hill, New York, 1972, pp. 610-611.

145. K. D. Schwartz, D. B. Milne, and E. Vineyard, Biochem. Biophys. Res. Comm., 40, 22 (1970).

146. H. A. Schroeder, J. J. Balassa, and I. H. Tipton, J. Chronic Dis., 17, 483 (1964).

147. R. A. Hiles, Toxicol. Appl. Pharmacol., 27, 366 (1974).

148. J. M. Barnes and H. B. Stoner, Pharmacol. Rev., 11, 211 (1959).

149. C. J. Benoy, P. A. Hooper, and R. Schneider, Food Cosmet. Toxicol., 9, 645 (1971).

150. A. P. DeGroot, V. J. Feron, and H. P. Til, Food Cosmet. Toxicol., 11, 19 (1973).

151. G. Prüll and K. Rompel, Clin. Neurophysiol., 29, 215 (1970).

152. I. M. Robinson, Food Cosmet. Toxicol., 7, 47 (1969).

153. H. G. Verchuuren, E. J. Ruitenberg, F. Peetoom, P. W. Hellman, and G. J. VanEsch, Toxicol. Appl. Pharmacol., 16, 400 (1970).

154. M. Nikonorow, H. Mazur, and H. Piekacz, Toxicol. Appl. Pharmacol., 26, 253 (1973).

155. K. H. Byington, R. Y. Yeh, and L. R. Forte, Toxicol. Appl. Pharmacol., 27, 230 (1974).

156. K. E. Moore and T. M. Brody, Biochem. Pharmacol., 6, 134 (1961).

157. J. B. Casals, Brit. J. Pharmacol., 46, 281 (1972).

158. R. E. Burr, A. M. Gotto, and D. L. Beaver, Toxicol. Appl. Pharmacol., 7, 588 (1965).

159. H. A. Schroeder, J. Buckman, and J. J. Balassa, J. Chronic Dis., 20, 147 (1967).

160. American Industrial Hygiene Association, Tellurium, Hygienic Guide, 1964.

161. M. H. H. Keall, N. H. Martin, and R. E. Turnbridge, Brit. J. Ind. Med., 3, 175 (1946).

162. F. A. Patty, in Industrial Hygiene and Toxicol (D. W. Fassett and D. D. Irish, eds.), 2nd Ed., Interscience, New York, 1963, pp. 871-910.

163. E. A. Cerwenka and W. C. Cooper, Arch. Environ. Health, 3, 189 (1961).

164. H. A. Schroeder and M. Mitchener, Arch. Environ. Health, 24, 66 (1972).

165. S. Duckett, Ann. N. Y. Acad. Sci., 192, 220 (1972).

166. M. L. Amdur, Arch. Ind. Health, 17, 665 (1958).

167. P. S. Chen, R. Terepka, and H. C. Hodge, Ann. Rev. Pharmacol., 1, 369 (1961).

168. H. A. Passow, A. Rothstein, and T. W. Clarkson, Pharmacol. Rev., 13, 185 (1961).

169. C. Voegtlin and H. C. Hodge (eds.), The Pharmacology and Toxicology of Uranium Compounds, Vol. 1-4, McGraw-Hill, New York, 1949-1951.

170. American Industrial Hygiene Association, Uranium (Natural) and Its Compounds, Hygienic Guide, 1969.

171. L. J. Leach, E. A. Maynard, H. C. Hodge, J. K. Scott, C. L. Yuile, G. E. Sylvester, and H. B. Wilson, Health Phys., 18, 599 (1970).

172. L. J. Leach, C. L. Yuile, H. G. Hodge, and G. E. Sylvester, Health Phys., 25, 239 (1973).

173. N. J. Tarasenko, in International Labour Office Encyclopaedia of Occupational Health and Safety, Vol. II, McGraw-Hill, New York, 1972, pp. 1452-1454.

TERATOGENICITY OF HEAVY METALS

Francis L. Earl and Theodore J. Vish
Food and Drug Administration
Washington, D. C.

The undesirable environmental effects of heavy metals and other toxic elements have been recognized for many years: first, in the workers of industrial factories; second, in people coming in contact with the effluence of
the factories (whether it be from stack emissions or water discharges in
the surrounding areas or downstream from the discharge); and finally, in
the consumer exposed to these products, such as lead paint. Occasionally
an imbalance in soil elements causes dietary problems associated with a
deficiency or an excess of heavy metals such as selenium, molybdenum, and
copper. At times, a more subtle and sinister effect occurs in the form of
terata (Gr terat-, teras monster) seen at birth in both the human and animal
population. Acute poisoning of humans and animals occurs occasionally from
industrial or agricultural accidents, but many of today's problems are the
result of long-term exposure to heavy metals as environmental contaminants.

The event of contamination is conditional upon the amount or concentration of a substance. The mere presence of a metal species does not constitute a threat. Indeed, the presence of a certain amount of some metals is
indispensable to the living cell. Iron and copper are required in various
respiratory pigments, e.g., hemoglobin, myoglobins, and hemocyanins, and in
oxidative enzyme systems required in metabolism. Cobalt requirement for
vitamin B12 synthesis and zinc requirement for carbonic anhydrase and dehydrogenases may vary with the organism. Higher plants which may ultimately
be consumed by both animals and humans require aluminum, boron, and vanadium.
Molybdenum is necessary in all organisms which derive nitrogen from inorganic
sources. Many other metals are commonly found in small quantities, but no
known biological function has been established for them. Other metals such

as antimony, arsenic, barium, beryllium, bismuth, cadmium, mercury, lead, silver, tellurium, and thorium have no known nutritive value and are commonly considered as toxicants [1].

MECHANISMS OF TERATOGENESIS

The above-mentioned metals usually produce toxicity in most animals when given chronically in sufficient amounts. Teratogenicity, on the other hand, cannot always be linearly correlated with dose. Some metals do not produce any teratogenic effects at sublethal doses, and the teratogenic potential of other metals can be altered by changing the species and the time and method of administration.

The specific mechanism of many teratogenic events remains a puzzle for the most part. Ferm [2] offers two hypotheses, however, that help explain why some teratogens act differently from others. One hypothesis is that the teratogen is nonspecific, i.e., the characteristics of a malformation depend primarily on the organogenetic event in progress at the time of the insult. Thus, a wide spectrum of malformations should result from a single teratogenic stimulus given at different periods of critical embryogenesis (broad-spectrum teratogens).

An alternative hypothesis suggests that certain teratogens might well prove to be site specific and induce malformations only in certain developing organ systems. This mechanism (site-specific teratogens) implies that a specific organ-teratogen relationship exists which could best be explained by interference with a particular physiologic event of development. If this hypothesis is correct, the metals should be good examples of site-specific teratogens, for metals enter into a variety of rather specific enzymatic reactions.

Early investigators used the egg to evaluate the effects of heavy metals on embryonic development [3-7]. However, the chick embryo has not proved to be an ideal model for the study of teratogenic effects; excessive concentrations of elements cause destruction and regression of organs already developed, rather than damaging the embryo in its early developmental stages. These effects produce acute toxicity which does not simulate natural exposure. Hence, in evaluating such data, it must be kept in mind that chick embryos can generate misleading results in which atrophy could be misinterpreted as teratogenesis.

Increased sophistication in teratological techniques has succeeded in eliciting a teratogenic response to a given agent from many species. Ideally,

it is desirable to have a species of animal that can be used to predict with
accuracy the teratogenic response which may be observed in humans. Unfortunately, the only animal that can do this unequivocally is the human him-
self. Thus investigators must rely on information derived from other animals
in making educated predictions when no information concerning exposure in
humans is available.

The difficulty of extrapolating animal teratogenic data to humans is
well recognized. The probability that a teratogen applied to a pregnant
mammal will produce malformations in the embryo depends on the agent, the
dose, the species, the genetic contribution of mother and embryo, and the
developmental stage of the embryo [8]. Demonstration of teratogenicity in
livestock and experimental animals can serve only as a warning of possible
teratogenic effects in humans and a guide to the types of malformations the
agent might produce. Conversely, failure to demonstrate teratogenic effects
experimentally does not prove a priori that the agent is harmless to the
human embryo.

ARSENIC

Inorganic

Arsenic trioxide and sodium arsenite were formerly used as "alterna-
tives and tonic" in various conditions in human medicine. They are no
longer extensively used, but acute exposure can result from arsenic-con-
taining pesticides, herbicides, and desiccants. Livestock, especially
cattle, are frequently poisoned by residual arsenic around dipping vats,
filling places of spraying and dusting rigs, and old orchards. Large quantities of arsenic (As) compounds have been introduced into the environment
for over 100 years through such processes as smelting, manufacturing, use
in paints and industrial chemicals, and agricultural applications. Chronic
exposure may occur from paint, dyes, cosmetics, and pesticides.

Egg inoculations with inorganic As can result in stunting, micromelia,
abdominal edema, and a high percentage of dose-related deaths [9,10].

The golden hamster is highly susceptible to intravenous injections of
sodium arsenate. This compound produces serious developmental malformations
(mild encephaloceles to complete exencephaly) when injected during the critical stages of embryogenesis. The effect of arsenic is considered site
specific in the hamster, related perhaps to the embryonic mesenchyme [11].

Hood and Bishop [12] found that sodium arsenate appeared to be a general, rather than site-specific, teratogen in mice, affecting several dif-

ferent systems. Dams treated by single intraperitoneal injection on one of days 6 to 10 of gestation gave birth to offspring with exencephaly, micrognathia, protruding tongue, and other defects. Both sodium arsenate and arsenite were shown to be embryocidal and teratogenic in mice [13]. Schroeder and Mitchener [14] observed that the feeding of As to pregnant mice elevated the ratio of males to females born. Five ppm of As in the drinking water of breeding mice did not significantly affect fertility or viability of offspring in a three-generation study.

Hamsters are the most sensitive to the teratogenic effects of sodium arsenate at 20-25 mg/kg [15]; rats are affected at 30 mg/kg [16] and mice at 45 mg/kg [12]. Skeletal malformations involving the ribs and the cranium occur in all three species. Vertebral defects have been found only in mice and rats and genitourinary abnormalities have been reported only in hamsters and rats. Other abnormalities occur in the above-noted species but less frequently. The time of induction of the above-mentioned malformations was similar in all three species (day 8-10). Bred ewes fed low doses of potassium arsenate exhibit no malformation of the lambs, but higher doses prove toxic and stunt fetal growth [17]. Lugo et al. [18] found no malformations following acute inorganic arsenic poisoning occurring late in human pregnancy.

Organic

Ancel [19] reported that methyl arsenate (1 mg) produced spina bifida in chick embryos. There are no reports of organic arsenicals causing teratogenesis in mammalian species. Underhill and Amatruda [20] were unable to produce any malformations in pregnant cats and rabbits by giving them organic arsenicals.

CADMIUM

Cadmium (Cd) is one of several "trace metals" existing in nature in small quantities that have no known nutritive value and are capable of producing a toxic effect. Cadmium ranks 67th of the 97 most common elements in the earth's crust and occurs in association with zinc (Zn) in a ratio of 1:445. Cadmium is a general cytotoxic agent with a particular affinity for sulfhydryl groups and, to a certain extent, for hydroxyl groups and ligands containing nitrogen. Cadmium is also a potent inhibitor of several enzyme systems. Evidently, excretion of Cd can occur within very narrow limits, and every increase in the normal intake results in an increased accumulation

primarily in nonosseous tissue. Little or no Cd is found in the tissues of
the newborn or the fetus [1].

Ribas and Schmidt [21] found that Cd, applied to the intravitelline
circulation of chick embryos, manifested teratogenic effects at the end of
the trunk and the "hind extremities." Microscopically, cells disassociated,
macrophages formed, and numerous cells "perished." Supravitelline application induced premature death of the embryo.

Cadmium induces serious facial malformations in hamster fetuses whose
dams are injected early in the eighth day of pregnancy [22]. Later treatment produces rib cage defects and limb bud abnormalities predominately [23].
The usual skeletal malformations are poor bilateral ossification of the
squamosal bones, retardation of ossification of vertebral bones, rib cage
fusion, and forelimb malformations [23]. Intravenous administration of
cadmium sulfate to hamsters causes 60% incidence of malformations (mainly
craniofacial) in the embryos [22]. Ferm et al. [24] found that radioactive
Cd was present in the embryos within 24 hr after the pregnant hamsters were
injected intravenously on day 8 of gestation. There was a relative decrease
in embryonic concentration of radioactive cadmium by day 12.

Mulvihill et al. [25] concluded that Cd has a marked effect on the
mesoderm of the head of the golden hamster, causing the production of numerous malformations including unilateral and bilateral cleft lip and palate.

Ferm et al. [24] state that Cd is known to cross the placental barrier
in the hamster. Friberg et al. [26], on the other hand, indicate that the
placenta constitutes a barrier against the transfer of small doses of Cd,
although larger doses may damage the barrier and enter the fetus. In human
newborns, the total content of Cd is small (less than 1 μg), which tends to
support the animal data [26]. Berlin and Ullberg [27] state that the placenta constitutes a barrier in the mouse, but the pattern of distribution
in the placenta indicates special uptake of Cd in some parts of the placenta
although no Cd was found in the fetus. Cd salts cause progressive pathological alterations of the placenta and ultimate death of Swiss albino mice
[28].

Schroeder et al. [29] found that Cd was present in the tissues of dams
given 5 ppm in the drinking water but no Cd was present in the carcasses of
five stillborn mice. Cadmium did cause a highly significant number of runts
and young deaths in the F_1 and F_2 generations of these mice. Maternal death
occurred in the F_3 generation and no offspring resulted. Cadmium sulfate or
chloride was teratogenic in Wistar rats with a spectrum of malformations

differing from that in hamsters and depending greatly upon the stock of rat used [30]. Subcutaneous cadmium chloride injections in rats have been shown to cause a dose-related rise in fetal deaths, fetal weights, and the number of abnormalities, including micrognathia, cleft palate, clubfoot, and small lungs. It is not known if the abnormalities result from a direct action on the fetus or indirectly from a maternal or placental influence or from a combination of these factors [31].

Flick et al. [32] concluded that the teratogenic effect of Cd in man is unresolved, although both acute and chronic intoxication have been reported.

COPPER

Acute and chronic copper (Cu) intoxication is not a significant problem today, largely because present-day manufacturing processes and uses of copper have reduced its potential as a major environmental contaminant. Copper sulfate, once used to treat parasitism in sheep, is no longer widely used.

Absorption of Cu is limited, which decreases its potency as a teratogen. However, laboratory experiments have demonstrated Cu teratogenicity in a few species. Copper salts injected intravenously into pregnant golden hamsters on the eighth day of gestation cause an increase in embryonic reabsorptions as well as developmental abnormalities. Malformations of the heart appear to be a specific result of the toxicity of copper compounds. Copper sulfate and citrate are teratogenic, and the citrate complex is the more teratogenic of the two. Radioactive copper citrate passes the placental barrier of hamsters, indicating that the metal may have a direct teratogenic effect on the developing embryo [33]. James et al. [17] demonstrated that copper sulfate given to pregnant ewes (10 mg/kg/day $CuSO_4$) for 45-146 days during pregnancy did not affect the newborn in three of four ewes. The remaining ewe aborted after 142 days.

LEAD

Common sources of lead (Pb) in the environment are Pb-base pigments in paints, Pb-containing pesticides, discarded wet cell batteries, shooting ranges or waterfowl hunting sites, putty, plumbing installations or repair sites, manufacturing fillers, untaxed whiskey, and liniments and lotions. Other sources of Pb contamination have been lead pipes used in wells or vegetation contamination resulting from heavy highway traffic or close proximity to a smelter.

The environmental contamination from Pb to date is not known to have caused any teratogenic effects. However, the treatment of chick embryos with Pb salts has been shown to produce a toxic effect on the morphogenesis of the lead primordium, hydrocephalus, and anterior meningoceles [34-36]. Sublethal doses of Pb ions have also produced an ectopic condition in chick embryos [9]. In golden hamsters, Pb salts induce malformations primarily localized within the sacral and tail vertebrae, characterized by varying degrees of tail malformation ranging from stunting to complete absence of the tail [37,38].

The addition of 25 ppm Pb to the drinking water of breeding mice can cause early deaths of the offspring, but no teratogenesis has been reported [39]. Lead was present in the tissues of dams receiving 5 ppm in the drinking water, but the metal was not detected in the carcasses of five stillborn mice [29]. McLellan et al. [40] found that high doses of lead chloride given to pregnant mice on day 9 of gestation caused a marked decrease in fetal weight (61%) with incomplete and/or delayed ossification in 73% of the fetuses. Infant mortality was 80% vs 25% in controls. Gross motor activity was 54% of the control values at day 35 postpartum, but the righting reflex was unaffected.

Lead levels in the fetal blood and amniotic fluid were found to be 55% of that of the maternal blood in a goat infused for 2 hr with lead chloride [40]. Two ewes fed 9 mg lead acetate/kg/day aborted on days 50 and 106, respectively, and death occurred from lead intoxication. However, two ewes given 5 mg/kg/day through day 45 of pregnancy were not affected and gave birth to two normal lambs at term [17]. Five mg lead acetate/kg/day produced lead toxicosis in pregnant cows, but their calves were unaffected [41].

Greenfield [42] reported one well-documented case of human exposure to low levels of Pb without effect on the fetus. However, it has been reported that severe exposure to a high level of Pb resulted in abortion [43,44]. Excessive exposure to industrial contamination is thought to cause symptoms of neurological disorder [45] and growth retardation [46]. Wilson [44] has reported that high levels of Pb in drinking water caused the birth of a stillborn infant and of an infant with congenital nystagmus and partial albinism. In the first case, fetal kidney and maternal blood contained high levels of Pb, and in the second case, the antenatal urine coproporphyrin output of the mother was increased. Barltrop [47] has reported that lead crosses the human placenta at high-level exposures. Palmisano et al. [46] noted that a woman gave birth to an infant that at 10 weeks of age showed evidence of neurological defects, intrauterine growth retardation, and

postnatal failure to thrive. The maternal history indicated a long-term
ingestion of untaxed whiskey.

Clegg [48] has questioned the value of teratogenic data concerning
human exposure to Pb, as the doses involved could not be calculated. Similarly, he considered that the route of administration and extremely high
doses involved in hamster teratogenicity experiments render extrapolation
to man almost impossible.

MERCURY

The more severe expressions of mercury teratogenicity in laboratory
animals are the result of intravenous injections of relatively large doses.
Oral dosing usually elicits more subtle and delayed reactions. This is an
important distinction when considering human exposure to mercury from environmental sources affecting food and water supplies.

Methyl mercury is the most common form of the metal as an environmental
contaminant. The majority of reports of human intoxication are the result
of methyl mercury or other organic compounds of mercury either working their
way up the food chain, as in Minamata Bay, or being directly consumed due to
mishandling of treated seed grain, as in Iraq. It is also possible, however,
for other forms of mercury to be converted to methyl mercury through micro-
bial action, thereby increasing the possible sources of methyl mercury pollution.

McLaughlin et al. [49] found that the inoculation of chick embryos with
0.5 mg HgCl caused the death of all embryos. Lower doses (0.25 mg) reduced
the hatchability by 80% [50]. Organic Hg-contaminated fertile eggs were
less successful in hatching; 85% died compared to 15% of controls. The hatch
time was prolonged 1-2 days and the body weight was less. No malformations
were found, but a slightly disturbed gait was noted. Histopathological
changes were occasionally observed in the neurons of the brain [51]. MeHgCl
is appreciably teratogenic in hamsters when given in single doses of 8 mg/kg
on various susceptible days of gestation or in daily injections of 2 mg/kg
throughout most of pregnancy [52]. These doses also cause overt signs of
maternal toxicity. Gale and Ferm [53] reported a small number of miscellaneous abnormalities in the golden hamster.

A single high dose or 16 low doses of MeHgOH had an embryo-toxic effect,
i.e., dose-related incidence of cleft palates and decreased behavioral emotionality and locomotor activity in mice [54]. Spyker and Smithberg [55]

found that methyl mercury caused growth retardation in the embryos of two
different strains of mice and was not embryocidal but was teratogenic. Their
results demonstrated that single doses of methyl mercury apparently did not
affect pregnant females, yet produced growth and developmental retardation
and congenital malformation. Differential effects were dependent on strain,
dose, and stage of development. The type and frequency of abnormalities
were also dependent on strain, dose, and treatment day. The placenta of
mice is no barrier to methyl mercury, as Hg is distributed in the fetus in
concentrations comparable to those found in maternal tissues [56]. A single
dose, one-fourth to one-third LD_{50}, injected in mice, resulted in a high
frequency of resorbed litters [57]. High oral doses of MeHgCl caused all
pups to be stillborn or to die as neonates. At lower doses, there was an
induced transitory inhibition of cerebellar cellular migration from the external granular layer and depressed reaction of oxidative enzymes [58].
Intraperitoneal injections of methyl mercury dicyandiamide before mating
reduced the incidence of pregnancies but not litter size. Injection on day
10 increased embryo mortality. Ethyl mercuric phosphate injected into pregnant mice on day 10 at 40 mg/kg caused reduced fetal weight and a 31.6%
incidence of cleft palate [59]. In the rat, 0.1 mg Hg/kg as methyl mercury
throughout pregnancy resulted in reduced birth weight and postneurological
disorders [60]. Rats given up to 0.25 mg methyl mercury/kg did not produce
offspring adversely affected. Postnatally, however, a histological condition
involving the eyelids, i.e., Harderian glands, the exorbital lachrymal gland,
and the parotid gland, was detected [58]. Ethyl mercury compounds were most
toxic in rats in respect to generative functions and offspring, and phenyl
mercury pesticides were less toxic with a less pronounced effect on generative functions [61].

Continuous low-dose exposure of MeHgOH in pregnant rats increased fetal
deaths, runting, and edema. No gross behavioral changes were noted during
the first 3 weeks postpartum in the pups [62]. A single injection of 8 mg
of methyl mercury per kg on day 10 or 11 has been shown to cause a decrease
in postpartum survival of neonates and teratogenic effects (skeletal abnormalities) in one of six litters. Behavioral effects were also observed only
in this group [54]. Moderate prolonged oral dosing with MeHgOH (4-5-6 mg/kg,
days 6-19 of pregnancy) in rats resulted in all pups being affected; effects
included abnormalities of the ribs (delayed calcification), brain, heart,
and testes [63]. Malformations of the cerebellum have been induced by

treatment of pregnant rats on days 9 to 11 of gestation with orally administered MeHgCl [64]. Newberne et al. [65] fed rats 12 µg of methyl mercury
per kg in fish protein concentrate with no adverse effects on conception or
pregnancy. This is the equivalent of 840 µg Hg in a 70-kg man, an amount
equivalent to eight times the average amount of fish consumed per capita in
the United States, according to Newberne's calculations. It was concluded
that the rat may not be the best model for providing data for extrapolation
to man. Yang et al. [66] found that fetal rat brains contained higher concentrations of Hg than their treated dams. Mansour et al. [67] found that
fetal uptake of methyl mercury was greater than that of mercury nitrate when
given to pregnant rats on days 15 and 20 of gestation.

Miller [68] observed that the Hg levels of brains of sows fed 50 µg
MeHgCl/kg/day for two years or longer were higher than those of their day-old
offspring. It should be underscored, however, that the 50 µg/kg/day regimen
was the lowest level at which sows showed overt signs of toxicity, viz.,
blindness. Swine fed low levels (25 µg/kg/day) of methylmercuric chloride
for 3 years showed no overt toxicity.

Pregnant cats have been given up to 0.75 mg/kg/day as MeHgCl from day
10-58 of pregnancy. At the high dose, overt toxicity and death of the queens
occurred. At 0.25 mg, there was an increased incidence of abortion and fetal
anomalies; in surviving fetuses a reduced neuronal population in the external
granular layer of the cerebellum was noticed. Specific areas of Hg concentration, in decreasing order, were fetal blood, maternal blood, and fetal
brain, with the Hg concentration of the dam's brain being equal to that of
her blood [69]. One of eight kittens from a queen treated with bis-ethyl
mercuric sulfide displayed an unsteady gait and a disturbance of posture
fixation 2 weeks after birth; it died 3 months later. Granular atrophy of
the cerebellum was present in the mother and the affected kittens [70].

Earl et al. [71] found that levels of 0.1 mg MeHgCl/kg/day given to
beagle dogs pregestationally and throughout pregnancy (av, 129 days) caused
one of 10 litters to be abnormally developed, i.e., omphalocele, cleft palate, patent fontanelles, superfluous phalanges and enlarged kidneys. The
incidence of stillborns was high in litters from dams given 0.1 and 0.25
mg/kg/day. No terata were seen in sows given 0.05 to 0.5 mg MeHgCl/kg/day,
but there was an increase in the percentage of stillborns up through the
0.25 mg level.

Cell cultures of lymphocytes from guinea pigs, rats, dogs, and man
treated with low concentrations of various Hg compounds produced lymphocyte

transformation and chromosome breaks, abnormal cell division, and vacuolization [72-75]. It is suggested that Hg is a nonspecific lymphocyte-stimulating agent [76].

The adverse effects of mercurial pollution have been reported from Minamata and Niigata, Japan, as Minamata disease in newborns [77-82]. Tejning [83] reported the passage of MeHg across the placenta in women and its possible preferential concentration in the fetus; human fetal erythrocytes showed 28% greater Hg concentration than maternal erythrocytes. Methyl mercury is more readily transferred across the placenta in mice than HgCl or phenylmercuric acetate [84].

Methyl mercury is an embryotoxic substance as seen in fetal Minamata disease. Exposure following placentation manifests clinical toxicity in the infant as congenital cerebral palsy. Miscarriages and true malformations were not found to have increased in the Minamata Bay area. However, the feeding of Hg-contaminated fish frequently produced miscarriages in rats and cats with no malformations [70,85]. The disease has two characteristic pathological features: neuropathologic findings associated with nonfetal infantile Minamata disease and the other related to the age (brain growth) at the time of fetal exposure, i.e., when the mother consumed the contaminated fish.

The disturbance of development in the cytoarchitecture of the brain suggests that the disease results from poisoning during the fetal period. The author does not mention that the clinical signs of congenital cerebral palsy might be the result of a teratogenic lesion. Changes represented as hypoplastic and dysplastic alterations in the central nervous system (CNS) were not identified as teratogenic lesions [86].

Twenty-three (6%) of 359 children born in the villages near Minamata Bay were affected with cerebral palsy-like disease. Several features are noteworthy in these cases: (a) the affected children had not eaten contaminated fish or shellfish, (b) the mothers apparently were not affected, and (c) clinical symptoms were more difficult to elicit and more varied than in cases of Minamata disease in adults and children [87]. Since the brains of these infants were still developing after birth, and since severe exposure to mercury also could have occurred through mother's milk, the term congenital (fetal) attached in these cases by Harada [88] and Takeuchi [86] may seem inappropriate [87].

Alkyl Hg poisoning of human fetuses has been observed in New Mexico. Treated seed wheat was fed to swine, the meat of which was consumed by the

farmer's family over a 3-month period. During the period in which the meat
was consumed a mother was in her second trimester of pregnancy. Upon delivery the child had tremulous movements and elevated urine Hg levels. At 6
weeks postnatally, the Hg levels were normal, but at 8 months the child displayed typical signs of methyl mercury poisoning. In utero exposure can
cause Hg poisoning even when the mother herself has no overt signs of exposure [89]. Human beings are believed to be most sensitive to methyl mercury
during the early stages of the life cycle, including both prenatal and postnatal periods. Observations indicate that hazardous amounts of methyl mercury can enter the fetus in utero [90]. Organic Hg seems to be more devas-
tating to the nervous system than inorganic Hg [89].

    In 1972, commercial interests sold seed wheat, treated with a mercurial
compound for weevil control, to the Iraqi government. Although marked with
the international sign for poison (a skull and crossbones), the wheat was
used for food and a catastrophic Hg poisoning of the population occurred.
Few data concerning teratology have yet evolved from this incident. It is
estimated that a relatively low number of pregnant females were affected,
and death occurred in almost half of these cases [90].

MOLYBDENUM

    Molybdenosis has appeared in many parts of the world due to industrial
molybdenum (Mo) contamination of nearby pastures. In addition, it has been
used as a growth promotant in pastures, and excesses have been found in the
plants. Molybdenum is not considered to be very toxic nor teratogenic in
the golden hamster. Ferm [91] found that Mo produced no embryocidal or
teratogenic effects up to 100 mg/kg. However, Schroeder [39] demonstrated
that 10 ppm in the drinking water of breeding mice caused a significant increase in young deaths in F_1 and F_3 generations and in dead litters in the
F_3 generation.

    Colmano [92] postulated that Mo may be an inhibitor of cellular fission,
evoking nuclear and chromosomal polyploidy and abnormal mitosis. He further
hypothesized that Mo may activate the uncontrolled patterns observed in some
neoplastic growths.

    Jeter and Davis [93] found no effect on the fertility nor gestation
of female rats given high doses of Mo. Mills and Fell [94] found severe
demyelinization of the CNS in newborn lambs from dams who, during pregnancy,
were maintained on diets high in Mo. However, affected lambs were also found
to have a low content of copper in their livers.

SELENIUM

Selenium, as a teratogen and a toxicant, is an evironmental hazard predominantly to grazing animals. The toxic effects of selenium (Se) in animals were observed in the 13th century by Marco Polo who correctly assigned the cause to the consumption of toxic plants [95]. This problem has become so prevalent that plants affected by Se have been classified into three categories: (a) the indicator plants, which need Se for growth; (b) secondary Se absorbers, which can grow without Se or will accumulate Se if is in the soil; and (c) nonaccumulators, which may or may not tolerate Se at all [96]. Selenium is an interesting element in that reproductive problems occur from both a deficiency and an excess of Se in the diet [97].

Laboratory investigators [9] as early as 1936 injected Se into the air sac of hen eggs and found that Se salts produced a large number of deaths and a high percentage of abnormalities. Other investigators [10,98] found that Se-inoculated eggs hatched a high percentage of monstrosities, bizarre abnormalities, and stunting. Underdevelopment of the beak and abnormalities of the feet and legs have also been seen, as well as fused or webbed feet of the lateral two toes [99].

Holmberg and Ferm [100] did not find Se teratogenic or embryolethal in the golden hamsters when given intravenously at one-half the lethal dose. Se has been shown to cross the placental barrier in the rat and cat [101], a finding further supported by the presence of Se in the offspring of rats, pigs [102], and sheep [103]. Foals and calves whose dams have grazed seleniferous rangelands have been born with deformed hoofs. Water containing 3 ppm Se given to bred mice resulted in a significant number of deaths in the F_1 generation and a significant number of runts in the F_1, F_2, and F_3 generations [39]. This author also reported that Se reduced the average number of litters and brought about a failure to breed in the third generation [14]. In rats, the addition of low concentrations of Se (1.5 and 2.5 ppm) to the drinking water of breeding rats for two generations had no effect on their reproduction. At the level of 2.5 ppm, Se did reduce the number of second-generation offspring reared, and 7.5 ppm prevented reproduction in the females [104].

Westfall et al. [101] fed inorganic Se salts at 15 ppm, or organic food Se at 8 ppm, and found that although Se was transferable through the placenta, deformities were not seen in rats and cats. Ten ppm of Se added to the diet of swine lowered the conception rate, increased the number of matings required for conception, and increased the percentage of pigs born dead; survivors were smaller and weak at birth. Also, fewer pigs were weaned and weaning weights were significantly reduced [102]. Pregnant ewes grazing on seleniferous range showed 75% incidence of malformations in lambs dying at birth and 10% in lambs dying between 3 and 5 months of age. The defective lambs that lived longer showed deformities of the eyes and extremities and hypoplasia of the reproductive organs [105]. Robertson [106] suspected that Se does not greatly interfere with the human reproductive processes on the basis of his observations of laboratory technicians exposed to selenite powder during preparation of bacterial media. Several pregnancies were terminated by miscarriages and one infant was born with bilateral club feet, but no abnormal occurrence of malformations from selenium exposure is postulated.

ZINC

The possibility of zinc (Zn) causing any significant teratogenic effects from an environmental hazard are considered rather remote at this time. Zinc is another substance wherein a deficiency is more detrimental to the embryo than an excess [107-110]. Halsted [111] suggested that some cases of dwarfism in man are undoubtedly caused by Zn deficiency.

Excess Zn does not cause malformations in hamsters even though it has been shown to cross the placenta in significant amounts [110,112]. Similar findings have also been reported in guinea pigs, sheep, and man [17,113]. In a multigeneration study in rats, 5000 ppm of $ZnCl_2$ increased the mortality of the offspring, a finding believed to be related to the destruction of the β-cells of the islets of Langerhans [114,115]. However, this level of ZnO caused very little increase in offspring mortality.

MISCELLANEOUS ELEMENTS

Lithium

Although lithium is not a heavy metal and does not constitute a contaminant of the environment, its wide use in treating mental disorders in man and its possible teratogenic effect deserve some mention. It has been shown to be teratogenic in chick embryos, frogs, toads, mice, and rats [116]. Shou and Amdisen [117] did not consider three malformed infants out of 60 born to lithium-treated mothers a great many more than would be found in the general population.

Manganese

Little is known about the embryotoxic effects of manganese (Mn). Ferm [91] reported that in preliminary experiments Mn in the pregnant golden hamster has been shown to be embryocidal but not teratogenic. Interestingly, a deficiency of Mn produced an ataxic condition characterized by incoordination, lack of equilibrium, and retracted head in the rat and guinea pig [118,119], and a peculiar screw-neck behavior in mink [120].

Nickel

Ferm [91] found that nickelous acetate was toxic to golden hamster embryos when 30 mg/kg was injected into pregnant mothers on day 8 of gestation. A few general malformations were induced in some of the surviving embryos. Nickel (Ni) added to the drinking water of breeding rats produced a significant number of young deaths in the F_1, F_2, and F_3 generations as well as runts in the F_1 pups [30]. Schroeder et al. [29] found Ni in the carcasses of five stillborn mice born from dams that had received 5 ppm Ni in the drinking water throughout life, indicating that Ni crossed the placental barrier.

Rhodium

Ridgway and Karnofsky [10] found that injection of rhodium onto the chorioallantoic membrane of egg embryos produced stunting, feather inhibition, micromelia, and mild edema.

Tellurium

Tellurium (Te) fed in the diet of rats has been shown to cause up to 100% hydrocephalus depending upon the level fed [121-123]. Placental transmission of radiotellurium in rats has been demonstrated in offspring of dams injected with the metal [123,124]. The critical period of hydrocephalus induction is day 9-10 of gestation in the rat [125]. Absorbed Te reached the fetal brain within minutes and presumably caused an arrest of the maturation of the telencephalic vesicles [126]. A single total insult of 50 mg Te on any one day did not produce hydrocephalus. No other abnormalities have been observed under the conditions studied [125]. James et al. [17] fed four pregnant ewes potassium tellurate 45 to 151 days and was unable to produce any abnormalities in their offspring.

Thallium

Thallium produced achondroplasia in chick embryos by injection on the chorioallantoic membrane on days 4 and 19 [10,127]. These findings were later confirmed by Hall [128] who showed that there was a defect in cartilage maturation and in the gross skeleton. The growth of the long bones was specifically affected; smaller bones contained less organic material and more water. The cartilage is the primary site of action. A similar finding has been observed in rats [129].

Titanium

Titanium in the drinking water of breeding rats caused a significant number of runts in the F_1, F_2, and F_3 generations [39]. A significant increase in the number of young deaths also occurred in the F_2 generation. There was a marked reduction in the number of animals surviving to the F_3 generation.

DELAYED TERATOGENIC EFFECTS OF HEAVY METALS

Insults to pregnant animals by environmental contaminants capable of crossing the placenta do not necessarily result in frank teratogenesis. This is especially true of agents which are potential CNS toxicants. Depletion of nerve cell populations and the decrease in the rate of brain protein synthesis caused by subtoxic doses of metals would become apparent only in periods of stress, long after termination of fetal development. Exposure to lead (Pb) by pregnant females could unmask itself in later life of the offspring as a learning deficiency. One might wonder if such toxic insults, which do not produce frank teratogenicity but which do result in a delayed toxicity, should be referred to as "delayed teratogenic effects." This conclusion seems to be a possible explanation for the observations reported by several investigators [66,130-132].

EFFECTS OF HEAVY METAL INTERACTION
ON TERATOGENESIS

The interaction of heavy metals from an environmental standpoint does not present a serious teratogenic problem. Although numerous toxic interrelationships of heavy metals are known, e.g., the intertwining of molybdenum with copper and sulfur, teratogenic effects of interactions have been demonstrated only in the laboratory.

Ribas and Schmidt [21] reported that supravitelline application of Cd on chick embryos resulted in malformations. The addition of Zn to the mixture prevented these malformations even though the dose of Cd was doubled. Mercuric acetate given with $CdSO_4$ intravenously on day 8 proved to be more detrimental to the embryos of golden hamsters than Hg with $ZnSO_4$ [133]. The severity of the toxicity to the embryo is dependent upon the method by which the metals are introduced and the dose level of Hg. The protective value also varies with the method of administration. The toxic effects of Hg and Zn on the embryo are much less severe than those of Hg and Cd. Lead also protects the embryo from Cd-induced facial defects [134]. Lead alone produced tail bud abnormalities in hamsters, but in combination with Cd it produced umbilical hernias and severe lower limb defects. Ferm [2] reported that Pb formed a complex interrelationship with Cd which delayed the Cd effect in the presence of Pb ions. The same inhibitory effect was seen with Zn and Se as well as As [100].

DISCUSSION

The exposure of an experimental model to the chronic effects of heavy metals can result in alterations in the various systems of the body as a result of inhibition or interference in various physiologic reactions. When the model happens to be a pregnant female, untoward effects which are hard to predict in advance arise from the interactions of heavy metals and various developing systems of the embryo. It has been shown that both a deficiency and an excessive exposure to heavy metals can have deleterious effects upon the zygote. The effect of heavy metal ions on enzymatic systems can easily alter the course of events. To date, a degree of sophistication has been achieved which allows a reasonable measure of predictability in a given species of animal. The projection of these data and the human application based on animal teratology remains to be confirmed. Chemical techniques are being developed to determine the sequential events that may produce these developmental aberrations.

Inducing teratogenesis in the laboratory is a necessary procedure if the mechanisms of developmental error are to be understood. The methodology usually involves injecting particularly susceptible animals with large doses at a time during gestation that is especially vulnerable to induced teratogenesis. It is a mistake, however, to project these results as probable reactions to environmental exposure. When evaluating the teratogenic hazard

of an environmental contaminant, the method of investigation must be designed
to parallel the circumstances of an actual insult to the population in its
natural habitat. Such an approach would yield data of much more practical
value for use in determining safe levels of human exposure.

Future studies will require refinement of existing techniques and development of other methods of detecting teratogenic defects. The concept
that teratology encompasses only morphological changes will have to be
broadened. Because of immaturity of the brain, many morphological abnormalities often do not manifest themselves until after weaning, during periods
of mental stress, or when increasing demands are placed upon the nervous
system. Many of these problems may arise from delayed and/or inhibited
brain maturation. Techniques must be developed to demonstrate these delayed
teratogenic effects in animals. This will require facilities to permit continuous observation of neonatal development to determine if "behavioral
teratology" is present in the animal model.

REFERENCES

1. R. Nilsson, Ecological Research Committee Bulletin No. 7, Swedish
    Natural Science Research Council, Stockholm, Sweden, 1969, p. 1.

2. V. H. Ferm, Biol. Neonate, 19, 101 (1971).

3. M. Ch. Fere, Comp. Rend. Soc. Biol., 45, 787 (1893).

4. F. S. Hammet and V. L. Wallace, J. Exp. Med., 48, 659 (1928).

5. W. Landauer, Poultry Sci., 8, 301 (1929).

6. C. R. Stockard, Amer. J. Anat., 28, 115, (1920-21).

7. C. M. Child, Protoplasma, 5, 447 (1928).

8. L. Fishbein, Sci. Total Environ., 1, 211 (1972).

9. K. W. Franke, A. L. Moxon, W. E. Poley, and W. C. Tully, Anat. Rec.,
    65, 15 (1936).

10. L. P. Ridgway and D. A. Karnofsky, Ann. N. Y. Acad. Sci., 55, 203
    (1952).

11. V. H. Ferm and S. J. Carpenter, J. Reprod. Fert., 17, 199 (1968).

12. R. D. Hood and S. L. Bishop, Arch. Environ. Health, 24, 62 (1972).

13. R. D. Hood and C. T. Pike, Teratology, 6, 235 (1972).

14. H. A. Schroeder and M. Mitchener, Arch. Environ. Health, 23, 102 (1971).

15. V. H. Ferm, A. Saxon, and B. M. Smith, Arch. Environ. Health, 22, 557
    (1971).

16. A. R. Beaudoin, Teratology, 10, 153 (1974).

17. L. F. James, V. A. Lazar, and W. Binns, Amer. J. Vet. Res., 27, 132
    (1966).

18. G. Lugo, G. Cassady, and P. Palmisano, Amer. J. Dis. Child., 117, 328 (1969).

19. P. Ancel, Arch. Anat. Microsc. Morphol. Exp., 36, 45 (1946).

20. F. P. Underhill and F. G. Amatruda, J. Amer. Med. Ass., 81, 2009 (1923).

21. B. Ribas and W. Schmidt, Gegenbaurs Morphol. Jahrb., 119, 358 (1973).

22. V. H. Ferm and S. J. Carpenter, Nature, 216, 1123 (1967).

23. T. F. Gale and V. H. Ferm, Biol. Neonate, 23, 149 (1973).

24. V. H. Ferm, D. P. Hanlon, and J. Urban, J. Embryol. Exp. Morphol., 22, 107 (1969).

25. J. E. Mulvihill, S. H. Gamm, and V. H. Ferm, J. Embryol. Exp. Morphol., 24, 393 (1970).

26. L. Friberg, M. Pascator, and G. Nordberg, Cadmium in the Environment, CRC Press, Cleveland, 1971, p. 110.

27. M. Berlin and S. Ullberg, Arch. Environ. Health, 7, 686 (1963).

28. J. Parizek, J. Reprod. Fert., 9, 111 (1965).

29. H. A. Schroeder, J. J. Balassa, and W. H. Vinton, Jr., J. Nutr., 83, 239 (1964).

30. M. Barr, Jr., Teratology, 7, 237 (1973).

31. N. Chernoff, Teratology, 8, 29 (1973).

32. D. F. Flick, H. F. Kraybill, and J. M. Dimitroff, Environ. Res., 4, 71 (1971).

33. V. H. Ferm and D. P. Hanlon, Biol. Reprod., 11, 97 (1974).

34. O. Catizone and P. Gray, J. Exp. Zool., 87, 71 (1941).

35. D. A. Karnofsky and L. P. Ridgway, J. Pharmacol. Exp. Ther., 104, 176 (1952).

36. E. M. Butt, H. E. Pearson, and D. G. Simonsen, Proc. Soc. Exp. Biol. Med., 79, 247 (1952).

37. V. H. Ferm and D. W. Ferm, Life Sci., 10, 35 (1971).

38. V. H. Ferm and S. J. Carpenter, Exp. Mol. Pathol., 7, 208 (1967).

39. H. A. Schroeder, in Essays in Toxicology (W. J. Hayes, Jr., ed.), Vol. 4, Academic, New York, 1973, p. 107.

40. J. S. McLellan, A. W. Von Smolinski, J. P. Bederka, Jr., and B. M. Boulos, Fed. Proc., 33, 288 (1974).

41. J. L. Shupe, W. Binns, L. F. James, and R. F. Keeler, J. Amer. Vet. Med. Ass., 151, 198 (1967).

42. I. Greenfield, N. Y. State J. Med., 57, 4032 (1957).

43. F. J. Taussig (ed.), Abortion, Spontaneous and Induced, Vol. 3, Klimpton, London, 1936, p. 354.

44. A. T. Wilson, Scot. Med. J., 11, 73 (1966).

45. C. R. Angle and M. S. McIntire, Amer. J. Dis. Child., 108, 436 (1964).

46. P. A. Palmisano, R. C. Sneed, and G. Cassady, J. Pediatr., 75, 869 (1969).

47. D. Barltrop, in Mineral Metabolism in Paediatrics (D. Barltrop and W. L. Burland, eds.), F. A. Davis Co., Philadelphia, 1969, p. 135.

48. D. J. Clegg, Food Cosmet. Toxicol., 9, 195 (1971).

49. J. McLaughlin, Jr., J. P. Marliac, M. J. Verrett, M. K. Mutchler, and O. G. Fitzhugh, Toxicol. Appl. Pharmacol., 5, 760 (1963).

50. S. Kuahara, J. Kumamoto Med. Soc., 44, 81 (1970); through T. Takeuchi, in Environmental Mercury Contamination (R. Hartung and B. Dinman, eds.), Ann Arbor Science, Ann Arbor, 1972, p. 302.

51. H. Kojima, personal communication, 1970; to T. Takeuchi, in Environmental Mercury Contamination (R. Hartung and B. Dinman, eds.), Ann Arbor Science, Ann Arbor, 1972, p. 302.

52. S. B. Harris, J. G. Wilson, and R. H. Printz, Teratology, 6, 139 (1972).

53. T. F. Gale and V. H. Ferm, Life Sci., 10, 1341 (1971).

54. G. T. Okita, M. Su, and M. S. Jacobson, private communication, 1974.

55. J. M. Spyker and M. Smithberg, Teratology, 5, 181 (1972).

56. M. Berlin and S. Ullberg, Arch. Environ. Health, 6, 610 (1963).

57. G. Lofroth, Ecological Research Comm. Bull. No. 4, Swedish Natural Science Research Council, Stockholm, 1968, p. 1.

58. K. S. Khera and S. A. Tabacova, Food Cosmet. Toxicol., 11, 245 (1973).

59. H. Oharazawa, Jap. J. Obstet. Gynecol., 20, 1479 (1968).

60. E. Fujita, J. Kumamoto Med. Soc., 43, 47 (1969).

61. G. A. Goncharuck, Gig. Sanit., 36, 32 (1971).

62. N. K. Mottet, Teratology, 10, 173 (1974).

63. L. G. Scharpf, Jr. and I. D. Hill, Nature, 241, 461 (1973).

64. H. Matsumoto, A. Suzuki, C. Morita, K. Nakamura, and S. Saeki, Life Sci., 6, 2321 (1967).

65. P. M. Newberne, O. Glaser, L. Friedman, and B. R. Stillings, Nature, 237, 40 (1972).

66. M. G. Yang, K. S. Krawford, J. D. Garcia, J. H. C. Wang, and K. Y. Lei, Proc. Soc. Exp. Biol. Med., 141, 1004 (1972).

67. M. M. Mansour, N. C. Dyer, L. H. Hoffman, J. Davies, and A. B. Brill, Amer. J. Obstet. Gynecol., 119, 557 (1974).

68. E. Miller, private communication, 1975.

69. K. S. Khera, Teratology, 8, 293 (1973).

70. N. Morikawa, Kumamoto Med. J., 14, 87 (1961).

71. F. L. Earl, E. Miller, and E. J. Van Loon, in The Laboratory Animal in Drug Testing (A. Spiegel, ed.), Gustav Fischer Verlag, Stuttgart, 1973, p. 233.

72. E. Schöpf and G. Nagy, Acta Hematol., 43, 73 (1970).

73. G. Fiskesjö, Hereditas, 64, 142 (1970).

74. B. L. Vallee and D. D. Ulmer, Ann. Rev. Biochem., 41, 91 (1972).

75. S. Skerfving, K. Hansson, and J. Lindsten, Arch. Environ. Health, 21, 133 (1970).

76. E. Schopf, K. H. Schulz, and I. Isensee, Arch. Klin. Exp. Dermatol., 234, 420 (1969).

77. L. A. Muro and R. A. Goyer, Arch. Pathol., 87, 660 (1969).

78. T. Takeuchi, Proceedings of the Seventh International Congress on Neurology, Rome, 1961, p. 1.

79. H. Matsumoto, G. Koya, and T. Takeuchi, J. Neuropathol. Exp. Neurol., 24, 563 (1965).

80. T. Takeuchi, International Conference of Environmental Mercury Contamination, Ann Arbor, Sept. 30-Oct. 2, 1970.

81. Report of an International Committee, Arch. Environ. Health, 19, 891 (1969).

82. K. Irukayama, Adv. Pollution Res., 3, 153 (1969).

83. S. Tejning, Rept. 68.02.20, Dept. Occup. Med., University Hospital, Lund, Sweden, 1961, p. 396.

84. T. Suzuki, N. Matsumoto, and T. Miyama, Ind. Health, 5, 149 (1967).

85. H. Matsumoto, G. Koya, and T. Takeuchi, Trans. Soc. Pathol. Jap., 54, 187 (1965).

86. T. Takeuchi, in Environmental Mercury Contamination (R. Hartung and B. Dinman, eds.), Ann Arbor Science, Ann Arbor, 1972, p. 302.

87. N. Nelson, Environ. Res., 4, 1 (1971).

88. Y. Harada, in Study Group of Minamata Disease, Kumamoto University, Kumamoto, Japan, 1968, p. 93.

89. R. D. Snyder, New Engl. J. Med., 284, 1014 (1971).

90. F. Bakir, S. F. Damluji, L. Amin-Zaki, M. Murtadha, A. Khalidi, N. Y. Al-Rawi, S. Tikriti, and H. I. Dhahir, Science, 181, 230 (1973).

91. V. H. Ferm, in Advances in Teratology (D. H. M. Woollam, ed.), Vol. 5, Logos Press, London, 1972, p. 51.

92. G. Colmano, Bull. Environ. Contam. Toxicol., 9, 361 (1973).

93. M. A. Jeter and G. K. Davis, J. Nutr., 54, 215 (1954).

94. C. F. Mills and B. F. Fell, Nature (London), 185, 20 (1960).

95. T. Sollmann, A Manual of Pharmacology, W. B. Saunders, Philadelphia, 1957, p. 1230.

96. E. G. C. Clarke and M. L. Clarke, Garner's Veterinary Toxicology, Bailliere, Tindall, and Cassell, 1967, p. 114.

97. H. A. Schroeder, J. Chronic Dis., 23, 227 (1970).

98. A. L. Moxon and M. Rhian, Physiol. Rev., 23, 305 (1943).

99. I. S. Palmer, R. L. Arnold, and C. W. Carlson, Poultry Sci., 52, 1841 (1973).

100. R. E. Holmberg, Jr. and V. H. Ferm, Arch. Environ. Health, 18, 873 (1969).

101. B. B. Westfall, E. F. Stohlman, and M. J. Smith, J. Pharmacol. Exp. Ther., 64, 55 (1938).

102. R. C. Wahlstrom and O. E. Olson, J. Anim. Sci., 18, 141 (1959).

103. I. Rosenfeld and O. A. Beath, J. Agr. Res., 75, 93 (1947).

104. I. Rosenfeld and O. A. Beath, Proc. Soc. Exp. Biol. Med., 87, 295 (1954).

105. I. Rosenfeld and O. A. Beath, Selenium, Academic, New York, 1964, p. 1.

106. D. S. F. Robertson, Lancet, 1, 518 (1970).

107. D. L. Blamberg, U. B. Blackwood, W. C. Supplee, and G. F. Combs, Proc. Soc. Exp. Biol. Med., 104, 217 (1960).

108. L. S. Hurley and H. Swenerton, Proc. Soc. Exp. Biol. Med., 123, 692 (1966).

109. J. Warkany and H. G. Petering, Teratology, 5, 319 (1972).

110. V. H. Ferm and D. P. Hanlon, J. Reprod. Fert., 39, 49 (1974).

111. J. A. Halsted, Lancet, 1, 1323 (1973).

112. V. H. Ferm and S. J. Carpenter, Lab. Invest., 18, 429 (1968).

113. J. Sternberg, M. M. Gelfand, and J. Kaneti, First Rochester Trophoblast Conference (H. A. Thiede, ed.), 1961.

114. V. G. Heller and A. D. Burke, J. Biol. Chem., 74, 85 (1927).

115. E. J. Underwood, Trace Elements in Human and Animal Nutrition, Academic, New York, 1962, p. 336.

116. H. T. Loevy and H. R. Catchpole, Proc. Soc. Exp. Biol. Med., 144, 644 (1973).

117. M. Schou and A. Amdisen, Lancet, 1, 1132 (1971).

118. L. S. Hurley, G. J. Everson, and J. F. Geiger, J. Nutr., 66, 309 (1958).

119. L. S. Hurley, E. Wooten, G. J. Everson, and C. W. Asling, J. Nutr., 71, 15 (1960).

120. L. C. Erway and S. E. Mitchell, J. Hered., 64, 111 (1973).

121. F. Garro and A. Pentschew, Arch. Psychiat. Nervenkr., 206, 272 (1964).

122. S. Duckett, Exp. Neurol., 31, 1 (1971).

123. W. F. Agnew, F. M. Fauvre, and P. H. Pudenz, Exp. Neurol., 21, 120 (1968).

124. S. Duckett and K. A. O. Ellem, Exp. Neurol., 32, 49 (1971).

125. W. F. Agnew, Teratology, 6, 331 (1972).

126. S. Duckett, A. Sandler, and T. Scott, Experientia, 27, 1064 (1971).

127. D. A. Karnofsky, L. P. Ridgway, and P. A. Patterson, Proc. Soc. Exp. Biol. Med., 73, 255 (1950).

128. B. K. Hall, Develop. Biol., 28, 47 (1972).

129. H. Nogami and Y. Terashima, Teratology, 8, 101 (1973).

130. J. M. Spyker, S. B. Sparber, and A. M. Goldberg, Science, 177, 621 (1972).

131. A. D. Beattie, M. R. Moore, A. Goldberg, Margaret Finlayson, Janet Graham, Elizabeth Mackie, Joan Main, D. A. McLaren, R. M. Murdoch, G. T. Stewart, Lancet, 1, 589 (1975).

132. P. J. Landrigan, R. H. Whitworth, R. W. Baloh, N. W. Staehling, W. F. Barthel, and B. F. Rosenblum, Lancet 1, 708 (1975).

133. T. F. Gale, Environ. Res., 6, 95 (1973).

134. V. H. Ferm, Experientia, 25, 56 (1969).

INTERACTIONS OF TRACE ELEMENTS

Eric J. Underwood
University of Western Australia
Nedlands, Western Australia

The absorption, utilization, and excretion of many trace elements, and therefore their physiological, pharmacological, or toxicological actions within the cells and tissues of the animal body, are greatly influenced by the extent to which other elements or compounds with which they interact are present or absent from the diet and from the body itself. There is thus no single minimum need of an essential trace element and no single safe dietary level of a toxic element. There is a series of such minimum needs or maximum tolerances depending upon the chemical form of the element, the duration and continuity of intake, and the nature of the rest of the diet, especially the amounts and proportions of other interacting elements and compounds.

Interactions among the trace elements are so pervading and so biologically influential that nutritional and toxicological studies carried out with single elements can be quite misleading unless the dietary and body tissue levels of interacting elements are known and the experimental conditions in these respects are clearly defined. With some elements, notably copper, interactions can be so dominant that a particular level of intake in the diet can lead to copper deficiency or copper toxicity in the animal depending upon the relative intakes, for example, of molybdenum and inorganic sulfate or of zinc and iron. Such interactions can be particularly important in monitoring the environment for the existence of marginal deficiencies of essential trace elements or of marginal toxicities from heavy metal pollution because potentially deficient elements are known to interact physiologically with potentially toxic elements, for example, zinc with cadmium and selenium with mercury. The adequacy of environmental levels of zinc and selenium can therefore be influenced by the degree of exposure to cadmium and mercury, respectively, and the safety of environmental levels of cadmium and mercury are similarly influenced by environmental intakes of zinc and selenium, respectively. Herbage contaminated with cadmium of industrial origin frequently carries coincidentally high concentrations of zinc and copper, which are cadmium antagonists. Possible adverse effects of the high-cadmium herbage upon animals may in this way be offset or reduced by the above-normal amounts of zinc and copper ingested, so long as these elements are in available forms. These and other interactions, and the mechanisms involved where such are known, are considered in the following sections of this review.

COPPER, MOLYBDENUM, AND SULFATE INTERACTIONS

The first indications of a physiological interaction between copper and molybdenum came more than 30 years ago from studies of a disease of grazing cattle, known locally as "teart," occurring in restricted areas in England. This disease, which is characterized by severe debilitating diarrhea and weight loss, was shown to be caused by excessive intakes of molybdenum from the herbage of the affected areas. The molybdenum levels in typical teart pastures range from 20 ppm to as high as 100 ppm (dry basis), compared with 3-5 ppm, or less, in nearby healthy herbage [1]. Following a report from Holland of a scouring condition in cattle responsive to copper therapy [2], treatment of teart with copper sulfate was tried by Ferguson and co-workers [3]. This treatment at the very high rate of 2 g/day for cows and 1 g/day for young stock, or the intravenous injection of 200-300 mg/day, effectively controlled the Mo-induced scouring. The mechanism of the protective effect of copper against the diarrhea is still obscure. There is no inflammation or local damage to the intestine and the molybdenum does not have to be ingested because the scouring can be induced by injections of molybdate over 2-3 weeks [4]. Depletion of tissue copper to deficiency levels occurs when high molybdenum intakes are prolonged, but the scouring and loss of condition that characterizes severe molybdenosis in cattle can occur without a concomitant hypocuprosis. Furthermore, hypocuprosis in cattle unassociated with high molybdenum intakes is not necessarily accompanied by diarrhea.

The quantitative nature of the physiological antagonism between copper and molybdenum is clearly apparent from a comparison of the conditions

under which teart and another naturally occurring disease of cattle known
as "peat scours" occur, and can be prevented or cured. This disease appears
in restricted areas in New Zealand where the pastures are (a) higher than
normal in molybdenum, but usually well below the levels typical of teart
herbage, and (b) subnormal in copper. In these circumstances the onset of
scouring is delayed until the tissue copper stores are depleted and control
of the scouring can be achieved merely by raising the copper content of the
pastures, or the copper intakes of the animals, to normal levels [5]. The
molybdenum intakes from peat scours pastures are not high enough to require
the very large copper supplements needed to control teart. Miltimore and
Mason [6] claim that the critical Cu/Mo ratio in animal feeds is 2.0 and
that feeds or pastures with lower ratios would be expected to cause conditioned copper deficiency. In a study of fodders and grains grown in British
Columbia these workers found an extremely wide Cu/Mo ratio, ranging from
0.1 to 52.7 in individual samples and with 19% of the samples having a Cu/Mo
ratio below 2.0. The nutritional implications of variations of environmental
origin of this magnitude are considerable, especially in relation to the
need for and extent of copper supplementation of diets. The results of a
study of "swayback" and other pastures in England carried out by Alloway
[7] also indicate the importance of the Cu/Mo ratio to the incidence of
copper deficiency in grazing sheep, but they suggest a higher critical ratio
than 2.0.

The interaction between copper and molybdenum revealed by the environmental problems just described is also apparent from experimental studies
with other species. For example, the addition of 80 ppm Mo as molybdate
inhibited growth and induced mortality in young rats fed a low-copper diet,
whereas no such disabilities arose when the copper content of the diet was
raised to 35 ppm with copper sulfate [8]. Similarly, young rats fed a diet
containing 77 ppm Cu grew poorly when molybdenum as sodium molybdate was
added at levels of 500 ppm and 1000 ppm Mo but grew normally when 200 ppm
Cu was supplied [9]. Dietary supplementation with copper has also been
shown to alleviate an Mo-induced growth depression in rabbits [10] and in
chicks [11].

Of particular interest in the present context is the finding that methionine and cystine can be as effective as copper in alleviating molybdenum
toxicity in rats [12] and in sheep [13] and that thiosulfate administration
is equally effective in sheep [13]. It seems that these substances, all of

which are capable of oxidation to sulfate in the tissues, act by reducing
molybdenum retention in the tissues. The potent influence of inorganic
sulfate upon molybdenum absorption and retention and upon the route of excretion of absorbed molybdenum is evident from the results of experiments
carried out by Dick [14]. Sheep fed a diet of oaten chaff (<0.1% sulfate)
plus 10 mg Mo/day excreted 63% of this molybdenum in the total excreta
during a period of 4 weeks, of which 3 to 4.6% appeared in the urine. When
fed a diet of alfalfa chaff (0.3% sulfate) plus 10 mg Mo/day, the recovery
in the excreta was 96%, of which 50-54% appeared in the urine. The administration of a single oral dose of potassium sulfate to the sheep on the
low-sulfate oaten chaff diet induced a rapid rise in urinary molybdenum
excretion (Fig. 1). The same effect on excretion at higher levels of molybdenum intake was subsequently demonstrated by Scaife [13]. This worker fed
sheep a low-sulfate diet and a high-sulfate diet plus 50 mg Mo/day in each
case. Only 5% of the molybdenum appeared in the urine on the low-sulfate
regimen, compared with 30-40% on the high sulfate.

The alleviation of molybdenum toxicity by sulfate does not appear to
be mediated entirely through its influence on the pattern of molybdenum

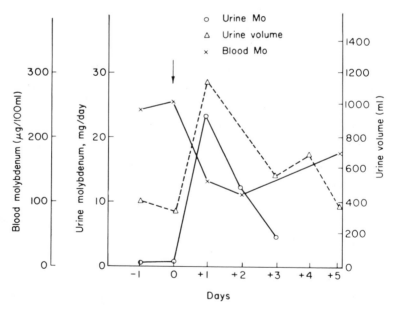

FIG. 1. The effect on blood and urine molybdenum of 11 g potassium sulfate
given by mouth, at the time indicated by the arrow on a diet of chaffed
oaten hay and a molybdenum intake of 10 mg/day. (Taken from Ref. 14 by
courtesy of the Australian Veterinary Association.)

excretion, or at least not in all species. In rats [15] and in cattle [16]
sulfate reduces molybdenum retention in the tissues as it does in the sheep,
but no such reduction is apparent in the chicks despite a marked beneficial
effect on the signs of molybdenum toxicity [17]. In the sheep, sulfate
limits molybdenum retention both by reducing intestinal absorption and increasing urinary excretion, the extent of each depending upon the previous
history of the animal with respect to molybdenum and sulfate intakes [13].

The increased urinary excretion of molybdenum induced by sulfate is
not a result of the greater urinary volume that occurs on high-sulfate diets
and is highly specific to sulfate. In sheep the effect on molybdenum excretion is not shared by tungstate, selenate, silicate, permanganate, phosphate malonate and citrate [13], and in rats the capacity of sulfate to
alleviate molybdenum toxicity is not shared by citrate, tartrate, acetate,
bromide, chloride, or nitrate [18]. Sulfate of endogenous origin can be
just as effective as dietary inorganic sulfate. This is indicated by the
effects of high-protein diets, by the catabolic breakdown of body tissue,
and by the administration of cystine, methionine, and thiosulfate to sheep,
as mentioned previously [13,19]. Dick [19] explains the influence of sulfate on molybdenum absorption and excretion on the hypothesis that inorganic
sulfate interferes with and, if its concentration is high enough, prevents
the transport of molybdenum across membranes. Such an effect would increase
urinary molybdenum excretion through the rise in the sulfate concentration
in the ultrafiltrate of the kidney glomerulus which follows the high sulfate
intakes, impeding or blocking reabsorption of molybdenum through the kidney
tubule. The mechanism of this postulated interference with membrane transport is unknown.

In the preceding paragraphs only the two-way interactions between copper and molybdenum and between molybdenum and sulfate have been considered.
The discovery of a three-way interaction between these three dietary constituents arose from studies of chronic copper poisoning in sheep in south-
eastern Australia (see Ref. 20). In certain areas the main pasture species
usually contain 10-15 ppm Cu and extremely low levels of molybdenum that
rarely exceed 0.1-0.2 ppm (dry basis). These conditions favor the development of a high copper status, especially a high liver copper status, and
lead to copper poisoning. Providing molybdate-containing salt licks to the
grazing sheep is highly effective in reducing liver copper levels and reducing mortality from the disease [21]. The environment to which the animals
are exposed and the treatment required can thus be considered as the reverse

of those in the occurrence and treatment of teart and peat scours, discussed
previously.

In further experimental studies designed to elucidate the factors influencing copper retention in the sheep, Dick [22] discovered that the limiting effect of molybdenum was exerted only when the diet also contained a
sufficient quantity of inorganic sulfate. For a given intake of molybdenum
the limitation of copper storage was found to be proportional to the sulfate
content of the diet (Fig. 2). This important discovery was subsequently
confirmed [23] and extensively studied [24].*

The complexity of the Cu-Mo-SO₄ interrelationship is illustrated by
the fact that molybdenum and sulfate can either increase or decrease the

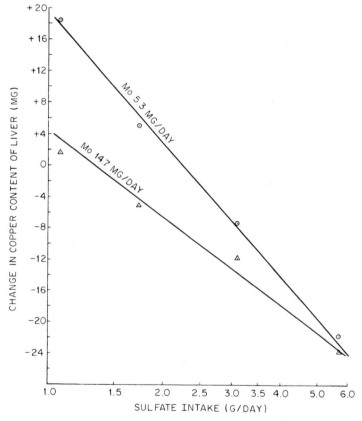

FIG. 2. The relation of the level of sulfate intake to the effect of molybdenum upon liver copper storage in the sheep. (Taken from Ref. 22 by courtesy of the Commonwealth Scientific and Industrial Research Organization,
Australia.)

*Later evidence obtained by N. F. Suttle [Brit. J. Nutr., 34, 411 (1975)]
indicates that total sulfur rather than inorganic sulfate is the more useful measurement in the Cu-Mo-S interrelationship.

copper status of an animal, depending on their intakes relative to that of
copper and by the existence of other factors, known and unknown, that have
a modifying influence. For example, Gray and Daniel [25] showed that when
the copper stores of rats were low and a copper-deficient diet was fed,
small amounts of molybdenum produced toxic symptoms which were intensified
by the addition of sulfate. When the copper stores were adequate, larger
amounts of molybdenum were required, as expected, to produce molybdenosis,
but in these circumstances sulfate completely prevented the effects of molybdenum. The direction of the sulfate effect on the Cu-Mo interaction can
thus actually be reversed by the copper status of the rat. Furthermore,
high manganese intakes can block or antagonize the limiting effect of molybdenum on copper storage in the sheep, even in the presence of adequate sulfate [26]. Other dietary differences can also affect the position. Thus
Mills and co-workers [27] were able to produce copper-deficient lambs by
feeding high amounts of molybdate and sulfate to sheep fed grass cubes,
whereas Butler and Barlow [28] found no such effect when the basal diet
consisted of hay and oats. Hogan et al. [29] similarly were unable to
reduce the copper status of lambs to deficiency levels by dosing their
mothers with molybdate and sulfate for 9 months. Subsequently they obtained
evidence of a dietary factor in a concentrate fed to penned sheep which
facilitated excessive copper storage in the liver. Feeding additional molybdate and sulfate reduced the effect of this unidentified factor, but did
not eliminate it.

Although it is over 20 years since the limiting effect of molybdenum
plus sulfate upon copper retention was first demonstrated and the problem
has been extensively studied since that time, no fully adequate explanation
of the mechanism or mechanisms involved has yet appeared. Mills [30] suggests that molybdate and sulfate restrict copper utilization in sheep by
depressing copper solubility in the digestive tract through the precipitation of insoluble cupric sulfide. Higher sulfide levels were observed in
the rumen of sheep fed molybdate and sulfate than in those fed sulfate alone,
and the concentration of soluble copper in this site was inversely related
to the sulfide level. Spais et al. [31] have also suggested that the sulfide formed in the rumen from high sulfate intakes acts by binding feed
copper to insoluble and unavailable copper sulfide. Increased ruminal sulfide concentrations and a decreased flow of copper to the omasum has, in
fact, been demonstrated in sheep when the intake of cystine-S or sulfate-S
was increased under steady-state feeding conditions [32]. A metabolic
interference with copper in the liver is also apparent from the experiments

of Marciless et al. [33], but the mechanism of this interference and the precise participation of the individual components of the $Cu-Mo-SO_4$ nexus are not revealed by this or the other experiments described.

A further hypothesis has recently been put forward [24] which proposes that copper becomes unavailable through two routes: (1) through interaction with molybdate to form a biologically unavailable Cu-Mo complex called cupric molybdate, previously described by Dowdy and Matrone [34] and Dowdy et al. [35] (This complex appears to be absorbed, transported, and excreted as a unit and appears to make both copper and molybdate less available.) and (2) through the formation of an insoluble cupric sulfide in the rumen, intestine, or in the tissues. Finally, Dick et al. [36] have produced evidence which supports the hypothesis that the essential steps in the control of copper storage are (1) reduction in the rumen of sulfate to sulfide, (2) the reaction at relatively neutral pH of the sulfide with the molybdate in the rumen to produce thiomolybdate, and (3) the reaction of the thiomolybdate with the copper to give the very insoluble copper thiomolybdate, $CuMoS_4$. The concept of the formation of a thiomolybdate ion and the tight complexing of this ion with copper represents a significant forward step involving for the first time a true three-way reaction.

INTERACTIONS OF COPPER WITH IRON AND ZINC

The interactions between copper, iron, and zinc are particularly apparent at very high dietary intakes of copper and at very high dietary intakes of zinc. Much of our knowledge of the former has come from studies designed to elucidate apparent discrepancies in observed responses to large copper supplements in growing pigs. In 1955 it was shown in England that the addition of copper, as copper sulfate, to a normal ration at the rate of 250 ppm Cu increased rate of weight gains in growing pigs [37]. In a later coordinated trial in that country, carried out in 21 centers and involving 245 pigs per treatment, such supplementation increased the mean daily liveweight gain by 9.7% and the efficiency of feed use by 7.9% [38]. These results were subsequently confirmed in a further trial which showed significant improvement from 150, 200, and 250 mg Cu/kg ration, but with the best performance and the highest increase in profitability from the largest copper supplement [39]. With the different basal rations predominant in the United States and Australia it was found that copper supplementation at a level of 250 ppm Cu can by contrast (a) reduce liveweight gains and efficiency of feed use [40], (b) lead to anemia and copper toxicosis in some animals [41,42], (c) cause mortality and result in skin lesions similar to those of parakeratosis or zinc deficiency and rectifiable by zinc supplements [43], and (d) include anemia preventable by increasing the iron content of the ration [44].

From the observations just cited, and particularly from the experiments of Suttle and Mills [45] on copper toxicosis in pigs, it appears that the discrepancies in the reported responses to copper can largely be explained by differences in the zinc and iron contents of the rations used and that copper supplements to promote growth and efficiency of feed use can be safely and satisfactorily exploited only if the zinc and iron contents of the pigs' diets are higher than those found adequate at lower copper intakes. If the zinc and iron intakes are sufficiently large pigs can be protected against copper levels much higher than the 250 ppm recommended as a practical procedure. For example, Suttle and Mills [45] showed that dietary copper levels of 425, 450, 600, and 750 ppm caused severe toxicosis, manifested by a severe depression in feed intake and growth rate, hypochromic microcytic anemia, and jaundice. All these signs of copper toxicosis were eliminated by simultaneously providing an additional 150 ppm Zn plus 150 ppm Fe to the diets containing 425 and 450 ppm Cu. Addition of 500 ppm Zn or 750 ppm Fe to diets containing 750 ppm Cu eliminated the jaundice and produced normal serum copper and aspartate aminotransferase (AAT) activities, but only iron protected against anemia.

Discrepancies in reported responses to copper in pigs may not always be due to differences in the intakes of iron and zinc, relative to those of copper, or to interactions confined to those three elements. Differences in the calcium content of the rations constitute a further factor of potential importance. Diets high in calcium have a lower zinc availability, thus enhancing copper toxicity and introducing a three-way interaction between Ca, Zn, and Cu [45]. Heavy copper supplementation of swine rations is clearly a matter of considerable nutritional complexity. It can also pose serious environmental problems because dietary copper is concentrated two- to threefold in animal wastes and may result in significant increases in soil and water copper concentrations when the wastes are discharged into bodies of water or onto the land [46]. Further consideration of this aspect of heavy metal contamination of the environment lies beyond the scope of this review.

Further interactions between copper, zinc, and iron have been revealed by studies of zinc toxicosis in rats. Rats fed diets containing 0.4% Zn

or more exhibit markedly depressed growth and appetite and an anemia of the
hypochromic, microcytic type develops [47,48], accompanied by subnormal
tissue levels of copper, iron, cytochrome oxidase, catalase, and δ-amino-
levulinate dehydratase [47,49-52]. The anemia and the accompanying biochemical changes can be partly overcome by dietary supplements of copper
[47,51,53] and completely overcome by supplements of copper plus iron [49,
50]. The anemia of zinc toxicity thus results from copper and iron deficiencies brought about by an interference with the utilization of these two
metals by the high zinc intakes.

There is now ample evidence that interference at the absorptive level
is the major or primary cause of the dietary interactions between copper,
zinc, and iron considered above. Direct evidence that high zinc intakes
depress copper absorption was obtained by Van Campen and Scaife [54], using
isolated duodenal segments of the rat. A depression of zinc absorption by
high levels of copper has similarly been demonstrated [55]. A mutual antagonism between zinc and copper in the absorptive process, taking place in
or on the intestinal epithelium, is thus apparent. A comparable mutual
antagonism between iron and copper in the absorptive process is evident from
recent studies of high copper intakes in pigs. Gipp et al. [56] showed con-
vincingly that the iron deficiency and hypochromic, microcytic anemia induced
by high dietary copper is due to impairment of iron absorption from the
gastrointestinal tract and that this impairment is ameliorated by ascorbic
acid. The precise site of the primary lesion(s) produced by the high dietary
copper was not disclosed by these studies. Nor is the exact mechanism of
the interaction apparent from this or other investigations. It is probable
that the elements compete for protein-binding sites involved in the absorptive process. Support for this hypothesis comes from the finding that zinc
and cadmium depress copper absorption in the chick by binding to and displacing copper from a duodenal mucosal protein with a molecular weight of
about 10,000 [57] and from evidence that at high zinc intakes zinc reduces
iron absorption by interfering with the incorporation of iron into and release from ferritin [57a].

INTERACTIONS OF CADMIUM WITH ZINC,
COPPER, AND IRON

A metabolic antagonism between cadmium and zinc might be expected from
the chemical similarities of the two metals. Such a mutual antagonism is
apparent from many studies with several animal species. The toxic effects

of cadmium can be ameliorated by appropriate dietary intakes of zinc, and the toxic effects of zinc can be inhibited by appropriate dietary intakes of cadmium. Furthermore, at marginally deficient intakes of zinc, cadmium can precipitate overt signs of zinc deficiency in the animal.

The mutual antagonism that exists between cadmium and zinc and important further interactions between cadmium and iron and copper have been clearly demonstrated in studies with the flour beetle, Tribolium confusum. High levels of zinc in the diet of that species were shown to reduce the toxicity of cadmium and additional copper slightly reduced the toxic effects of both cadmium and zinc. The zinc requirements of the beetle were thus considerably raised and the copper requirements slightly raised by cadmium feeding [58]. Comparable interactions involving cadmium, zinc, iron, and copper have been demonstrated in mice and rats [59]. The reduced weight gains induced by 100 ppm Cd in the diet were largely overcome by additional zinc and copper.

The interaction between cadmium and zinc can be explained by competition for protein-binding sites both at the mucosal cell level and in the tissues. Reduced absorption of ^{65}Zn has been achieved in the chick by cadmium feeding [60] and the intracellular distribution of ^{65}Zn in mouse liver cells influenced by injected cadmium or by cadmium feeding [61]. The competition between zinc and cadmium for protein-binding sites presumably includes the zinc metalloenzymes. It certainly includes metallothionein which can vary in cadmium and zinc contents while the sums of the two elements remain constant [62]. Although the simultaneous presence of Cd, Zn, and even Hg in a low-molecular-weight protein isolated from kidney cortex was demonstrated many years ago [63], the biochemical function of this compound (metallothionein) is still not clear. However, since there is a rapid rise in metallothionein synthesis following the oral or intraperitoneal administration of cadmium to rabbits [64], rats [65], and chicks [66], it seems that one important action is the decontamination of the organism from harmful cadmium ions.

The metabolic antagonism between cadmium and zinc at the tissue level, as distinct from the effects on absorption, is further apparent from the protection afforded by injected zinc against the remarkable toxic effects of injected cadmium on the testes [67] and on pregnant rats [68]. Rats protected by zinc salts show no reduction in blood cadmium comparable to that brought about by selenium, as discussed later, and the concentration of cadmium in the liver is actually increased [67]. This raises the possibility that zinc reduces cadmium toxicity by increasing the excretion of cadmium from the organism by kidneys, intestine, or biliary tract.

Cadmium feeding does not consistently reduce the zinc concentrations in the tissues, nor does zinc feeding consistently reduce the cadmium concentrations, even though each element ameliorates the toxic effects of the other [59,69]. Furthermore, cadmium feeding can have a greater effect on the copper status of animals than it has on their zinc status, indicating that cadmium is an even more powerful metabolic antagonist of copper than of zinc. This is well illustrated by the experiments of Mills and Dalgarno [70] with sheep and of Campbell and Mills [70a] with weanling rats. Little reduction in plasma zinc was observed in the Cd-fed lambs, but there was a marked reduction in whole blood copper and ceruloplasmin activity. The influence of the cadmium feeding upon the liver zinc concentrations of ewes and lambs was similarly small or nonsignificant, whereas the copper concentrations in these organs in ewes and particularly in lambs were greatly reduced, especially at the higher cadmium intakes (Table 1). The experiments with rats strikingly demonstrate how a relatively small increase in cadmium intake can adversely affect copper metabolism when copper intake is marginal. Dietary cadmium intakes at the rate of 6.1 mg/kg was as effective in reducing plasma ceruloplasmin activity over a 9-week period as 1000 mg/kg of dietary zinc [70a]. A depression in blood and liver copper levels in sheep fed cadmium as $CdCl_2$ at the rate of 7.5 mg Cd/day or 15.0 mg Cd/day has also been observed by Lee and Jones [71]. In an experiment with chicks fed 75 ppm Cd, by contrast, iron utilization, and to a lesser extent zinc utilization, was more affected than was copper compared with control chicks. Serum zinc was depressed, liver zinc concentration slightly elevated, and liver copper level unchanged. On the other hand, the concentrations of iron in the livers and kidneys of the Cd-fed chicks were decreased and the hematocrit and hemoglobin levels reduced [73].

A metabolic antagonism between cadmium and iron, as well as between cadmium and zinc and copper, is apparent from the preceding experiments. With iron and copper this antagonism is particularly prominent at the site of absorption. High dietary levels of cadmium have been shown directly to depress copper uptake from the duodenum [74,75]. In recent experiments with Japanese quail 1% ascorbic acid alleviated or prevented almost all aspects of toxicity in birds fed 75 ppm of dietary cadmium, including the anemia characteristic of cadmium toxicosis [76]. Since ascorbic acid enhances the absorption of iron [77,78] and depresses the absorption of copper [79], it seems that in the circumstances of this experiment the antagonism between cadmium and iron was more pronounced than the antagonism between cadmium

TABLE 1. Trace Metal Content (ppm dm) of Livers of Ewes and Lambs Given Diets Differing in Cadmium Content During Late Pregnancy and Early Lactation[a]

	Cadmium Content of Diet (ppm dm)				Significance of Treatment Effects
	0.7	3.5	7.1	12.3	
Ewe liver (at termination of experiment)					
Cadmium	0.95 ± 0.37[b]	2.01 ± 0.27	3.50 ± 0.95	11.20 ± 1.17	P < 0.001
Copper	185 ± 51	174 ± 32	131 ± 56	59 ± 19	P < 0.05
Zinc	109 ± 11	106 ± 11	107 ± 4	114 ± 7	N.s.[c]
Number of livers analyzed	4	4	4	4	
Lamb liver (at termination of experiment)					
Cadmium	0.14 ± 0.01	1.57 ± 0.48	3.49 ± 1.36	10.95 ± 1.00	P < 0.001
Copper	101 ± 31	22 ± 3	62 ± 35	13 ± 2	P < 0.01
Zinc	135 ± 8	96 ± 5	103 ± 3	94 ± 6	P < 0.01
Number of livers analyzed	5	5	4	6	
Lamb liver (at birth)					
Cadmium	<0.14	<0.14	<0.14	<0.14	N.s.
Copper	183 ± 91	213 ± 47	115 ± 27	73 ± 38	N.s. (0.1 > P > 0.05)
Zinc	178 ± 81	266 ± 72	137 ± 25	148 ± 55	N.s.
Number of livers analyzed	3	3	8	5	

[a]Reprinted from Ref. 70 by courtesy of Nature, London.

[b]Standard error of mean.

[c]N.s., not statistically significant (P > 0.05).

and copper. The anemia induced by high dietary cadmium can therefore be ascribed primarily to a depression in iron absorption, or in copper absorption, or in both iron and copper absorption, depending upon the iron and copper status of the diets and of the experimental animals.

The metabolic interactions just described should be taken into account in any consideration of possible toxicity to animals and man from industrial contamination of the environment. Herbage so contaminated with cadmium generally also contains abnormally high concentrations of zinc and copper [70,72]. Since, as we have seen, both these elements are cadmium antagonists in the animal body, the adverse effects of any one of the three elements could be offset or reduced by the presence of sufficient quantities of the others. In this respect, Mills and Dalgarno [70] have stated that "their (i.e., cadmium and zinc) adverse effects as Cu antagonists may be offset by the high levels of Cu often encountered in such herbage, if this copper is also in an available form."

INTERACTIONS OF SELENIUM WITH ARSENIC, CADMIUM, AND MERCURY

Selenium-Arsenic Interactions

The two naturally occurring diseases of livestock known as "blind staggers" and "alkali disease," which were shown in 1935 to be manifestations of acute and chronic selenium poisoning, respectively (see Ref. 80), presented formidable difficulties in prevention and control until the effect of arsenic was discovered. In 1938 Moxon [81] showed that 5 ppm As in the drinking water prevented all signs of selenosis in rats. Arsenic has since been used successfully to alleviate selenium poisoning in pigs, dogs, chicks, and cattle. Sodium arsenite and arsenate are equally effective, arsenic sulfides are ineffective, and various organic forms of arsenic provide partial protection [82-85].

The mechanism by which arsenic protects against selenium poisoning is incompletely understood. When subacute injections of arsenic are given with the selenium, pulmonary exhalation of selenium is diminished and excretion of selenium into the gastrointestinal tract via the bile fluid is increased, resulting in decreased retention in the tissues [86-88] (Table 2). Such effects of arsenic on selenium metabolism are not shared by mercury, thallium, and lead [89] or by cadmium [86], as discussed in the following section of this review. Presumably, the enhanced loss of selenium from the

TABLE 2. Effect of Diet, Arsenic, and Cadmium on the Retention of Selenium 10 hr After the Injection of Selenite[a]

	Se (mg/kg)	Retention[b] (% of dose)		
		Control	+ Arsenic[c]	+ Cadmium[c]
Experiment 2				
Purified diet	2.0	51.9	40.3	
Crude diet	2.0	35.6	32.6	
Experiment 3				
Purified diet	1.5	61.7	41.5	79.9
Crude diet	1.5	49.2	36.0	73.0

[a]Reprinted from Ref. 86 by courtesy of American Institute of Nutrition.

[b]Retention = total recovery minus total elimination (air + GI tract + urine).

[c]Intraperitoneal injection of As or Cd in the form of sodium arsenite or cadmium chloride preceded the selenite injection by 10 min.

body induced by arsenic constitutes a partial reason for its protective effect against selenosis. Perhaps, as Frost [90] has suggested, arsenic reacts directly with Se in vivo, possibly as Se^{2-} to form As^+Se^- complexes of particle size and solubility that favor biliary excretion. The similarity of Se and As, which differ by only one atomic number and one electron in the outer ring, is probably relevant to their metabolic interaction, in accord with the concept of Hill and Matrone [91] that trace elements with similar electron structures such as Se^{4+}, As^{3+}, and Te^{4+} are likely to be biological antagonists. In this connection, Hill [92] has recently produced evidence that selenate is effective in counteracting the effect of arsenate in uncoupling oxidative phosphorylation and that the basis for this interaction is the reciprocal inhibition of uptake of these two ions by respiring mitochondria.

Selenium-Cadmium Interactions

The first evidence of a biological interaction between selenium and cadmium emerged from studies carried out initially by Parizek [93,94] demonstrating a drastic testicular necrosis in rats given single small injections of cadmium chloride. Several substances were later shown to protect the animal against the toxic effects of cadmium on the testes. These included zinc, as already mentioned, and selenium [95,96]. The severe toxic effects of injected cadmium on the male are paralleled, in certain circumstances, by equally severe effects on the female, notably massive hemorrhagic necrosis in the nonovulating ovaries of young rats [97], complete destruction of the pars fetalis of the placenta, and high mortality in pregnant rats [98,99]. The cadmium-induced toxemia of pregnancy can be completely prevented by injections of sodium selenite or selenate in a slightly higher than equimolar proportion to cadmium [100]. Selenium thus emerges as a protective agent against cadmium toxicity effects on the testes, on the ovaries of prepubertal rats, and on pregnant rats.

The biochemical basis for the detoxification of cadmium by mercury is becoming clear. The protective effects appear to be connected with changes in the chemical reactivity and distribution of cadmium in the animal. Thus Parizek et al. [101] showed that Se increased the levels of Cd and of Se in rat tissues when high levels of salts of both elements were administered. Similarly, a series of experiments by Gunn et al. [102] revealed that Se, far from preventing Cd from reaching the testes, actually led to higher testicular levels. It was concluded that an inert Se-Cd complex was formed in the testis, thus accounting for the inactivation of the cadmium. Ganther et al. [110] have taken the problem further and have produced evidence suggesting that the 10,000 molecular weight Cd-binding protein fraction in testicular homogenates may be a target of cadmium related to its damaging effects, and that selenium forms selenoprotein derivatives of the bulk testicular proteins that have a high affinity for cadmium and complex it, thus diverting cadmium from its usual target.

The metabolic antagonism between selenium and cadmium disclosed by the studies of cadmium toxicity just described is similarly evident from dietary studies of selenium toxicity carried out by Hill [103]. This worker showed that the growth retardation and mortality brought about by feeding selenium dioxide to chicks could be partially alleviated by inclusion of cadmium sulfate in the diet. Alleviation of selenium toxicity was also achieved in these experiments by supplementary copper and mercury, considered below. When the reaction product of cadmium and selenium, containing 36% Se and approximating to cadmium selenite, was fed to chicks, it was found to be less toxic than SeO_2 fed at comparable selenium levels. This suggests that cadmium inhibits selenium toxicity, at least in part, by forming a compound or compounds with selenium in the intestinal tract which are of low availability and therefore poorly absorbed. On the other hand, cadmium administered daily as $CdCl_2$ in a drench at the rate of 7.5 mg or 15.0 mg Cd/day to sheep containing Se pellets in their rumens had no limiting effect over a period of 6 months upon the increased Se concentrations in blood, liver, kidney, and muscle induced by the pellets. A tendency for the selenium to depress cadmium storage was evident in these experiments [71]. Further studies designed to elucidate the mechanisms involved and the reasons for apparent discrepancies in experimental findings are clearly necessary.

Selenium-Mercury Interactions

The first evidence of a metabolic antagonism between selenium and mercury came from studies by Parizek et al. [104] showing that selenite protected against the renal necrosis and mortality in rats caused by injected mercuric chloride. The same group also showed that selenium counteracts the placental transfer of mercury and can increase the levels of Hg and Se in rat tissues when high levels of Hg and Se are administered [101,105,106]. The whole question of Se:Hg interactions assumed a new dimension when Ganther et al. [107] demonstrated a protective effect of dietary selenium against the chronic toxic effects of mercury. Rats given a diet to which sodium selenite was added at a level of 0.5 ppm Se grew better and survived longer than rats not so treated with selenium when methyl mercury was added to the drinking water of both groups. Similarly, Japanese quail given 20 ppm Hg as methyl mercury in diets containing 17% by weight of tuna fish (approximating 2-3 ppm Se) survived longer than quail given this concentration of mercury in a corn-soya (low-Se) diet [107]. This important discovery suggests that the relatively high content of selenium in tuna lessens the danger to man of the mercury in tuna. It suggests, further, that the maximum permissible or "safe" levels of mercury in fish and other foods would be influenced by actual environmental intakes of selenium and the optimal or desirable intakes of selenium by man would be influenced, in turn, by the extent of his exposure to mercury.

The preceding findings have been confirmed and extended in several investigations. Thus Potter and Matrone [108] fed rats diets containing methyl mercury and mercuric chloride with and without sodium selenite supplements. The selenite supplements induced an enhanced growth rate with both forms of mercury, altered tissue mercury levels and the percentage distribution of mercury among several tissues, and, in addition, protected against the mortality and neurotoxicity caused by dietary methyl mercury. In the experiments of Hill [103] referred to in the previous section, the toxic effects of selenium, fed as selenium dioxide to chicks, were shown to be partially alleviated by the inclusion of mercuric chloride and of phenyl-mercuriacetate in the diet (see Table 3). The molar ratio of Hg to Se for the most effective counteraction of selenium toxicity when the two elements were fed in the inorganic form was 1:1. For counteracting the toxicity of phenylmercuriacetate by diphenylselenium the most effective ratio was 4:1, indicating that the mechanisms on which the interactions are based are different in the two instances.

So far, the biochemical mechanisms involved in the amelioration or prevention of mercury toxicity by selenium or of selenium toxicity by mercury remain largely obscure. It seems clear that the protection afforded by selenite to mercury poisoning is not due to increased mercury excretion. Indeed, most of the evidence suggests that there is an increase in mercury retention, or at least a redistribution of retained mercury resulting in increased levels in some tissues but not in others. It is known also that the protection afforded by mercury against selenium toxicity is not dependent upon either element being in the inorganic form [103]. Unlike mercuric chloride, dietary methyl mercury is not found on metallothionein and combines

TABLE 3. Effect of Phenylmercuriacetate on Growth Retardation of Selenium-Fed Chicks[a]

Diet	3-wk Gain $(g \pm Se)$[b,c]
Control	322 ± 7.0[*]
Se 10 ppm[d]	276 ± 27.1[†]
Se 20 ppm	91 ± 8.1[‡]
PMA[e], $\approx$ 25 ppm Hg	310 ± 7.0[*]
PMA, $\approx$ 50 ppm Hg	282 ± 9.5[†]
Se 10 ppm + PMA $\approx$ 25 ppm Hg	281 ± 7.2[†]
Se 20 ppm + PMA $\approx$ 50 ppm Hg	247 ± 8.1[†]

[a]Reprinted from Ref. 103 by courtesy of American Institute of Nutrition.
[b]Each mean represents the mean of three lots of 10 chicks each.
[c]Weights followed by the same superscript are not significantly different.
[d]Se fed as SeO_2.
[e]PMA = phenylmercuriacetate.

poorly with this compound in vitro. Furthermore, dietary selenite does not
increase the amount of mercury in thionein when this mercury is fed as
methyl mercury [109]. This indicates that selenite does not ameliorate
methyl mercury toxicity by increasing the rate of methyl mercury breakdown.

INTERACTIONS OF MANGANESE WITH IRON

High levels of dietary manganese have been shown to interfere with iron
metabolism and to depress hemoglobin formation in sheep [111,112], cattle
[113], rabbits, and pigs [114]. Hemoglobin regeneration was greatly retarded and serum iron depressed in anemic lambs fed diets containing 1000
ppm or 2000 ppm Mn. In normal lambs similar effects were produced by higher
levels up to 5000 ppm Mn, accompanied by decreased concentrations of iron
in the liver, kidney, and spleen [111]. Older sheep (8-9 months of age)
grazing normal pastures and given much smaller manganese supplements, e.g.,
daily pellets equivalent to 250 or 500 mg Mn/day, suffered from depressed
growth and exhibited significantly lower iron levels in heart and plasma,
compared with untreated controls [112]. It should be noted that the pastures
contained 154-160 ppm Mn on the dry basis, so that the total manganese intakes of the sheep, assuming they consumed 1 kg dm/day, were approximately
400 and 650 mg Mn/day, equivalent to 400 and 650 ppm of the dry diet. Ma-
.ture rabbits and baby pigs fed diets containing 1250 and 2000 ppm Mn revealed
impaired hemoglobin formation which was not apparent when a dietary supplement of 400 ppm of iron was given [114].

Little is known of the precise mechanism by which manganese affects
iron metabolism and hemoglobin formation, although an interference with iron
absorption rather than with hematopoiesis accords with the experimental data
so far obtained. The levels of manganese used in the experiments with lambs,
pigs, and rabbits, described above, are so high that they are never likely
to be achieved except under the most abnormal conditions of environmental
contamination with manganese. However, Matrone et al. [114] estimate that
the minimum level of dietary manganese capable of adversely affecting hemoglobin formation is only 45 ppm for anemic lambs and lies between 50 and
125 ppm for mature rabbits and baby pigs. Such manganese levels are quite
common in ordinary livestock diets, suggesting that the Mn:Fe interaction
may have wider significance than is commonly conceived.

Whether the metabolic antagonism between Mn and Fe evident from very
high Mn-to-Fe dietary ratios is a mutual antagonism, i.e., whether high iron

intakes would similarly interfere with manganese utilization does not appear
to have been studied.

INTERACTIONS OF SILVER WITH
SELENIUM AND COPPER

Evidence of an interaction between silver and selenium may be said to
have appeared in 1951 when Shaver and Mason [115] showed that soluble salts
of silver could accentuate vitamin E deficiency in rats, although the nexus
between selenium and vitamin E was unknown at the time. This observation
was subsequently confirmed with chicks [116]. Later Bunyan et al. [117]
showed that the greenish exudate produced in chicks given 0.15% silver acetate in the drinking water could be prevented by supplementary vitamin E or
selenium, and Petersen and Jensen [118] found that the growth depression
and high mortality induced in chicks by adding 900 ppm Ag (as AgNO$_3$) to a
diet marginal in vitamin E and selenium could be prevented by including
either 1 ppm Se or 100 IU vitamin E. Adding 100 ppm Ag (as silver acetate)
to the drinking water of rats fed purified casein diets low in vitamin E
and selenium was also found to promote liver necrosis characteristic of se-
lenium-vitamin E deficiency [110]. This effect was not observed with either
cadmium or methyl mercury similarly administered, which implies a rather
specific complexing of silver with some biologically active form of selenium.
Ganther et al. [110] suggest that glutathione peroxidase might be this specific molecular target of silver, which binds to this enzyme in the liver
to inhibit peroxide decomposition by glutathione peroxidase and thus bring
about liver necrosis. Such a hypothesis is consistent with the observations
mentioned above, that either selenium, vitamin E, or antioxidants prevent
Ag-induced lesions since all of these agents have complementary roles in
preventing oxidative damage.

An interaction between silver and copper is well established but not
well understood. Thus Hill et al. [119] observed that silver accentuated
the copper deficiency induced by a low-copper basal diet. Jensen et al.
[120] found that the depressed growth rate, reduced packed cell volume,
slightly reduced hemoglobin level, and cardiac enlargement induced in turkey
poults by adding 900 ppm of silver to practical diets could be prevented by
50 ppm of supplementary copper. Adding silver to a practical diet for chicks
also resulted in reduced growth and cardiac enlargement [121]. The cardiac
enlargement was completely prevented by 50 ppm copper, but growth retardation
was only partially corrected, presumably because of an inadequate level of
selenium and vitamin E relative to the high intakes of silver, as discussed

in the preceding paragraph. The manner in which silver interferes with
copper metabolism remains to be determined. Apparently, this interference
is not primarily at the absorptive level since Van Campen [75] found silver
to have little effect on the uptake of ^{64}Cu from the intestine of the rat.

INTERACTIONS OF COBALT
WITH IRON AND SELENIUM

A mutual antagonism between cobalt and iron in absorption has been
demonstrated directly using isolated segments of rat intestine [122].
Thomson et al. [123] also reported that the interaction between these two
elements results from the competition for intestinal transport mechanisms,
and Chetty [124] found that the addition of cobalt to an iron-deficient
diet resulted in a greater degree of anemia when the chicks were fed equal
amounts of feed. That cobalt acts as an iron antagonist comparable to the
action of manganese, as mentioned on page 659 of this review, could be pre-
dicted on the basis of the similarity of their electronic structures if the
concept of Hill and Matrone [91] is accepted that trace elements with similar electron structures are likely to be biological antagonists.

Many years ago cobalt was reported to be one of the cations which enhances the toxicity of selenium when added to a seleniferous diet [81].
Much more recently Burch et al. [125] fed rats a low-protein diet supplemented with selenium at the rate of 10 µg/g of diet as selenium nitrate and
with selenium at this rate plus 10 µg/g cobalt as cobaltous chloride. The
rats on the supplemented diets grew poorly and showed cardiac and hepatic
enlargement and increased tissue selenium concentrations. These concentrations were enhanced in the cobalt-treated rats in all tissues studied except
the spleen. It is of interest in the overall context of this review that
the supplements of selenium and of selenium plus cobalt were associated with
decreased tissue manganese and copper levels. This implies metabolic interactions between these elements which warrant further investigation. The
results of these experiments imply further, as the authors point out, that
selenium toxicity could be one of the contributing factors in the development of the heavy beer drinkers' cardiomyopathy in man which ensued following the addition of cobalt to beer.

EFFECT OF LEAD ON COPPER METABOLISM

The anemia of lead intoxication has long been believed to be caused or
enhanced by a lead inhibition of heme synthesis. The possibility that this

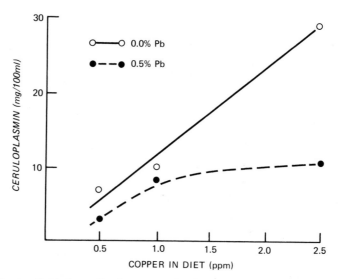

FIG. 3. Effect of dietary lead on ceruloplasmin levels in plasma of male rats as a function of dietary copper: control groups (open circles), lead-treated groups (closed circles). (Taken from Ref. 126 by courtesy of Environmental Trace Substances Center, University of Missouri.)

anemia is related also to an interference by lead with copper metabolism, or the dietary absorption of copper, must now be considered. Klauder et al. [126] found that 0.5% lead (as lead acetate) in the diets of male rats caused a growth inhibition which was inversely related to the dietary copper levels. A reciprocal antagonism between lead and copper at the absorptive level is suggested by their finding that the dietary lead resulted in reduced plasma copper and ceruloplasmin levels (Fig. 3) and that erythrocyte lead levels were reduced as the dietary copper was increased. The possibility that the lead-copper interaction revealed by these studies is significant in relation to the incidence of swayback in lambs in parts of England and of other disorders of environmental origin is pertinently raised by the authors.

GENERAL CONCLUSIONS

It is apparent from the foregoing sections of this chapter that metabolic interactions occur among a wide range of trace elements and that these are particularly powerful among the heavy metals which are of most concern as environmental contaminants. Extrapolation to the environment from interactions demonstrated experimentally with the highly available soluble salts of the elements mostly employed needs to be made with considerable caution.

Little is known of the chemical forms of the elements as they are ingested, or inhaled, from a contaminated environment, so that they may be in forms of quite different availability or biological reactivity. Further studies are needed of the nature of such chemical forms of the trace elements and the extent of their interactions in the animal, among themselves and with the major elements.

Most of the research on trace element interactions is so recent that additional interactions appear inevitable as research proceeds. This research should be aimed particularly at quantifying these interactions and at identifying the precise mechanisms and loci of their action within the body. Research of this nature could do a great deal to further illuminate the mode of action of the trace elements and to define the conditions under which deficiencies or toxicities in animals and man are likely to arise. It cannot be stressed too strongly that metabolic interactions among the trace elements can be so powerful that environmental studies involving single elements can lead to dangerously erroneous conclusions.

REFERENCES

1. A. H. Lewis, J. Agr. Sci., 33, 52, 58 (1943).

2. F. Brouwer, A. M. Frens, P. Reitsma, and C. Kaleswaart, Versl. Land-bouwk, Onderzoek., 44C, 267 (1938).

3. W. S. Ferguson, A. H. Lewis, and S. J. Watson, Nature, 141, 553 (1938); J. Agr. Sci., 33, 43 (1943).

4. R. Allcroft and G. Lewis, Landbouwk. Tijdschr., 68, 711 (1956).

5. I. J. Cunningham, in Symposium on Copper Metabolism (W. D. McElroy and B. Glass, eds.), Johns Hopkins Press, Baltimore, 1950, p. 246.

6. J. E. Miltimore and J. L. Mason, Can. J. Anim. Sci., 51, 193 (1971).

7. B. J. Alloway, J. Agr. Sci., 80, 521 (1973).

8. C. L. Comar, L. Singer, and G. K. Davis, J. Biol. Chem., 180, 913 (1949).

9. J. B. Nielands, F. M. Strong, and C. A. Elvehjem, J. Biol. Chem., 172, 431 (1948).

10. L. R. Arrington and G. K. Davis, J. Nutr., 51, 295 (1953).

11. D. Arthur, I. Motzok, and H. D. Branion, Poultry Sci., 37, 1181 (1958).

12. R. Van Reen and M. A. Williams, Arch. Biochem. Biophys., 63, 1 (1956).

13. J. F. Scaife, N. Z. J. Sci. Technol., 38A, 285, 293 (1963).

14. A. T. Dick, Aust. Vet. J., 28, 30 (1952); 29, 18, 233 (1953); 30, 196 (1954).

15. R. F. Miller, N. O. Price, and R. W. Engel, J. Nutr., 60, 539 (1956).

16. I. J. Cunningham, K. G. Hogan, and B. M. Lawson, N. Z. J. Agr. Res., 2, 145 (1959).

17. R. E. Davies, B. L. Reid, A. A. Kurnich, and J. R. Couch, J. Nutr., 70, 193 (1960).

18. R. Van Reen, J. Nutr., 68, 243 (1959).

19. A. T. Dick, in Inorganic Nitrogen Metabolism (W. D. McElroy and B. Glass, eds.), Johns Hopkins Press, Baltimore, 1956, p. 445.

20. E. J. Underwood, Trace Elements in Human and Animal Nutrition, 3rd Ed., Academic Press, New York, 1971.

21. A. T. Dick and L. B. Bull, Aust. Vet. J., 21, 70 (1945).

22. A. T. Dick, Aust. J. Agr. Res., 5, 511 (1954).

23. K. G. Hogan, D. F. L. Money, and A. Blayney, N. Z. J. Agr. Res., 11, 435 (1968).

24. J. Huisingh, G. G. Gomez, and G. Matrone, Fed. Proc., 32, 1921 (1973).

25. L. F. Gray and L. J. Daniel, J. Nutr., 84, 31 (1964).

26. A. T. Dick, Soil Sci., 81, 229 (1956).

27. B. F. Fell, C. F. Mills, and R. Boyne, Res. Vet. Sci., 6, 10 (1965).

28. E. J. Butler and R. M. Barlow, J. Comp. Pathol. Ther., 73, 208 (1963).

29. K. G. Hogan, D. R. Ris, and A. J. Hutchinson, N. Z. J. Agr. Res., 9, 691 (1966).

30. C. F. Mills, Rowett Res. Inst. Collect. Pap., 17, 57 (1961).

31. A. G. Spais, T. K. Lazaridis, and A. G. Agiannidis, Res. Vet. Sci., 9, 337 (1968).

32. P. R. Bird, Proc. Aust. Soc. Anim. Prod., 8, 212 (1970).

33. N. A. Marciless, C. B. Ammerman, R. M. Valsecchi, B. G. Dunavant, and G. K. Davis, J. Nutr., 99, 177 (1969).

34. R. P. Dowdy and G. Matrone, J. Nutr., 95, 191, 197 (1968).

35. R. P. Dowdy, G. A. Kunz, and H. E. Sauberlich, J. Nutr., 99, 491 (1969).

36. A. T. Dick, D. W. Dewey, and J. M. Gawthorne, J. Agr. Sci., 85, 567 (1975).

37. R. S. Barber, R. Braude, and K. G. Mitchell, Brit. J. Nutr., 9, 378 (1955).

38. R. Braude, M. J. Townsend, G. Harrington, and J. G. Rowell, J. Agr. Sci., 58, 251 (1962).

39. R. Braude and K. Ryder, J. Agr. Sci., 80, 489 (1973).

40. B. Bass, J. T. McCall, H. D. Wallace, G. E. Combs, A. Z. Palmer, and J. E. Carpenter, J. Anim. Sci., 15, 1230 (1956).

41. H. D. Ritchie, R. W. Luecke, B. V. Baltzer, E. R. Miller, D. E. Ullrey, and J. A. Hoefer, J. Nutr., 79, 117 (1963).

42. H. D. Wallace, J. T. McCall, B. Bass, and G. E. Combs, J. Anim. Sci., 19, 1155 (1960).

43. P. J. O'Hara, A. P. Newman, and R. Jackson, Aust. Vet. J., 36, 225 (1960).

44. R. J. Bunch, V. C. Speers, V. M. Hays, and J. T. McCall, J. Anim. Sci., 22, 56 (1963).

45. N. F. Suttle and C. F. Mills, Brit. J. Nutr., 20, 135, 149 (1966).

46. G. K. Davis, Fed. Proc., 33, 1194 (1974).

47. D. R. Grant-Frost and E. J. Underwood, Aust. J. Exp. Biol. Med. Sci., 36, 339 (1958).

48. E. A. Ott, W. H. Smith, R. B. Harrington, and W. M. Beeson, J. Anim. Sci., 25, 414, 419 (1966).

49. D. H. Cox and D. L. Harris, J. Nutr., 70, 514 (1960).

50. A. C. Magee and G. Matrone, J. Nutr., 72, 233 (1960).

51. R. Van Reen, Arch. Biochem. Biophys., 46, 337 (1953).

52. I. J. Witham, Biochem. Biophys. Acta, 11, 509 (1963).

53. S. E. Smith and E. J. Larson, J. Biol. Chem., 163, 29 (1946).

54. D. R. Van Campen and P. U. Scaife, J. Nutr., 91, 473 (1967).

55. D. R. Van Campen, J. Nutr., 97, 104 (1969).

56. W. F. Gipp, W. G. Pond, F. A. Kallfelz, J. B. Tasker, D. R. Van Campen, L. Krook, and W. J. Visek, J. Nutr. 104, 532 (1974).

57. B. Starcher, J. Nutr., 97, 321 (1969).

57a. C. T. Settlemire and G. Matrone, J. Nutr., 92, 153 (1967).

58. J. C. Medici and M. W. Taylor, J. Nutr., 93, 907 (1967).

59. C. R. Bunn and G. Matrone, J. Nutr., 90, 395 (1966).

60. J. G. Lease, J. Nutr., 96, 294 (1969).

61. G. C. Cotzias and P. S. Papavasilou, Amer. J. Physiol., 206, 787 (1964).

62. P. Pulido, J. H. R. Kagi, and B. L. Vallee, Biochemistry, 5, 1768 (1966).

63. M. Margoshes and B. L. Vallee, J. Amer. Chem. Soc., 79, 4813 (1957).

64. G. F. Nordberg, M. Nordberg, M. Piscator, and O. Vesterberg, Biochem. J., 126, 491 (1972).

65. D. R. Winge and K. V. Rajagopalan, Arch. Biochem. Biophys., 153, 755 (1972).

66. U. Weser, F. Donay, and H. Rupp, FEBS Lett., 32, 171 (1973).

67. J. Parizek, J. Endocrinol., 15, 56 (1957).

68. J. Parizek, I. Benes, J. Kalowskova, A. Babicky, and J. Lener, Physiol. Bohemoslov., 18, 89 (1969).

69. A. Hennig and M. Anke, Arch. Tierernahr., 14, 55 (1964).

70. C. F. Mills and A. C. Dalgarno, Nature, 239, 171 (1972).

70a. J. K. Campbell and C. F. Mills, Proc. Nutr. Soc. (Cambridge), 33, 15A (1974).

71. H. J. Lee and G. B. Jones, personal communication, 1974.

72. J. V. Lagerwerff, D. L. Brouwer, and G. T. Biersdorff, Trace Substances in Environmental Health, VI (D. D. Hemphill, ed.), University of Missouri, Columbia, Mo., 1972, p. 71.

73. J. H. Freeland and R. J. Cousins, Nutr. Rep. Int., 8, 337 (1973).

74. C. H. Hill, G. Matrone, W. L. Payne, and C. W. Barber, J. Nutr., 80, 227 (1963).

75. D. R. Van Campen, J. Nutr., 88, 125 (1966).

76. M. E. Richardson, M. R. Spivey Fox, and B. E. Fry, Jr., J. Nutr., 104, 323 (1974).

77. L. Hallberg and L. Solvell, Acta Med. Scand., 181, 335 (1967).

78. G. Pirzio-Biroli, T. H. Bothwell, and C. A. Finch, J. Lab. Clin. Med., 51, 37 (1958).

79. D. R. Van Campen and E. Gross, J. Nutr., 95, 617 (1968).

80. A. L. Moxon, S. Dakota Agr. Exp. Sta. Bull., 311, 1937.

81. A. L. Moxon, Science, 88, 81 (1938).

82. C. M. Hendrick, H. L. Kleig, and O. E. Olson, J. Nutr., 51, 131 (1953).

83. K. L. Kuttler and D. W. Marble, Amer. J. Vet. Res., 22, 422 (1961).

84. E. Leitis, I. S. Palmer, and O. E. Olson, Proc. S. Dakota Acad. Sci., 35, 189 (1956).

85. R. C. Wahlstrom, L. D. Kamstra, and O. E. Olson, J. Anim. Sci., 14, 105 (1955).

86. H. E. Ganther and C. A. Baumann, J. Nutr., 77, 210 (1962).

87. O. A. Levander and C. A. Baumann, Toxicol. Appl. Pharmacol., 9, 98, 106 (1966).

88. K. P. McConnell and D. M. Carpenter, Proc. Soc. Exp. Biol. Med., 137, 996 (1971).

89. O. A. Levander and L. C. Argrett, Toxicol. Appl. Pharmacol., 14, 308 (1969).

90. D. V. Frost, C. R. C. Crit. Revs. Toxicol., October (1972).

91. C. H. Hill and G. Matrone, Fed. Proc., 29, 1474 (1970).

92. C. H. Hill, in Trace Elements in Human Health and Disease, II (A. S. Prasad, ed.), Academic Press, New York, 1976, p. 281.

93. J. Parizek and Z. Zahor, Nature (London), 177, 1036 (1956).

94. J. Parizek, J. Endocrinol., 15, 56 (1957).

95. A. B. Ka and R. P. Das, Proc. Nat. Sci. India, Part B, 29, Suppl. 297 (1963).

96. K. E. Mason, J. O. Young, and J. E. Brown, Anat. Rec., 148, 309 (1964).

97. J. Parizek, Proceedings of the Second International Congress on Endocrinology (London, 1964), P. H. Vuysje, Amsterdam, 1965.

98. J. Parizek, J. Reprod. Fertil., 7, 263 (1964).

99. J. Parizek, J. Reprod. Fertil., 9, 111 (1965).

100. J. Parizek, I. Ostadalova, I. Benes, and A. Babicky, J. Reprod. Fertil., 16, 507 (1968).

101. J. Parizek, D. Benes, I. Ostadalova, A. Babicky, T. Benes, and T. Lenar, Physiol. Bohemoslov., 18, 95 (1969).

102. S. A. Gunn, T. C. Gould, and W. A. D. Anderson, Proc. Soc. Exp. Biol. Med., 128, 591 (1968).

103. C. H. Hill, J. Nutr., 104, 593 (1974).

104. J. Parizek, I. Benes, I. Ostadalova, A. Babicky, J. Benes, and J. Pitha, in Mineral Metabolism in Pediatrics (D. Barltrop and W. L. Burland, eds.), Blackwell, Oxford, 1969.

105. J. Parizek and I. Ostadalova, Separatum Experention, 23, 142 (1967).

106. J. Parizek, J. Ostadalova, J. Ralovskova, A. Babicky, L. Paulik, and R. Bibz, J. Reprod. Fertil., 25, 57 (1971).

107. H. E. Ganther, C. Gondie, M. L. Sunde, M. J. Kopecky, P. Wagner, S. Hoh, and W. G. Hockstra, Science, 175, 1122 (1972).

108. S. Potter and G. Matrone, J. Nutr., 104, 638 (1974).

109. R. W. Chen, H. E. Ganther, and W. G. Hockstra, Biochem. Biophys. Res. Commun., 51, 383 (1973).

110. H. E. Ganther, P. A. Wagner, M. L. Sunde, and W. G. Hoekstra, in Trace Substances in Environmental Health, VI (D. D. Hemphill, ed.), University of Missouri, Columbia, Mo., 1973, p. 247.

111. R. H. Hartman, G. Matrone, and G. H. Wise, J. Nutr., 57, 429 (1955).

112. N. D. Grace, N. Z. J. Agr. Res., 16, 177 (1973).

113. N. W. Robinson, S. L. Hansard, D. M. Johns, and G. L. Robertson, J. Anim. Sci., 19, Proc. 1290 (1960).

114. G. Matrone, R. H. Hartman, and A. J. Clawson, J. Nutr., 67, 309 (1959).

115. S. L. Shaver and K. E. Mason, Anat. Rec., 109, 382 (1951).

116. H. Dam, G. K. Nielsen, I. Prange, and E. Sundergaard, Experientia, 14, 291 (1958).

117. J. Bunyan, A. T. Diplock, M. A. Cawthorne, and J. Green, Brit. J. Nutr., 22, 165 (1968).

118. R. P. Peterson and L. S. Jensen, personal communication, 1975.

119. C. H. Hill, B. Starcher, and G. Matrone, J. Nutr., 83, 107 (1964).

120. L. S. Jensen, R. P. Peterson, and L. Falen, Poultry Sci., 53, 57 (1964).

121. R. P. Peterson and L. S. Jensen, Poultry Sci., 54, 771 (1975).

122. W. Forth and W. Rummel, in Intestinal Absorption of Metal Ions, Trace Elements, and Radionuclides (S. C. Skoryna and D. Waldron-Edward, eds.), Pergamon Press, Montreal, Canada, 1971, p. 173.

123. A. B. R. Thomson, L. L. Valberg, and D. G. Sinclair, J. Clin. Invest., 50, 2384 (1971).

124. K. N. Chetty, Ph.D. thesis, North Carolina State University, 1972 (cited by Hill, Ref. 92).

125. R. E. Burch, R. V. Williams, and J. F. Sullivan, in Trace Substances in Environmental Health, VII (D. D. Hemphill, ed.), University of Missouri, Columbia, Mo., 1973, p. 257.

126. D. S. Klauder, L. Murthy, and H. G. Petering, in Trace Substances in Environmental Health, VI (D. D. Hemphill, ed.), University of Missouri, Columbia, Mo., 1972, p. 131.

REGULATORY ASPECTS OF TRACE ELEMENTS
IN THE ENVIRONMENT

<hr>

William A. Rader* and John E. Spaulding
U.S. Department of Agriculture
Washington, D. C.

For many years the United States Department of Agriculture (USDA) has been aware of the presence of detectable levels of trace elements[†], including heavy metals, in edible tissues of animals and poultry [1]. Surveys are routinely conducted to determine the levels of trace elements in edible tissues of animals. Regulatory action is taken when the residue level detected exceeds the norm for that species of animal in that geographic region [2].

METHODS OF CONTROLLING TRACE ELEMENTS IN EDIBLE TISSUE

The determination of acceptable levels of trace elements presents a unique challenge to USDA and the Department of Health, Education, and Welfare (DHEW). It has been shown that the normal ("background") levels of trace elements in soils and animal feeds vary in various areas of the United States and the world from severely deficient to toxic [3,4]. Trace element imbalances in these materials are common, creating an additional problem in interpretation of results [3]. Animal tissues reflect the levels of trace elements in their environment; therefore, the normal background levels in edible animal tissue should reflect the area in which the animal was raised.

Regulatory Policy

The data available indicate that establishing a uniform national level for any trace element in edible animal tissue would be difficult; therefore,

<hr>

*Present Address: 4638 Bayshore Road, Sarasota, Florida.
†The term <u>trace elements</u> will be used throughout the chapter since "heavy metals" has limited regulatory connotation.

regulatory policy must be broad enough to allow for regional variation in trace element residue levels. The policy now used in the USDA is reflected in the following statement: "The acceptable level of a trace element in edible animal tissue must be within the normal range for the geographic area from which the animal originated." Generally speaking, the smallest geographic area from which adequate data are available is a state.

Defining this acceptable residue level requires sound scientific judgment and adequate background data. The following general logic is used in these determinations: Is the source of the trace element a normal environmental condition? Is the residue level within the acceptable range for the area? Can this residue level be altered by good agricultural practices?

Regulations

When the level of a trace element is above that normally acceptable in edible animal tissue from a specific geographic region in the United States, it can usually be attributed to a source not normally found in the animal's environment. The amounts added from this source, then, are considered added to the natural levels present in food, water, or air and are considered a "food additive" by the DHEW, as defined in Section 409 of the Food, Drug, and Cosmetic Act (FDC) [5].

The term food additive is defined as

> any substance the intended use of which results, or may reasonably
> be expected to result, directly or indirectly, in its becoming a
> component or otherwise affecting the characteristics of any food
> (including any substance intended for use in producing, manufactur-
> ing, packing, processing, preparing, treating, packaging, transport-
> ing, or holding food), if such substance is not generally recognized
> among experts qualified by scientific training and experience to
> evaluate its safety, as having been adequately shown through scien-
> tific procedures (or, in the case of a substance used in food prior
> to January 1, 1958, through either scientific procedures or experi-
> ence based on a common use in food) to be safe under the conditions
> of its intended use.

The term safe as used in the DHEW Food, Drug, and Cosmetic Act [5] has reference to the health of man and animal.

The Federal Meat Inspection Act [6], the Poultry Products Inspection Act [7], and the DHEW Food, Drug, and Cosmetic Act [5] define adulterated product with essentially the same words and require adulterated products to be condemned. An adulterated food is defined as one that "bears or contains any poisonous or deleterious substance which may render it injurious to health; but in case the substance is not an added substance such food shall not be considered adulterated if the quantity of such substance in

such food does not <u>ordinarily</u> render it injurious to health." It can be
concluded that any trace element present in amounts which are judged ordinarily to render the product injurious to health would make the edible
animal tissue adulterated, no matter what the source of the trace element.
All edible animal tissues considered adulterated are subject to condemnation
by the Meat and Poultry Products Inspection Acts.

Distinction Between Naturally Occurring and Added Poisonous Substances

The DHEW Food and Drug Administration (FDA) has made a distinction
between food additives and naturally occurring poisonous and deleterious
substances and has established action levels for the latter substances.
Part 122.3 of the Code of Federal Regulations 21 states:

> A 'naturally occurring poisonous or deleterious substance' is an
> inherent natural constituent of a food and is not the result of
> environmental, agricultural, industrial, or other handling or con-
> tamination.
>
> An 'added poisonous or deleterious substance' is a poisonous or
> deleterious substance that is not a naturally occurring poisonous
> or deleterious substance. When a naturally occurring poisonous
> or deleterious substance is increased to abnormal levels through
> mishandling or other intervening acts, it is an added poisonous
> or deleterious substance to the extent of such increase.
>
> 'Food' includes human food, substances migrating to food from
> food-contact articles, pet food, and animal feed. [10]

The authority for this distinction is given to the FDA under Section 402(a)
of the FDC Act [5]. This is the food adulteration section of the law and
applies to all poisonous and deleterious substances whether naturally occurring or added. The broad scope of the section has been shown by the fact
that substances are exempted from Section 402(a) [1] only if they are covered by regulations set under Section 406 (tolerances) for poisonous or
deleterious substances, Section 408 for pesticides, Section 409 for food
additives, or Section 512 for new animal drugs, all of which may contain
trace elements [8]. In addition, the Environmental Protection Agency (EPA)
has authority under the Federal Insecticide, Fungicide, and Rodenticide Act
[9] to set tolerances for trace elements regulated by the act.

Tolerances for Unavoidable Food Contaminants

The levels (tolerances) for unavoidable food contaminants can be established under Section 406 of the FDC Act. The FDA interpretation of this
section of the act is as follows:

"...except for substances whose deleterious nature is inherent to the natural state of the food, all poisonous or deleterious components are 'added' within the meaning of the FDC Act. Moreover, when a naturally occurring poisonous or deleterious substance is increased to abnormal levels through mishandling or other intervening acts, it is 'added' to the extent of the increase. Whenever a food contaminant is unavoidable, and tolerances cannot be set under Section 409 (food additive) of the act, a procedure to establish a tolerance under Section 406 of the act will come into play" [10].

An example of this is lead. It cannot be the subject of a food additive regulation because lead serves no functional purpose. Therefore, a tolerance would necessarily have to be established under Section 406 of the act. Under this authority a tolerance was established for lead in evaporated milk at 0.3 ppm [10].

As can be seen, such tolerances are used in relatively static circumstances and are set at a level necessary for the protection of the public health, taking into account the extent to which the substance cannot be avoided [10].

The use of certain arsenical compounds as pesticides [10] and animal drugs [11] resulted in tolerances being established and regulated in edible animal tissues under Title 40, Part 180 and Title 21, Part 135 of the Code of Federal Regulations.

Establishment of Action Levels

Under certain circumstances an "action level" can be established. An action level must meet the same criteria as a tolerance, except that it is temporary and remains in effect only until additional scientific evidence makes a formal tolerance appropriate. Section 306 of the act has been interpreted to permit the FDA to establish action levels in implementing the adulteration provisions of the act.

Action levels have been established for trace elements, i.e., mercury at 0.5 ppm in fish. All action levels for unavoidable poisonous or deleterious substances are to be published in Title 21, Part 122 of the Code of Federal Regulations, along with the circumstances that require the use of informal action [10].

Mixing of Food Containing
Above-Tolerance Levels

The DHEW has ruled that, in general, the mixing of a poisonous or deleterious substance in the amount above the tolerance or action level with another food is not permitted and renders the final food unlawful regardless of

the amount of poisonous or deleterious substance in the final food [10].
This applies to trace elements that exceed their background levels in edible
tissues from food-producing animals. There are provisions under the Poultry
Products Inspection Act to dispose of specific organs or tissues by condemnation, as long as the remaining tissues are within the acceptable levels.

Difficulty in Establishing a
Tolerance for Trace Elements

A specific tolerance for naturally occurring trace elements in edible
animal tissues is very difficult to establish because

Each region or area in the United States contains certain well-
established background levels of trace elements.

Livestock raised, grown, or fed in a specific area or region will
reflect the background levels of trace elements.

Livestock raised, grown, or fed in a specific area or region will
reflect the background levels of trace elements in the soil,
feed, or water (environment).

There is a considerable vital organ variation as well as a species
variation.

A single numerical tolerance for trace elements in the United States
could allow misuse of the element in certain regions, while in
other regions the tolerance could restrict livestock production
due to the high levels that are normal in the environment in
that region.

This reasoning has been well documented in environmental and epidemiological
investigations and by evidence gathered by regulatory surveillance of specific incidents by the FDA, EPA, and USDA [1,16].

PRACTICAL METHODS OF CONTROLLING TRACE
ELEMENTS IN FOOD-PRODUCING ANIMALS

Factors Influencing the Level of
Trace Elements in Edible Tissues

There are many other factors that may affect the level of trace elements
in edible tissues. Extremely low levels may be caused by dehydration, parasitism, disease, diarrhea, or confinement without proper supplementation.
Excessive levels can occur, environmentally, from industrial or agricultural
practices in which trace elements are involved, e.g., painted walls (lead),

waste disposal grounds, misplaced pesticides (lead, arsenic, and mercury),
trace mineral supplements, consumption of sprayed or treated plants, improper application of pesticides (arsenic, lead, or copper), or feeding
treated seed grains (lead, arsenic, mercury).

When agricultural chemicals contain trace elements, contamination can
also occur from intentional misuse of approved chemicals, intentional misuse
of unapproved chemicals, accidental exposure to excessive levels of approved
chemicals, industrial accidents, or environmental exposure to effluents from
manufacturing and processing facilities, refineries, and mine tailings.
These sources can contaminate soil, pastures, plants, and feed through the
air, water, and soil.

Other sources are disposal of these chemicals by burning, dust from
cleanup operations in manufacturing plants, from warehouse or factory fires,
and indiscriminate dumping of refuse that contains trace elements. The list
can be as long as the classic toxicology textbook. Any cause of excessive
levels of trace elements is of great concern to regulatory agencies [5-7].

Biological Magnification of Trace Elements

The concern for biological magnification of trace elements has been a
worldwide concern for many years. The National Academy of Sciences [14],
scientists [15], the USDA [18], the EPA, The International Organization for
Economic Cooperation and Development, and the DHEW have been involved in
many studies and discussions. Simply stated, biological magnification refers to the buildup of trace elements in plants, animals, and the environment.

Magnification is more pronounced in animals than in plants, water,
soil, or other components of the environment because animals are the final
recipients of the concentration in the ecosystem [14]. In general, the
levels of the trace elements accumulating in various food-producing animals
are influenced by the amount ingested, the age, species, sex (state of gestation or lactation in females), and physical condition of the animal, the
time period over which the trace elements are ingested, and the storage
capability in specific tissue in an animal [15,23]. This process depends
on the amount of contamination, chemical form of trace element, operable
routes of translocation [15,25], plant and animal species differences, the
plant and animal food nutrients, and environmental extremes at each level
of trace element in the chain.

Individual variation can also occur due to parasitism, disease, pathology in certain tissues or organs, and metabolic disturbances. In addition, the rate of metabolism (turnover rate), method of excretion, and degree of chelation, biological availability, and tissue binding of trace elements play an important role in biomganification commonly occurring with mercury, lead, cadmium, selenium, arsenic, copper, and molybdenum.

Regulatory agencies are faced with biological magnification and its many facets. Toxicologists dealing with regulatory control of trace elements must consider all the preceding facts in the decision-making process.

Translocation of Trace Elements

Translocation of trace elements from one part of a plant system to another is also a great concern to the scientific and regulatory community. Under normal conditions, this process depends primarily on the amount and availability of the trace element in the soil. The plant assimilates the trace element from the soil and then through its metabolic pathway redistributes it from the roots to other parts of the plant, i.e., leaves, seeds, seed pods, stems, and branches. This process is dependent upon atmospheric conditions, amount of nutrients available in the soil, stages of development of the plant when sampled, operable routes of translocation, and the growing season. In addition, some species of plants are "accumulators" of specific trace elements.

It has been suggested [15] that further emphasis should be placed on translocation of trace elements in the following areas: quantitative determination of specific chemical forms of trace elements and their biological availability, long-term health effects resulting from low-level exposures, increased surveillance of chemicals in all foods, epidemiological studies to determine the health of animal and human populations when environmental contamination is evident, and more in-depth understanding of the interrelationships that exist among trace elements.

USDA Approach to Controlling Excessive
Levels of Trace Elements

An extensive survey was conducted by the USDA in 1971 to determine the background level of five trace elements in cattle from all geographic locations in the United States [13]. Muscle, liver, and kidney tissues from 2176 animals were analyzed for arsenic, cadmium, mercury, lead, and copper. The ranges for these tissues, as well as the mean values in those

TABLE 1. Trace Elements in Cattle. National Summary of 2176 Animals Sampled, 1971[a]

Trace Elements		Average of Positive Samples (ppm)	Range (ppm)	Incidence of Positive Samples (%)	Location of High Level (State) Including Range Within the State
Arsenic	Liver	0.09	0.02-0.22	6.7	Arizona (0.11-0.22)
	Kidney	0.08	0.05-0.17	7.1	New York (0.05-0.17)
Mercury	Liver	0.02	0.01-1.79	18.2	Ohio (0.01-1.79)
	Muscle	0.03	0.01-1.85	26.0	Colorado (0.01-1.85)
	Kidney	0.03	0.01-5.25	66.9	Ohio (0.01-5.25)
Copper	Liver	34.92	1.30-123.00	99.9	Wisconsin (11.30-123.00)
	Muscle	1.82	0.03-29.90	99.9	Illinois (0.90-29.90)
	Kidney	4.18	0.08-24.20	99.9	Nebraska (0.49-24.20)
Lead	Liver	0.54	0.01-3.74	99.1	Missouri (0.06-3.74)
	Muscle	0.36	0.01-2.96	95.6	Iowa (0.01-2.96)
	Kidney	0.63	0.02-4.90	100.0	Louisiana (0.27-4.90)
Cadmium	Liver	0.21	0.01-3.17	97.5	Mississippi (0.12-3.17)
	Muscle	0.08	0.01-1.00	81.1	Louisiana (0.01-1.00)
	Kidney	0.55	0.01-7.82	98.8	Kansas (0.05-7.82)

[a]From Ref. 13.

tissues with detectable levels, are listed in Table 1. The limit of detection was in the range of 0.01 to 0.05 ppm (wet-tissue basis). The incidence is the percentage of animals showing detectable levels of the trace elements.

This chart demonstrates the wide variation of trace elements in cattle tissues in the United States. Data from individual states indicate the high and low areas of the United States for each trace element in edible animal tissue. These data are critical for regulatory control of trace elements.

The highest mercury level in cattle was found in Ohio in only one animal. This individual had been exposed to mercury in its diet. By looking at the national average for mercury in kidney (0.03 vs the high level of 5.25) and the national average in liver (0.02 vs the high level of 1.79), it is easy to judge that there was something unusual in this instance. Moreover, mercury was found in only 26.0% in bovine muscle to 66.9% in the kidney tested. Therefore, the excessive level became obvious.

Conversely, when considering cadmium, lead, and copper, a high incidence rate and wide ranges are found. The high level of lead (4.90 ppm) reported in the kidney in Louisiana was found among 17 head of cattle in one parish; however, levels up to 1.0 ppm in kidney are not uncommon throughout the United States. Copper is found in edible tissue of cattle at levels above 80 ppm in several geographic regions in the United States and is as high as 123 ppm in Wisconsin. The incidence rate for copper is nearly 100% in all tissues (Tables 2 and 3).

Data for other species of animals indicate similar patterns (Tables 4-8). However, there is a considerable variation in organs from species to species.

TABLE 2. Trace Elements in Heifers. National Summary of 119 Samples, 1974[a]

Trace Element		Average of Positive Samples (ppm)	Range (ppm)	Incidence of Positive Samples (%)
Arsenic	Liver	0.09	0.05-0.30	14
	Muscle	0.05	0.05	8
	Kidney	0.15	0.05-0.40	35
Mercury	Liver	0.05	0.05-0.10	9
	Muscle	0.06	0.05-0.10	7
	Kidney	0.05	0.05	18

TABLE 2 (Continued)

Trace Element		Average of Positive Samples (ppm)	Range (ppm)	Incidence of Positive Samples (%)
Copper	Liver	35.36	0.20-152.00	100
	Muscle	2.36	0.10-5.50	100
	Kidney	5.18	0.15-15.00	100
Lead	Liver	0.45	0.5-1.45	76
	Muscle	0.33	0.05-1.6	70
	Kidney	0.49	0.05-2.73	88
Cadmium	Liver	0.29	0.05-4.23	93
	Muscle	0.12	0.05-0.85	68
	Kidney	0.57	0.10-2.50	98
Iron	Liver	45.75	36.00-72.50	100
	Muscle	37.08	28.00-50.00	100
	Kidney	55.96	42.00-78.50	100

[a]From Ref. 1.

TABLE 3. Trace Elements in Steers. National Summary of 161 Animals, 1974[a]

Trace Element		Average of Positive Samples (ppm)	Range (ppm)	Incidence of Positive Samples (%)
Arsenic	Liver	0.08	0.01-0.30	14
	Muscle	0.08	0.01-0.20	10
	Kidney	0.09	0.01-0.20	31
Mercury	Liver	0.08	0.01-0.40	9
	Muscle	0.07	0.01-0.20	7
	Kidney	0.07	0.01-0.70	27
Copper	Liver	38.13	0.65-108.00	100
	Muscle	3.36	0.01-5.50	100
	Kidney	5.47	0.15-10.80	100
Lead	Liver	0.54	0.02-1.60	84
	Muscle	0.42	0.02-1.70	78

TABLE 3 (Continued)

Trace Element		Average of Positive Samples (ppm)	Range (ppm)	Incidence of Positive Samples (%)
	Kidney	0.56	0.02-2.20	93
Cadmium	Liver	0.20	0.01-0.85	95
	Muscle	0.16	0.01-3.25	65
	Kidney	0.54	0.01-4.90	95
Iron	Liver	53.90	36.00-88.50	100
	Muscle	37.33	22.50-64.00	100
	Kidney	57.33	39.50-74.50	100

[a]From Ref. 1.

TABLE 4. Trace Elements in Swine. National Summary of 763 Samples, 1975[a]

Trace Element		Average of Positive Samples (ppm)	Range (ppm)	Incidence of Positive Samples (%)
Arsenic	Liver	1.62	0.01-6.30	36
	Muscle	0.46	0.01-0.30	35
	Kidney	0.67	0.01-4.60	45
Mercury	Liver	0.04	0.01-0.05	21
	Muscle	0.06	0.01-0.10	37
	Kidney	0.04	0.01-0.05	44
Copper	Liver	6.77	2.03-26.42	100
	Muscle	0.98	0.55-3.70	100
	Kidney	5.51	0.50-19.26	100
Lead	Liver	0.33	0.15-0.60	100
	Muscle	0.24	0.15-0.40	100
	Kidney	0.28	0.10-0.70	100
Cadmium	Liver	0.14	0.01-0.30	100
	Muscle	0.10	0.01-0.50	100

[a]From Ref. 1.

TABLE 5. Trace Elements in Lambs. National Summary of 16 Animals, 1974[a]

Trace Element		Average of Positive Samples (ppm)	Range (ppm)	Incidence of Positive Samples (%)
Arsenic	Liver	0.04	0.01-0.05	19
	Kidney	0.04	0.01-0.05	13
Mercury	Liver	0.05	0.05	31
	Muscle	0.06	0.05-0.10	33
	Kidney	0.06	0.01-0.10	60
Copper	Liver	49.21	7.91-98.68	100
	Muscle	1.11	1.11-1.87	100
	Kidney	3.39	2.62-3.92	100
Lead	Liver	0.45	0.15-1.34	100
	Muscle	0.21	0.10-0.35	100
	Kidney	0.29	0.20-1.03	100
Cadmium	Liver	0.15	0.05-0.25	100
	Muscle	0.09	0.05-0.15	93
	Kidney	0.19	0.10-0.30	100

[a]From Ref. 1.

TABLE 6. Arsenic in Poultry. National Summary, 1974[a]

Tissue	No. of Samples	Average of Positive Samples (ppm)	Range (ppm)	Incidence of Positive Samples (%)
Young chickens				
Liver	952	0.70	0.01-4.70	89
Muscle	26	0.12	0.01-0.20	77
Mature chickens				
Liver	77	0.64	0.01-5.50	52
Young turkeys				
Liver	274	0.35	0.01-2.76	45

[a]From Ref. 1.

TABLE 7. Zinc in Cattle Tissue in Three Geographic Locations. National Summary, 1971[a]

Geographic Location	No. of Samples	Average of Positive Samples (ppm)	Range (ppm)	Incidence of Positive Samples (%)
Liver				
Louisiana	64	45.52	20.40-105.30	97.0
Los Angeles	50	39.86	20.60-71.40	100.0
Wisconsin	32	45.63	20.00-123.00	100.0
Muscle				
Louisiana	64	42.52	27.30-63.70	97.0
Los Angeles	50	42.35	36.60-63.70	100.0
Wisconsin	32	47.13	26.60-69.30	100.0
Kidney				
Louisiana	64	25.85	18.70-40.10	97.0
Los Angeles	50	24.24	16.70-41.60	100.0
Wisconsin	32	25.76	17.80-45.10	100.0

[a]From Ref. 13.

TABLE 8. Trace Elements in Hair from Cattle in Four Geographic Locations, 1971 Survey[a]

Trace Element	No. of Samples	Average of Positive Samples (ppm)	Range (ppm)	Samples Containing Trace Elements (%)
Los Angeles area				
Arsenic	50	0.19	0.07-0.37	18.0
Cadmium	50	0.27	0.05-0.57	100.0
Mercury	50	0.20	0.04-1.13	100.0
Lead	50	5.03	1.00-11.50	100.0
Copper	50	13.22	6.00-70.50	100.0
Zinc	50	135.50	100.30-237.90	100.0
Louisiana area				
Arsenic	65	0.13	0.05-0.29	7.6
Cadmium	65	0.23	0.03-1.28	95.5
Mercury	65	0.13	0.01-0.54	95.5
Lead	65	4.40	1.10-9.45	97.0

TABLE 8 (Continued)

Trace Element	No. of Samples	Average of Positive Samples (ppm)	Range (ppm)	Samples Containing Trace Elements (%)
Copper	65	12.92	6.50-33.40	97.0
Zinc	65	127.18	94.50-193.50	97.0
Wisconsin area				
Arsenic	32	0.25	0.09-0.79	15.6
Cadmium	32	0.15	0.03-0.30	100.0
Mercury	32	0.20	0.01-0.74	100.0
Lead	32	2.51	0.35-14.90	100.0
Copper	32	9.10	3.30-25.80	100.0
Zinc	32	104.85	62.30-162.50	100.0
New York State area				
Arsenic	45	0.23	0.17-0.49	11.1
Cadmium	45	0.18	0.02-0.80	97.8
Mercury	45	0.28	0.02-0.53	80.0
Lead	45	0.84	0.02-2.40	77.8
Copper	45	6.05	1.80-56.80	100.0

[a]From Ref. 13.

THE IMPORTANCE OF THE REGULATORY CONTROL OF TRACE ELEMENTS

Mercury

Mercury has been recognized as an environmental problem since the early 1940s [17] with poisoning episodes occurring in Japan, Sweden, Pakistan, Iraq, Guatemala, and the United States [14]. High levels of mercury can be caused by the use of treated seed as animal feed, by environmental exposure, from manufacturing plants using mercury, through wood preserving, from chlorine and caustic soda manufacturing, through electrical uses, and from drugs [18]. It has been speculated that Napoleon, Ivan the Terrible, and Charles II of England died of mercurial poisoning [17].

The most noticeable effects of poisoning episodes are an increased public and regulatory concern over mercury in the environment. This has resulted in an awareness of industry to the problem, the banning of the use

of mercury in some agricultural and industrial uses, and the recycling of
wastes that were earlier disposed of through the air, water, and in waste
disposal areas.

These efforts have decreased the possibility of exposure of food-producing animals to mercury. The greatest regulatory concern is that so little
knowledge exists regarding the chemical forms or combinations of mercury
found in nature, body tissues, and food [15]. Therefore, any increase in
background levels in edible tissues of animals is given careful consideration by the USDA. The greatest single regulatory problem is the feeding of
mercury-containing food substances, especially seed grains treated with
mercurial compounds, to food-producing animals.

The influence of mercury on the absorption and transport of other trace
elements, such as copper, zinc, and cadmium [15], is also of concern to
regulatory agencies.

Lead

For years lead has been recognized as a health hazard to man and animals. Lead occurs naturally and is distributed widely at varying levels in
soils, plants, and animal tissues [19,20,22,26,27]. It is also found in
insecticides, paints, food containers, water pipes, auto exhausts, used
motor oil, and in plants and soils along highways [3]. Mine tailings in
some states contain large amounts of lead and therefore create regulatory
problems when animals are grazed on downwind pastures (dust contamination)
or drink water from streams and wells (leaching of lead). Smelters and
lead recycling plants are also a constant source of environmental lead.

Monitoring for excessive levels of lead in edible animal tissue remains
essential since low levels in the diet of children and animals are thought
to produce neurological changes [20]. It is interesting to note that lead
is found in all tissues of cattle at ranges from 0.01 to 2.96 ppm in the
muscle, 0.01 to 3.74 ppm in the liver, and 0.01 to 4.90 ppm in the kidney
(Table 1).

Cadmium

Although cadmium has been recognized as a toxic element for many years
[24], it was not until recently that concern was expressed over the possible
effects on human health from long periods of exposure at low concentrations.
Data on cadmium in soils near the sources of emission, such as smelters and
metallurgical plants, indicate high concentrations of cadmium fallout.

Sewage sludge and phosphate fertilizers also contain notable amounts of cadmium [21].

Cadmium background levels in edible animal tissues reflect wide ranges in different tissues. In cattle cadmium ranges in kidney from 0.01 to 7.8 ppm, in liver from 0.01 to 3.1 ppm, and in muscle from 0.01 to 0.08 ppm. The sporadic high levels in kidney and liver are of regulatory concern since the average for the two tissues is 0.55 and 0.21, respectively. Highest levels are found mostly in the central and southern parts of the United States (Kansas, Mississippi, and Louisiana) [1].

Cadmium in the environment is continuing to be studied by the Environmental Protection Agency [23,26,27].

Arsenic

Inorganic arsenical compounds are used widely as rat poisons and in insecticides, paints, and dyes [15,20]. Organic arsenical compounds are used in poultry and swine feeds as growth promotants and are also employed therapeutically in swine [20].

Poisonings from various arsenical compounds are frequent and, when detected, cause considerable regulatory difficulty. However, excessive use of organic arsenicals in animal feeds and improper observation of the approved withdrawal period consistently create great regulatory problems in poultry and swine [2].

The approved regulatory method of analysis for both the organic and inorganic forms is the dry ash atomic absorption method, which detects the elemental arsenic. A tolerance has been established by both the FDA and the EPA for poultry and swine [11,12]. The tolerance for arsenic in chickens and turkeys is 0.5 ppm in uncooked muscle and 2.0 ppm in uncooked edible by-products. The tolerance for edible tissue in swine is 2.0 ppm in liver and kidney and 0.5 ppm in uncooked muscle tissue and by-products other than liver and kidney.

Copper

The trace element copper is unique from both the regulatory and toxicology standpoints. From the regulatory standpoint, copper is a normal component of all tissues and fluids in all animal species. However, the levels vary greatly from tissue to tissue and species to species. From a toxicity standpoint, there is also great species variation. Sheep become toxic when levels reach approximately 200 ppm in the liver, producing a fatal intravascular hemolysis [20]. Swine receiving 200 ppm over several months in the feed for growth promotion show no ill effects. Cattle may carry up to 123 ppm in the liver (i.e., the high normal background level) with no apparent ill effects.

Under grazing conditions toxicosis may occur due to naturally high levels in soils and from smelters and mine tailings. In addition, medications and forage sprays which have copper as the main ingredient have resulted in excessively high levels in edible animal tissues.

Zinc

Elemental zinc is relatively nontoxic to birds and mammals, with a wide margin between normal background levels and those that will produce toxicosis. Zinc is found in all body tissues and fluids; however, the prostate appears to be the accumulator in man and rats.

From a regulatory standpoint, zinc poses little difficulty except when animals are grazed near smelters or metal refineries or are exposed to drinking water containing zinc, zinc-coated watering troughs, or zinc phosphide [28]. Lambs and feeder cattle are somewhat less tolerant to high zinc intakes than pigs and poultry [3]. The half-life of the element is 322 days in the human [3]. Liver is the organ of choice for analyses in food-producing animals [28].

Selenium

Selenium has been considered a controversial tissue element from a regulatory standpoint. While selenium has been shown to be toxic to all food-producing animals, it is also an essential trace element in most species of animals [3,28]. It has been suspected of being a carcinogen in laboratory animals.

Selenium has been approved for use as a feed additive by the FDA for the prevention of selenium deficiency in poultry and swine [12]. The geological distribution of selenium in soils and the toxicosis and deficiency syndromes are well reviewed in the literature and elsewhere in this volume.

CONCLUSION

The amount of trace elements in edible animal tissue is determined by the amount of environmental contamination plus the background level [16]. The purpose of laws passed by Congress is to assure that edible animal products consumed by man are free from contamination.

The greatest sources of this contamination are generally manmade. These include industry, agriculture, waste disposals (dumps or incinerators),

accidental use, and deliberate misuse of trace elements. By various mechanisms, trace elements accumulate in edible animal tissues. These include
direct contamination of the diet, biological magnification, translocation
of trace elements in the ecosystem, and environmental effects.

Regulations implemented to enforce the current laws are explicit enough
to reasonably assure that edible animal products will be free from trace
element contamination from any source.

REFERENCES

1. U.S. Department of Agriculture, Trace Element Survey (1969-1974),
    unpublished data.

2. U.S. Department of Agriculture, Regulatory Actions for Trace Elements
    (1965-1974), unpublished data.

3. E. J. Underwood, Trace Elements in Human and Animal Nutrition, 3rd Ed.,
    Academic, New York, 1971, pp. 1-12.

4. W. H. Allaway, Agronomic Controls over the Environmental Cycling of
    Trace Elements, Adv. Agron., 20, 235-274 (1968).

5. Federal Food, Drug, and Cosmetic Act, as Amended, U.S. Department of
    Health, Education, and Welfare, Washington, D. C., 1972.

6. Federal Meat Inspection Act, as Amended, Public Law 90-201, 90th Con-
    gress, H. R. 12144, December 15, 1967.

7. Poultry Products Inspection Act, as Amended, Public Law 90-492, 90th
    Congress, H. R. 16363, August 18, 1968.

8. Louis Rothschild, Jr. (ed.), Poisonous or Deleterious Tolerance Rules
    Proposed by FDA, Food Chemical News, 16 (38), 21-27 (1974).

9. Federal Insecticide, Fungicide, and Rodenticide Act, as Amended, Public
    Law 92-516, 92nd Congress, H. R. 10729, October 21, 1972.

10. Poisonous or Deleterious Substances in Food, Federal Register, 39,
    42743-42748 (1974).

11. Code of Federal Regulations, Title 40, Section 180. Revised as of
    April 1, 1974, Office of the Federal Register, National Archives and
    Records Service, G. S. A., Washington, D. C.

12. Code of Federal Regulations, Title 21, Section 135. Revised as of
    April 1, 1974, Office of the Federal Register, National Archives and
    Records Service, G. S. A., Washington, D. C.

13. U.S. Department of Agriculture, Trace Element Survey in Cattle (1971),
    unpublished data.

14. E. G. Hunt, Biological Magnification of Pesticides, in Scientific
    Aspects of Pest Control, Publication 1402, NAS-NRC, Washington, D. C.,
    1966, pp. 251-262.

15. C. P. Stewart and A. Stolman, Toxicology, Mechanisms and Analytical
    Methods, Vol. 1, Academic Press, New York, 1960, pp. 202-222.

16. C. R. Donn and P. E. Phillips, Translocation of Heavy Metals in Human
    Food Chains, Proc. 77th Annual Meeting, U.S. Animal Health Association,
    1973, pp. 267-281.

17. A. Ahlmark, Poisoning by Methyl Mercury Compounds, Brit. J. Ind. Med.,
     5, 117-119 (1948).

18. P. Montague and K. Montague, Mercury, How Much Are We Eating?, Saturday
     Review, February 1971, pp. 50-55.

19. U.S. Department of Agriculture, The Nature and Fate of Chemicals Applied
     to Soils, Plants, and Animals, ARS 20-9, September 1960, pp. 48-115.

20. W. B. Buck, G. D. Osweiler, and G. A. Van Gelder, Veterinary Toxicology
     Notes, Iowa State University, Ames, 1971, pp. 83-90.

21. M. Fleischer, A. F. Sarofim, D. W. Fassett, P. Hammond, H. T. Shack-
     lette, Ian C. T. Nisbet, and S. Epstein, Environmental Impact of Cad-
     mium: A Review by the Panel on Hazardous Trace Substances, Environ-
     mental Health Perspectives, Experimental Issue, 7, 253-323 (May 1974).

22. J. McCaull, Building a Shorter Life, Environment, 13 (7), 3-41 (1971).

23. L. Friberg, M. Piscator, G. Nordberg, and T. K. Jellstrom, Cadmium in
     the Environment, II, Office of Research and Monitoring, U.S. Environ-
     mental Protection Agency, Washington, D. C., EPA-R2-73-190, February
     1973, pp. 29-59.

24. H. A. Schroder and J. J. Balassa, Abnormal Trace Metals in Man: Cad-
     mium, J. Chron. Dis., 14 (2), 236-258 (1961).

25. G. Young and J. P. Blair, Threat to Man's Only Home, National Geo-
     graphic, 138 (6), 739-780 (1970).

26. Phase I, Administrative and Scientific Report: Toxic Substances Data
     Collection and Analysis for Pennsylvania and Colorado, M 74-110, Vols.
     1 and 2, Office of Toxic Substances, Environmental Protection Agency,
     Washington, D. C., December 1974, pp. 21-99.

27. Technical Summary Report, Second Quarter, Toxic Substances Data Col-
     lection and Analysis in Massachusetts, New Jersey, New York, and
     Missouri, M 75-3, Office of Toxic Substances, Environmental Protection
     Agency, Washington, D. C., January 1975, pp. 47-92.

28. R. J. Garner, Veterinary Toxicology, 2nd Ed., The Williams and Wilkins
     Company, Baltimore, 1961.

BENEFICIAL EFFECTS OF TRACE ELEMENTS

Raymond J. Shamberger
The Cleveland Clinic Foundation
Cleveland, Ohio

CHROMIUM

Chemistry of Chromium

Although chromium is widely dispersed in natural deposits, it is never found in the uncombined state. Chromite ($FeO \cdot Cr_2O_3$) is the only important ore of chromium. Approximately 0.03% of the igneous rock in the earth's crust is chromium.

Chromium is one of the transition elements appearing in the sixth group of the periodic table. Its atomic number is 24 and it has an atomic weight of 51.996. Natural isotopes include ^{50}Cr, ^{52}Cr, ^{53}Cr, and ^{54}Cr. The most prevalent valence states are 2, 3, and 6.

Aqueous HF, HCl, HBr, and HI slowly dissolve chromium. Dilute sulfuric acid slowly dissolves chromium with the evolution of hydrogen while the metal liberates SO_2 in boiling concentrated acid. At room temperature, fuming nitric acid and aqua regia have no effect on chromium. Chromium is only slightly attacked by acetic acid and not at all by formic, citric, or tartaric acids. Chromium reacts with the anhydrous halogens, hydrogen chloride and hydrogen fluoride, at temperatures of $600°$ C or higher.

Chromium is used mainly as an additive to iron, nickel, and other metals to increase their strength and corrosion and oxidation resistance. Chromium is also added to other metals to form a refractory. Chrome chemicals are used in pigments, as mordants in the textile industry, in chrome tanning, for hardening photographic films, in photoengraving, in plating metal surfaces, and in corrosion control.

Essentiality

Schwartz and Mertz [1] first observed impaired glucose tolerance in
rats fed various diets. The impaired glucose tolerance was unrelated to
the selenium-responsive necrotic liver degeneration that occurred on these
diets. A new dietary agent was postulated and designated GTF (glucose tolerance factor). The active component was subsequently shown to be trivalent
chromium [2]. Several trivalent chromium compounds administered at dose
levels of 20 to 50 µg Cr/100 g body weight completely restored tolerance to
injected glucose, whereas hexavalent chromium and some forms of trivalent
chromium were either inactive or less active. Chromium deficiency is characterized by impaired growth and longevity and by disturbances in glucose,
lipid, and protein metabolism. Rats fed diets low in chromium (less than
0.1 ppm Cr) and protein also develop a corneal lesion in one or both eyes.
The cornea also becomes opaque and the iridal vessels become congested [3].

Chromium stimulation of growth and biotin synthesis in Aerobacter
aerogenes has also been observed [4].

Rats require a diet containing a minimum of 100 ppb chromium to avert
features of deficiency [5]. The corresponding figure for man has not been
established. Reports of average chromium intake for adults in this country
range from 52 [6] to 78 [7] µg daily, but it is not certain if this is adequate to maintain optimal chromium nutrition. In comparison with intakes
reported from other countries including Italy, Japan, Egypt, India, and
South Africa, the average intake in the United States is low [5]. In the
United States there is a wide individual variation in intake ranging from
5 to 115 µg/day in diets which are otherwise well balanced. The variation
is dependent largely on the source of protein; for example, fish is a poor
source of chromium, whereas beef and liver have a relatively high chromium
content.

In two studies with diabetics and old people [8,9], some responses to
chromium supplementation were obtained when the daily intake was estimated
to be as low as 50 µg Cr/day. These intakes are very much lower than those
reported for two adults by Tipton et al. [10], namely 330 and 400 µg Cr/day,
in a comprehensive spectrographic study of trace elements in diets and excreta.

Drinking water can be a significant source of chromium in some areas.
The municipal water supplies of 24 United States cities were found to contain from 0.001 to 0.010 ppm Cr [11]. A chromium level of 0.001 ppm has

been reported in Egyptian tap water and 0.0005 to 0.0016 ppm in different
areas of Jordan [13]. Marked differences in chromium content of potable
water from different parts of the United States have been reported by
Schroeder [7].

Prevention of chromium deficiency cannot be achieved by supplementing
food staples with inorganic chromium, which is not an acceptable substitute
for the biologically active chromium glucose tolerance factor occurring
naturally in some but not all food materials. In addition to its greater
biological activity, chromium in GTF is much better absorbed than inorganic
chromium; at least 10% of chromium GTF is absorbed, compared with 1% or less
of ingested inorganic chromium [14]. Therefore, diets cannot be evaluated
adequately by measurement of total chromium content. Knowledge of the "biologically meaningful" chromium in foods is needed [15]. Toepfer et al. [15]
have found no correlation between total chromium concentration of a variety
of different foods and the relative GTF biological activity of these foods,
determined by CO_2 production from oxidation of glucose 1-14 C by epididymal
fat tissue in the presence of 100 μU insulin/flask. If the food nutrients
were extracted with 50% ethanol, which extracts GTF but only part of the
total chromium, a highly significant relationship was observed between
chromium concentration of the extracts and biological activity.

Foods containing chromium but virtually no biological activity were
primarily fruits and vegetables, but they also included egg yolk which contains large amounts of chromium. For the remaining foods, the percentage
of extractable chromium ranged from 14% for flour to 100% for beer and
black pepper. The greatest amounts of ethanol-extractable chromium were
found in brewer's yeast, black pepper, liver, beef, bread, mushrooms, and
beer. The lowest concentration was found in skimmed milk, haddock, flour,
and chicken breast.

Metabolism

The absorption, distribution, and excretion of chromium by animals and
man at levels well beyond normal ingestion have been well investigated [16].
At these levels, orally administered trivalent chromium is absorbed to the
extent of only about 1% or less, regardless of dose or of dietary chromium
status [17-19]. Soluble chromates are poorly absorbed and appear mainly
in the feces in soluble complex form [20]. Chromic oxide is so insoluble
that it is used as a "marker" for determining the digestibility of dietary
components and of feed intakes by grazing stock [21-22]. Chromium has also
been used as a marker in human metabolic balances [23-24].

Hexavalent chromium is better adsorbed than trivalent chromium [17,25]. There is a greater blood radioactivity following intestinal administration of hexavalent ^{51}Cr than after trivalent ^{51}Cr. Patients with pernicious anemia and achlorhydria absorbed significantly more hexavalent chromium than did the controls. Acid gastric juice may reduce the hexavalent chromium to the poorly absorbable Cr^{3+} ions.

Hexavalent chromium readily passes through the membrane of red blood cells and becomes bound to the globin fraction of hemoglobin. Trivalent chromium is unable to pass the membrane and combines with the β-globulin fraction of the plasma. It is transported to the tissues bound to siderophilin [26-27]. This property of trivalent chromium led to the development of effective labeling for erythrocytes, platelets, and plasma proteins to determine their life span or survival time [27-33].

Although the main part of absorbed or injected chromium is excreted mainly in the urine [34-35], tissue uptake is quite rapid. The plasma is cleared of a dose of ^{51}Cr within a few days [19,34]. The bones, spleen, testis, and epididymis retained more ^{51}Cr after 4 days than the heart, lung, pancreas, or brain. Because various tissues retain chromium longer than the plasma suggests that there is no equilibrium between tissue stores and circulating chromium. Tissue chromium uptake is dependent on age [36]. Older mice had about half the injected ^{51}Cr in liver, stomach, epididymal fat pad, thymus, kidney, and especially the testes than younger animals. Mertz has suggested [5] that these observations might offer an explanation for the declining tissue chromium levels with age, detected in a survey of the United States population [7].

The chromium entering the tissues is distributed in an unusual way among the subcellular fractions. Edwards and co-workers [37] found that 49% was concentrated in the nuclear fraction, 23% occurred in the supernatant, and the remainder was divided equally between the mitochondria and the microsomes. The concentration of chromium in the nucleus may indicate that chromium may be important for nucleic acid metabolism or structure or both [5,38,39]. In rat liver in vitro dietary chromium stimulated the conversion of L-gulonolactone to L-ascorbic acid [40]. Increases of ascorbic acid in rat spleen and adrenal glands were also observed.

Glucose administration mobilizes chromium from body stores. Plasma chromium levels of five healthy subjects were sharply elevated in parallel to glucose levels and fell as the glucose levels declined [41]. Injections of insulin raises circulating chromium in rats [18]. The elevation of chromium is not observed when the subject is in the fasting state [41], indicating that body reserves may be low or depleted.

Rat studies have failed to detect any [19,42,43] significant transfer of ^{51}Cr from the mother into the fetus [29,30] despite measurable amounts of stable chromium in the newborn [7,42], in human embryos [44,45], and newborn infants [7]. However, trivalent ^{51}Cr extracted from brewer's yeast readily crossed the placenta indicating that chromium might be in the form of a natural complex.

Votava et al. [46] have partially characterized the ^{51}Cr complex from brewer's yeast. The complex is a peptide that contains at least six amino acids. Gel-filtration chromatography showed a single radioactive peak which was eluted at a volume suggesting a molecular weight of approximately 400-600 daltons.

Health Effects

Glucose Metabolism. The earliest detectable and most prominent feature of chromium deficiency in rats [47] and other animals [48] is an impairment of glucose tolerance. After a few weeks on a torula yeast diet, glucose removal rates declined almost 50%. The defect can be reversed rapidly by one oral dose of 20 µg or an intravenous dose of 0.25 µg/100 g body weight of trivalent chromium [18,49].

A more severe degree of chromium deficiency leads to a syndrome indistinguishable from mild diabetes mellitus, including glycosuria and fasting hyperglycemia [50].

Since 1966, evidence for a human nutritional requirement for chromium has been looked at in patients with an impairment of glucose tolerance including "maturity onset" diabetes, middle-aged and elderly subjects with chemical evidence of impaired glucose tolerance, and infants with protein-calorie malnutrition. The first therapeutic trial [8] included six maturity-onset diabetics. Administration of 180 to 1000 µg of chromium as $CrCl_3 \cdot 6H_2O$ for periods of 7 to 13 weeks significantly improved four patients. Shorter periods of chromium supplementation did not improve glucose utilization. Sherman et al. [51] treated 10 adult diabetics with 150 µg daily for 16 weeks and observed no improvement of glucose tolerance. In another study, 4 of 12 diabetics treated with 1 mg chromium daily for 6 months had improved glucose tolerance, but 16 treated for a shorter period of time with 150 µg chromium daily did not improve [52]. In 10 elderly patients over 70 [6] treated with 150 µg of chromium for periods up to 4 months, glucose tolerance was restored to normal in four. No improvement was observed in six. Fifty percent of a group of middle-aged subjects treated with 150 µg daily for 6 months had a marked improvement in glucose tolerance [53].

The "diabetogenic" effect of pregnancy is characterized by impairment of peripheral glucose metabolism, decreased glucose tolerance, and an exaggerated insulin excretion in response to glucose challenge. Davidson et al. [54] suggested that the diabetogenic effect is related to a significantly lower chromium plasma of pregnant women.

Recently, human polymorphonuclear leukocytes from patients with diabetes mellitus have been reported [55] to have a requirement for insulin during chemotaxis, which can be measured by an in vitro technique [56]. Because chromium has a physiological role in every insulin-dependent system that has been investigated [5], this suggests [57] that the effects of chromium deficiency on an insulin-dependent system in man could be studied with a peripheral venipuncture. Preincubation of the cell suspension with trivalent chromium results in a significant improvement in chemotaxis of leukocytes from children with insulin-dependent diabetes [58].

Morgan [59] has evaluated hepatic chromium content from postmortem examinations in elderly patients with diabetes, with ischemic heart disease, with hypertensive cardiovascular disease, and without disease. The control group had a hepatic chromium content of 12.7 µg/g. The arteriosclerotic group had 9.96 µg/g and the hypertensive group 10.2 µg/g. Diabetic subjects had 8.59 µg/g. The diabetic group was significantly decreased in regard to the control population (p = 0.05). This study suggests that further consideration of chromium deficiency as a cause of diabetes in elderly subjects might be worthwhile.

Lipid Metabolism. Chromium addition to a low-chromium diet suppressed cholesterol levels in rats and inhibited the tendency of these levels to increase with age. Male rats fed 1 µg Cr/ml and females fed 5 µg/ml in the drinking water had significantly depressed serum cholesterol [60-61]. Schroeder [62] later confirmed these experiments. Brown sugar which contains chromium also lowered serum cholesterol. Serum cholesterol levels were relatively elevated and increased with age in the rats receiving white sugar, which is low in chromium [62-63]. A significant decline of serum cholesterol was seen in institutionalized patients fed 2 mg Cr for 5 months. Other patients treated similarly showed no response [52].

A significantly lower (2%) incidence of spontaneous plaques [60] were observed in the chromium-fed animals than the chromium-deficient animals

(19%). Lowered amounts of stainable lipids and of fluorescent material in the aorta were observed [60]. A similar picture is observed in man in that diabetes is associated with an increased incidence of vascular lesions [64]. Mertz et al. [65] have observed that chromium plus insulin significantly increased glucose uptake and incorporation of glucose into epididymal fat in chromium-deficient rats. Curran [66] has observed that trivalent chromium enhances the incorporation of acetate into cholesterol and fatty acids.

Protein Synthesis. Rats fed diets deficient in chromium and protein have an impaired capacity to incorporate α-amino isobutyric acid, glycine, serine, and methionine into heart protein [3,67]. No such effect of chromium was observed with lysine, phenylalanine, and a mixture of 10 other amino acids. Insulin in vivo also enhanced the cell transport of an amino acid analog to a greater degree in rats fed a low-protein, chromium-supplemented diet than it did in Cr-deficient controls [68].

Several studies indicate that protein-calorie malnutrition may be complicated by chromium deficiency. Studies in Jordan [69], Nigeria [70], and Istanbul [71] indicated that chromium administration to infants increased the mean glucose removal rate by three- to fivefold. On the other hand, chromium did not enhance the mean glucose removal in Egyptian infants [72]. Regional differences could account for these effects. In the Nile valley of Egypt no evidence of chromium deficiency is seen, whereas chromium deficiencies have been observed in Nigerian food. A common food staple for Nigerian children is maize pap, which contains only about 10 ppb chromium.

Birth Effects, Growth, and Longevity. The mean hair chromium level of newborn infants was found to be significantly higher than that of older children [73]. This corresponds with the higher chromium levels in other newborn tissues [74]. The mean hair chromium concentration of premature newborn (30 to 36 weeks gestation) was significantly lower than that for term newborn; the mean for a small group of newborn with evidence of intrauterine growth retardation was also significantly lower [75]. Bone ash chromium concentration from the human fetus varied directly with gestational age [45]. Thus, the low-birth-weight infant may be at particular risk from a low-chromium state. Hair chromium levels of parous women [76] and of children with insulin-dependent diabetes [77] were significantly lower than those of nulliparous women and of normal children, respectively. Changes in hair chromium have been studied retrospectively by analyzing sections of hair shaft at increasing distances from the scalp. The mean hair chromium content was found to vary directly with the distance from the scalp, demonstrating that the proximal, more recently grown hair in later infancy had less chromium than the more distal hair shaft which had been formed in the hair follicle at a younger age [73].

Mertz and Roginski [78] have shown that raising rats in plastic cages on a low-protein, low-chromium diet results in a moderate depression of growth which can be alleviated by chromium supplementation. When the animals were subjected to controlled exercise or blood loss, the low-chromium state was aggravated. On a diet of rye, skim milk, and corn oil (containing 0.1 ppm Cr), with added vitamins and minerals, male mice and rats receiving 2 or 5 ppm Cr(III) in the drinking water grew significantly better than their controls [79-87]. This effect was associated with decreased mortality. Gurson and Saner [83] have provided evidence that chromium deficiency is a cause of impaired growth in addition to glucose intolerance in man.

Male rats given chromium in water from the time of weaning lived to greater ages than those not so fed [79-80]. The median age of male mice at death was 99 days longer when they were fed chromium than when they were not, and the mean age was 91 days longer [79-80]. No such differences in longevity due to chromium were observed in female mice or rats.

Diagnostic Uses of Chromium. Labeled trivalent chromium is used as an effective agent for determining the life span or survival time for erythrocytes, platelets, and plasma proteins [27-29,30-33]. Radiochromate has also been used to study the kinetics of blood lymphocytes in chronic lymphocytic leukemia [84]. Thyroglobulin antibodies can be determined by using chromic chloride as a coupling reagent for a passive hemagglutination reaction [85, 86]. Chromium chloride is not absorbed well and is used as a marker of digestibility of dietary components in studies of human metabolic balances [23,24]. In addition, [^{51}Cr]albumin is used as a gastric marker to determine gastric loss in patients with exudative gastropathy [87].

COBALT

Chemistry of Cobalt

Cobalt is classified in Group VIII of the periodic table between iron and nickel. Cobalt closely resembles these metals in both its pure and combined states. The atomic weight is 58.9332 and the atomic number is 27. Cobalt is widely diffused but makes up only 0.001% of the igneous rocks of the earth's crust. The important cobalt minerals are sulfides, arsenides, and oxidized compounds. The sulfide ores include carrollite, linnaeite, or siegenite. Cobalt arsenides include smaltite, safflorite, and skutterudite. Asbolite and heterogenite are two of the important oxide ores.

The main valence states of cobalt are 2+ and 3+. In coordination complexes, cobalt prefers the trivalent states, and numerous ammonium compounds with cobalt have been described. In general, cobalt is present in the 2+ state in most compounds. Cobalt is not attacked by air or water at ordinary temperatures. The metal is readily attacked by sulfuric, hydrochloric, and nitric acids, but slowly by hydrofluoric acid, ammonia, and sodium hydroxide.

Cobalt is used in magnetic alloys, hard-facing alloys, cutting and wear-resistant alloys, high-speed steels, glass-to-metal seals, dental and surgical alloys, spring alloys, maraging steels, and low-expansion and constant-modulus alloys. Cobalt is used in cemented carbides, electroplating, in glasses, as a stain in ceramics, and as a catalyst of economic importance.

Essentiality of Cobalt

Sheep and cattle grazing on certain types of pastures became weak, emaciated, and progressively anemic and usually died. Various local names were given to these maladies such as "pining," "vinquish," "salt-sick," "nakuruitis," "bush sickness," "wasting disease," and "coast disease." Aston [88-91] first postulated that bush sickness in cattle was due to an iron deficiency. Several investigators noted that it took large and variable amounts of iron to cure bush sickness. In one of the iron compounds tested, the potency was found to be due to the cobalt it contained [92]. Normal growth and health of sheep and cattle were obtained on the deficient pastures by the administration of small doses of a cobalt salt [93].

The discovery in 1948 [94,95] that the antipernicious anemia factor in liver contained 4% cobalt led to the discovery of vitamin B12. Within 3 years of its original discovery as a cobalt compound, Smith et al. [96] found that B12 injections completely alleviated cobalt deficiency in lambs.

Efforts to produce cobalt deficiency have failed per se in animals other than ruminants. Cobalt also plays an essential role in nitrogen fixation by the root nodules of legumes [97,98]. Significant growth responses to cobalt in pasture legumes have been demonstrated in certain areas [99,100].

Tipton et al. [101], estimating by emission spectroscopy, have obtained daily intakes of 160-170 μg Co for the diets of two individuals measured over 30-day periods. Schroeder et al. [102], using both atomic absorption

and emission spectroscopy, obtained a range of 140 to 580 µg Co/day with a
mean adult diet of 300 µg Co/day. Green leafy vegetables are the richest
and most variable sources of cobalt, and dairy products and cereals, especially refined cereals, are the poorest [103,104]. Except for milk and cereals
which were much higher, similar food levels were reported by Schroeder et al.
[102].

When the concentration of cobalt in the bacteria-free rumen fluid falls
below about 20 pg/ml [105], the rate of B12 synthesis is reduced below the
animal's needs. When the stores of vitamin B12 laid down by the liver fall
below 0.10 µg/g wet weight [106] and when plasma B12 falls below a critical
level of 0.2 ng/ml, characteristic signs of cobalt deficiency begin to appear in most lambs and calves.

Although the human cobalt requirement is not known, several estimates
have been made for sheep and cattle. Early evidence from Australia [107-
110] and New Zealand [111] indicated that 0.07 or 0.08 ppm Co in the dry
diet was adequate. Two other studies indicated that 0.11 ppm or more would
probably exclude the likelihood of cobalt deficiency [106,112]. Lee and
Marston [113] estimated 0.08 mg/day Co along with three cobalt supplements
weekly were the minimal requirements. Deficiency can be prevented in low-
cobalt areas by topdressing of the soil, direct administration of cobalt to
stall-fed animals, placing cobalt in salt licks, or dosing sheep with 2 or 7
mg of cobalt weekly [114].

Metabolism

Comar and co-workers [115,116] gave radioactive cobalt orally and by
injection to several species of animals. After oral administration to rats,
80% of the radioactivity was found in the feces, 10% in the urine, with
little in the tissues, except the liver. With cattle, 80% was also found
in the feces but only 0.5% in the urine, indicating a greater initial retention by the tissues. Injected cobalt is excreted principally in the
urine, with a small fraction present in the bile to become part of the fecal
cobalt. About 65% of the injected radiocobalt appeared rapidly in the urine,
and 7-30% in different experiments in the feces.

Tipton et al. [101], who found daily intakes of 160-170 µg Co, reported
mean daily urinary excretions of 140 and 190 µg Co and fecal losses of 40
and 60 µg. In another diet balance study with preadolescent girls, Engel
et al. [117] found 90% of the excreted cobalt in the feces and only 10% in
the urine.

Methylmalonyl-CoA isomerase was found to be a vitamin B12-requiring enzyme. The isomerase catalyzes the conversion of methylmalonyl-CoA succinyl-CoA [118,119], and the activity of this isomerase is severely depressed in the livers of vitamin B12-deficient rats [120,121]. Marston et al. [105] suggested that a breakdown in propionate utilization might be the primary defect in Co-vitamin B12 deficiency in ruminants, and that the depression of appetite might be due to an increased blood level of propionate. Examination of liver homogenates from sheep [105] revealed that in the B12-deficient animal (a) there is a failure to convert propionate efficiently to succinate, (b) there is an accumulation of the intermediate methylmalonyl-CoA, and (c) this accumulation can be prevented by the addition of methylmalonyl-CoA isomerase.

Increased concentrations of pantothenic acid or CoA occur in the livers of B12-deficient sheep [122,123]. The cause is unknown but is apparently not primarily due to accumulation of methylmalonyl-CoA.

Deficiencies of either B12 or folic acid can cause an increase in the excretion of formiminoglutamic acid (FIGLU) in humans [124,125], in rats [126,127], in chicks [128], and in sheep [129]. Vitamin B12 may participate in the methyltetrahydrofolate-homocysteine transmethylase reaction, thus regulating the availability of tetrahydrofolic acid, and thereby indirectly affects FIGLU catabolism [130,131].

Health Effects of Cobalt

B12 Absorption Diagnostic Tests. The physiological absorption of vitamin B12, i.e., the gastric intrinsic factor (GIF)-mediated vitamin B12 absorption, may be evaluated in man by orally administering 0.5 to 2.0 µg of labeled B12 and measuring the amount of radioactivity that appears in the urine, plasma, or stool, concentrated in the liver or retained by the whole body at an appropriate time interval after dosing [132]. Although all five methods provide adequate assessment of vitamin B12 absorption and in fact have been shown to correlate rather well [133], each method has its advantages or disadvantages. The selection of one particular method over another depends on the familiarity of the physician with a technique and the availability of appropriate counting apparatus.

The urinary excretion test originally described by Schilling [134] is the method most commonly employed. After labeled vitamin B12 is fed to the patient, an injection of unlabeled vitamin B12 is administered to block out all potential vitamin B12 binding tissue sites. This allows the labeled vitamin B12 to be flushed out in the urine. Katz et al. [135] suggested a modification of this technique whereby [^{57}Co]vitamin B12 and GIF-[^{60}Co]vitamin B12 complex are both administered simultaneously to the patient. This latter procedure shortens the time required to detect GIF deficiency. Studies depending on urinary excretion require accurate urine collections and are, of course, unreliable in patients with renal disease.

After the oral administration of labeled B12, one can also do a plasma absorption test by collecting a plasma sample 8 hr later [136]. A "flushing" dose is not necessary. Although some investigators have failed to find a good correlation between the urinary excretion and the plasma level of labeled vitamin B12 [137], others find the test useful.

In the fecal excretion test [138], stools are collected until less than 1% of the orally administered labeled vitamin B12 appears on 2 consecutive days of fecal collections. The method takes from 3 to 8 days. The main limitation of this method is the difficulty in obtaining complete stool collections.

The hepatic uptake test [139] requires external counting over the liver 5 to 7 days after the oral administration of labeled vitamin B12. Although this technique avoids the need for a urine or a fecal collection, the lag period of 1 week before obtaining the results is a major limitation. In addition, hepatic uptake may be impaired in patients with liver disease.

In the whole body counting method [140] the procedure is similar in principle to the hepatic uptake method and has the same disadvantages. In addition, whole body counters are not readily available in most hospital laboratories.

Determination of B12. Serum B12 was previously determined by a microbiological assay using Lactobacillus leichmanni or Euglena gracilis. Lau et al. [141] have described a relatively simple method of employing the principle of radioisotope dilution and the absorptive properties of coated charcoal. The free form but not the bound form of ^{57}B12 can be removed by coated charcoal. In another approach, sephadex is used to separate ^{57}B12 bound to intrinsic factor from unbound ^{57}B12 [142].

Levels of serum B12 from 0 to 150 pg/ml are considered low. The normal range is 150-900, and B12 levels over 900 pg/ml are considered to be elevated. Advantages of the radioimmunoassays over the bioassay are as follows: The radioimmunoassay is more rapid and has greater accuracy and precision; the radioactive assay is not inhibited by antibiotics which are sometimes present in the sera of hospital patients; the Euglena gracilis method is

linear only to 900 pg/ml, whereas the radioassay method is linear to 2000
pg/ml; and the radioassay seems to be diagnostically better.

Malabsorption Problems. Vitamin B12 deficiency secondary to inadequate
intake is rare in the western world except among Seventh Day Adventists,
food faddists [143-148], and infants breast-fed by mothers who are vegetar-
ians [149]. B12 deficiency occurs only after a prolonged period of inadequate intake since such subjects secrete adequate quantities of GIF and thus
continue to efficiently reabsorb B12 that is secreted into the small intestine via bile. Patients with pernicious anemia (PA) develop a deficiency
after a shorter depletion period and are also unable to reabsorb endogenous
vitamin B12 excreted into the bile because of the lack of GIF.

When normal gastric function exists, the release of vitamin B12 from
dietary protein does not restrict the rate of B12 absorption. However, when
acid-peptic digestion is depressed, such as may occur in gastric atrophy or
after subtotal gastrectomy, the release of free vitamin B12 from dietary
sources may be impaired.

Vitamin B12 may fail to attach to GIF. The most common cause is the
lack of GIF associated with Addisonian pernicious anemia. As part of the
generalized atrophy of the acid-pepsin portion of the stomach, GIF secretion is markedly depressed. Patients with idiopathic gastric atrophy or
after gastric surgery may have depressed secretion of GIF in the basal
state. GIF antibodies may also occur, but are rarely found in diseases
other than PA and are virtually diagnostic of this disease. A few patients
with diabetes mellitus [150], adrenal insufficiency [151], thyrotoxicosis
[152], and hypothyroidism [150,153,154] have serum GIF antibodies.

Another group of malabsorptive diseases are associated with the passage
of the GIF-vitamin B12 complex down the small intestine. The blind loop
syndrome has been noted in various diseases associated with bacterial over-
growth. The absorptive defect appears to result from the intraluminal competition of the bacteria with the host for the dietary B12. The mechanism
of B12 malabsorption after infestation with the fish tapeworm Diphylloboth-
rium latum has not been clarified. Unexplained malabsorption of B12 has
been observed in several patients with pancreatic exocrine insufficiency
[155,156]. A pH of greater than 5.6 was necessary for the optimal uptake
of GIF-vitamin B12 complex by the mucosa of the small bowel of rats [157].
Veeger et al. [158] have postulated that a damaged pancreas would not be
able to buffer the gastric acid output of the stomach and would impair B12

absorption. Both sodium bicarbonate and pancreatic extract correct the B12 malabsorption.

Certain B12 malabsorptive diseases are associated with the passage of B12 through the ileal epithelial cell. It has been suggested that children with familial selective vitamin B12 malabsorption (Imerslund or Grasbeck syndrome) [166,167] lacked the specific ileal receptors for the GIF-vitamin B12 complex. However, MacKenzie et al. [168] have suggested that the abnormality occurred after the GIF-vitamin B12 complex attached to the ileal mucosa and before B12 was bound to transcobalamin II.

Malabsorptive disease may be associated with the exit of B12 from the epithelial cell. Transcobalamin II deficiency has been described by Hakami et al. [169]. A number of therapeutic agents have been shown to interfere with the absorption of B12 including p-aminosalicylic acid [170-173], colchicine [174], alcohol [175], metformin [176], and neomycin [177].

Elevated B12 Conditions. Serum B12 levels well over 1000 pg/ml of serum are suggestive of either liver disease or a myeloproliferative disorder (such as polycythemia vera, myeloid metaplasia, or granulocytic leukemia); levels above 4000 pg/ml are unusual in liver disease but common in myeloproliferative disorders [178-180].

Hyperglycemia and Erythropoietic Factor. Injection of cobaltous chloride causes a hyperglycemia in fowl [181] and rabbits [182]. Triglyceride levels were increased in the experiments with rabbits [182]. Cobalt also increases erythropoietic factor and the kidney hydroxylases cathepsins A and B [183].

COPPER

Chemistry of Copper

Copper lies between nickel and zinc and is in subgroup IB of the periodic table. It has an atomic number of 29 and a molecular weight of 63.54. Copper occurs in rock and soils as well as in oceanic clays and in river silts. Copper comprises about 0.007% of the earth's crust. Some copper occurs as native copper. Some occurs as the sulfide ores chalcocite (Cu_2S), covellite (CuS), chalcopyrite ($CuFeS_2$), bornite ($CuFeS_4$), enargite (Cu_3AsS_4), and tetrahedrite (Cu_3SbS_3). Oxide ores include cuprite (Cu_2O), tenorite (CuO), malachite [$CuCO_3 \cdot Cu(OH)_2$], azurite [$2CuCO_3 \cdot Cu(OH)_2$], chalcanthite ($CuSO_4 \cdot 5H_2O$), and brochantite [$CuSO_4 \cdot 3Cu(OH)_2$].

The most common valence number of copper is 1+ or 2+. Copper lies
below hydrogen in the electromotive series of the elements and consequently
does not replace hydrogen from solutions. Although copper is not soluble
in acids with the evolution of hydrogen, it is readily soluble in oxidizing
acids such as nitric acid, hot sulfuric acid, or sulfuric acid and ferric
sulfate. Copper is also soluble in ammonia and ammonium salts in the presence of air and in sodium and potassium cyanide. Cuprous ion is unstable
in aqueous solution; its salts readily decompose to form the metal and
cupric salts:

$$2Cu^+ \rightarrow Cu + Cu^{2+}$$

Copper is widely used in alloys such as cupronickels, aluminum bronze,
silicon bronze, beryllium copper, and manganese bronze. Copper is also
widely used in copper wire, sheet, and strip and in standard electrolytic
copper. The major portion of the world's production of copper is utilized
by the electrical industries in generators, light bulbs, telephones and
telegraphs, light and power lines, and other rods and wires.

Essentiality of Copper

Copper supplements as low as 0.005 mg Cu/day give a growth and hemoglobin response in young rats fed a milk diet [184]. Supplements of 0.01
to 0.05 mg Cu/day were optimum. Solid diets containing 1 ppm or less brings
a rapid copper deficiency in young rats. A diet containing only 0.3-0.4 ppm
Cu established the following tentative minimum requirements for 70-g rats
fed a 10-g diet daily: for hemoglobin production, 1 ppm; for growth, 3 ppm;
for melanin production in hair, 10 ppm [185].

As long ago as 1928, Evvard et al. [186] associated an improvement in
the growth of pigs when their normal ration was supplemented with copper
sulfate. Ullrey and co-workers observed no significant differences in
growth rate, food use efficiency, or of blood copper levels when baby pigs
were fed copper levels of 6, 16, and 106 ppm. The Agricultural Research
Council of Great Britain [187] came to the conclusion that 4 ppm Cu was
probably adequate for growing pigs up to 90 kg live weight.

There are no definitive data on the minimum copper requirements of
chicks for growth or hens for egg production [188]. Nor is there any evidence that poultry have high copper requirements relative to mammals, as
as they have for manganese. Diets containing 4-5 ppm are probably adequate.

All rations composed of normal feeds are likely to contain more than 5 ppm of this element.

The minimum copper requirement of cross-bred sheep can be maintained at intakes of 1 mg Cu/day or less [189]. Merino sheep [190-192] grazing on the calcareous soils of South Australia require close to 10 mg/day or about 10 ppm of the diet. Molybdenum intakes as low as 0.5 mg/day [189] can adversely affect copper retention in sheep, provided the sulfate intake is high. Excess sulfate in the herbage in certain parts of Greece in the presence of normal levels of copper and molybdenum has been associated [193, 194] with copper deficiency and ataxia in lambs. Certain English pastures having 7-14 ppm Cu or more and normal levels of molybdenum and sulfate may result in subnormal copper status in cattle [195,196] and in sheep, along with ataxia in lambs [196-202]. Three methods of preventing copper deficiency in grazing sheep and cattle are employed [188]. Addition of 5-7 lb/acre of copper-containing fertilizers has proved effective in Australia. Salt licks containing 0.5-1.0% copper sulfate have been employed. Dosing and drenching of animals or subcutaneous or intramuscular injections of some safe and slowly absorbed organic copper complex have been employed [203-207].

Estimates of the human requirements at different ages have been made from balance studies. Scoular [208] reported that the average 3- to 6-year-old child weighing up to 20 kg requires 1.0-1.6 mg Cu daily. Engel et al. [209] estimated in a study on 36 preadolescent girls, aged 6-10 years, that 1.3 mg Cu/day was necessary for balance. They suggested a daily allowance of 2.5 mg. Copper balance is maintained in adults on an intake of about 2 mg/day [210,211] or less [212].

The actual human daily copper intake lies between 2 and 4 mg [211,213, 214], with lower estimates for certain Dutch [215] and poor English and Scottish diets [216]. Indian adults consuming rice and wheat diets ingest 4.5-5.8 mg Cu/day [217]. In 4200-cal/day diets fed to 16- and 19-year-old North American boys, the overall average copper intake was found to be 3.8 mg [218]. The recommended daily intake for adults is 2 to 5 mg/day. The recommended intake for infants and children is 80 mcg/kg/day [219].

The amount of copper ingested daily is determined mainly by the selection of foods making up the diet and the water source. Schroeder et al. [213] have observed a progressive increase in the copper in water from brook to reservoir to hospital tap or private homes. Soft waters with their capacity to corrode metallic copper could raise intakes by as much as 1.4 mg per day, whereas hard waters would reduce this copper source to 0.05 mg or

less. The richest sources of copper are crustaceans and shellfish, especially oysters, and the organ meats (liver, kidney, and brain), followed by
nuts, dried legumes, dried vine and stone fruits, and cocoa [213,220,221].
These foods contain from 20 to 400 ppm. The poorest sources of copper are
dairy products (milk, butter, and cheese) and white sugar and honey, which
rarely contain more than 0.5 ppm Cu. Nonleafy vegetables, most fresh fruits,
and refined cereals have a content of less than 0.5 ppm Cu. The copper content of leafy vegetables frequently reflects the copper status of the soil
upon which they have grown. However, malnutrition attributable to a lack
of dietary copper has not been observed in areas with copper-poor soils.
The refining of cereals for human consumption results in a significant loss
of minerals, including copper. North American hard wheat may contain as
much as 5.3 ppm, but after refining the white flour made from these wheats
averaged only 1.7 ppm [222].

Metabolism of Copper

Copper is absorbed from different parts of the intestine or stomach,
depending on the species. In dogs [223], copper is absorbed from the upper
jejunum, but in pigs [224], it is absorbed from the small intestine and the
colon. In man [214] and chicks [225], it is mainly absorbed from the duodenum. In the rat, copper is absorbed to about the same extent from the
stomach as from the small intestine [226].

In most species [224,227], copper is not well absorbed, but in man up
to 32% of the copper is absorbed [228,229]. A copper-binding protein has
been demonstrated by Starcher [225] in the mucosal cells of the chick duodenum. Marked depression in copper absorption can be brought about by high
dietary intakes of calcium carbonate and of ferrous sulfide [189]. Different compounds of copper may be absorbed well, partially absorbed, or unabsorbed by anemic rats [230-232], pigs [224], or sheep [233]. Zinc [234-237]
and molybdenum [238,239] and high levels of cadmium [237,240] also depress
copper absorption. Zinc and cadmium may be displacing copper from a duodenal
mucosal protein with a molecular weight of about 10,000 [225]. Molybdenum
may interfere with copper absorption by complexing with copper to form a
complex, probably $CuMoO_4$, of low absorptivity [241].

Organic complexes are also important to copper absorption. Phytate
can reduce the assimilation of copper [242]. High dietary ascorbic acid
increased the severity of copper deficiency in chicks [243] and in rabbits
[244]. Copper entering the blood plasma from the intestine becomes loosely

bound to serum albumin to form the small, direct-reacting pool of plasma copper, in which form it is distributed widely to the tissues and can pass readily into the erythrocytes [245]. The Cu-albumin serum also receives copper from the tissues. The copper in ceruloplasmin appears to be tightly bound and not so available for exchange or for transfer.

The copper reaching the liver is incorporated into the mitochondria, microsomes, nuclei, and soluble fraction of the parenchymal cells in proportions which vary with the age [246-248], the strain [249,250], and the copper status [246,251] of the animal. The copper is stored in the liver particulates or released for incorporation into erythrocuprein and ceruloplasmin and the various copper-containing enzymes of these cells. Ceruloplasmin is synthesized in the liver [252-253] and is secreted into the serum. Erythrocuprein is probably synthesized in normoblasts from the bone marrow [245]. Hepatic copper is also secreted into the bile and excreted via the route back to the intestinal contents. Some copper passes directly from the plasma into the urine or through the intestinal wall.

Most of the ingested copper consists of unabsorbed copper, but active excretion via the bile occurs in all species. The biliary system is the major pathway of excretion in humans [254], pigs and dogs [223,255], mice [256,257], and ducks and fowl [258]. Changing the body temperature of rats $40°$ to $30°$ decreases the biliary excretion of copper 14-fold, indicating that bile excretion of copper is temperature dependent in the rat [258]. Of the 2-5 mg Cu ingested daily by adult man, 0.6-1.6 mg (32%) is absorbed, 0.5-1.3 mg is excreted in the bile, 0.1-0.3 mg passes directly into the bowel, and 0.1-0.6 mg appears in the urine [228,229]. Small amounts of copper are excreted daily in the urine. Giorgio et al. [260] has estimated the mean 24-hr excretion of copper in the urine of 20 normal adult persons to be 21 ± 5.2 μg. Others have reported variable amounts ranging from 9 μg/24 hr for 10 Utah subjects [261] to 18 [262], 30 [254], and 60 μg/24 hr [213]. Negligible amounts of copper are lost in the sweat [263] and comparatively small amounts are lost in the normal menstrual flow [211]. The loss of copper in the milk at the height of human lactation is somewhat greater (0.4 mg/day). There is no evidence that this loss imposes any nutritional hazard.

Copper deficiency does prevent the induction of liver microsomal enzyme activity by phenobarbital [264]. Phenobarbital administration significantly increased microsomal copper in rats receiving a normal copper intake and increased both whole liver and microsomal copper concentration in copper-deficient rats. The normal developmental increase in liver aniline hydroxylase and hexobarbital oxidase activities with age was delayed in the offspring of female rats maintained on a copper-deficient diet.

There are numerous copper-activated enzymes and cuproproteins in plants and animals. The list is summarized in Table 1.

TABLE 1. Cuproenzymes and Cuproproteins

Enzyme or Protein	Source
Hemocyanin	Molluscs, arthropods
Mitochondrocuprein	Neonatal bovine and human liver
Pink copper protein	Human erythrocytes
Ceruloplasmin	Human plasma
Uricase	Porcine liver
Cytochrome c oxidase	Bovine heart
Monoamine and diamine oxidase	Bovine plasma and liver, porcine kidney, pea seedlings
Lysine oxidase	Mammalian connective tissue
Dopamine β-hydroxylase	Adrenal glands
Ascorbic acid oxidase	Squash, cucumber
Laccase	Latex of lacquer tree
D-galactose oxidase	Dactylium dendroides
Phenolase (tyrosinase)	Neurospora crassa, mushrooms, mammalian tissues, melanomas
Ribulose diphosphate carboxylase	Spinach
Quercetinase (dioxygenase)	Aspergillus flavus
Azurin	Pseudomonas aeruginosa and Bordetella pertussis
Stellacyanin	Spinach, Phaseolus vulgaris, Chemopodium album
Mung bean pigment	Mung bean seedlings
Umecyanin	Horseradish root
Proteins containing both copper and zinc	
Superoxide dismutase (cytocuprein, cerulocuprein, erythrocuprein, hepatocuprein)	Brain, erythrocyte, and human, equine, and bovine liver

Health Effects of Copper

Copper and Anemia. A blood copper level of 0.10 to 0.12 µg/ml has
been found to limit blood formation in the sheep [191,192,265,266], and 0.2
µg/ml has been suggested as the minimal level for normal hematopoieses to
take place in the pig [267].

The morphological characteristics of the anemia of copper deficiency
vary in different species. In rats, rabbits, and pigs, it is hypochromic
and macrocytic [267-269]. In lambs, the anemia is also hypochromic and
macrocytic [270-273], and in chicks [274] and dogs [275-277], normocytic
and normochromic. Copper is probably concerned with the erythrocyte maturation process because copper-anemic pigs and dogs contain a lower percentage of reticulocytes in their blood than those with iron anemia [267,275-
277]. When copper is added to the diet of rats, rabbits, and pigs suffering
from a combined iron and copper deficiency anemia, copper elicits a reticulo-
cyte response, whereas iron has little effect [267,268,278]. Survival time
of the erythrocytes is shorter than normal in the Cu-deficient pig [279].
Copper, therefore, may be an essential component of adult red cells.

The defect in hemoglobin synthesis of copper deficiency could arise
from abnormalities in the biosynthesis of protoporphyrin and heme, or of
globin, or from abnormalities in iron metabolism. Protein synthesis is
generally normal [280,281], and Lee et al. [282] were unable to demonstrate
any abnormality in the heme biosynthetic pathway in Cu-deficient pigs. In
hypocupremic chicks, however, addition of copper normalizes the reduced rate
of glycine incorporation into heme [283]. Chase et al. [284,285] reported
that copper increased radioiron absorption in rats and that Cu-deficient
pigs have a decreased ability to absorb iron, to mobilize iron from the
tissues, and to utilize iron in hemoglobin synthesis [286]. Lee et al.
[287] confirmed this observation and also found that intramuscular injections of iron were observed in the reticuloendothelial system, the hepatic
parenchymal cells, and the normoblasts of copper-deficient pigs. This accumulation of iron may reflect a lack of ability to release iron to the
plasma. Iron cannot be incorporated into hemoglobin and, instead, accumulates as nonhemoglobin iron.

Malnourished infants [288-292] with anemia and neutropenia caused by
copper deficiency have been reported. In general, copper is widely distributed in foods and it is virtually impossible for severe copper deficiency to develop on a nutritional basis in the adult. Dunlap et al. have

reported a copper deficiency in an adult woman and an adolescent girl who
had experienced extensive bowel surgery and received long-term parenteral
hyperalimentation [293]. A similar case was reported for a 56-year-old
woman on intravenous hyperalimentation [294]. The megablastoid changes in
the bone marrow of one of the patients were seen in some of the infants
[288,290]. This abnormality was corrected by copper, which implies an
effect on RNA/DNA synthesis in the de nova pathway of deoxyuridine to thy-
mine. The neutropenia, which is thought to be the most constant sign of
copper deficiency [289], was clearly reversed in both patients by copper
therapy. Neutropenia has been reported in all of the copper-deficient infants [288-292] and has also been reported in swine [295].

Copper and Bone Formation. Bone abnormalities have been reported in
Cu-deficient rabbits [296], chicks [297-299], pigs [267,300,301], dogs [275-
277], foals [302,303], and mice [304]. A low incidence of spontaneous bone
fractures have been observed in sheep and cattle feeding on Cu-deficient
pastures [209,305,306]. In severely copper-deficient dogs, fractures and
severe deformities occur in many of the animals [275-277]. The weakness in
bone structure may be related to collagen solubility. Collagen extracted
from the bones of Cu-deficient chicks contains less aldehyde and is more
solubilized than collagen from control bones [299]. Collagen, like elastin,
contains intramolecular cross-links and its solubility is inversely related
to cross-linking [307,308]. Copper may be involved in promoting the structural integrity of bone collagen.

Copper and Neonatal Ataxia. A nervous disorder of lambs characterized
by incoordination of movement has been given local names in various parts
of the world such as swayback, lamkruis, renguera, and Gingin rickets.
Bennetts and Chapman [309] showed this condition to be associated with subnormal pasture levels of copper. The ataxia could be prevented by copper
supplementation of the diet. Neonatal ataxia has also been reported in Cu-
deficient goats [310-312] and has been demonstrated experimentally in the
newborn guinea pig [313]. Ataxia has been observed in young pigs [314,315].
The Cu-deficient pigs had demyelination of the spinal cord. Neural lesions
have been observed in the offspring of female rats fed a Cu-deficient diet
[316].

The lambs may be born paralyzed, but in some cases ataxia is not seen
for several weeks. Incoordinated movements of the hind limbs, a stiff and
staggering gait, and swaying of the hindquarters are evident as the disease
develops.

The primary lesion in swayback may be a low brain content of copper, leading to a deficiency of cytochrome oxidase in the motor neurones [317]. Investigators have observed lowered copper levels in the heart, liver, and bone marrow of the Cu-deficient rat [318,319]; in the heart and liver of Cu-deficient pigs [320]; and in the brain, heart, and liver of Cu-deficient rats [280,281]. Inhibition of cytochrome oxidase can lead to demyelination [321]. Therefore, severe deficiency of this enzyme should produce the same effect.

Copper and Pigmentation of Hair and Wool. Achromotrichia occurs in the Cu-deficient rat, rabbit, guinea pig, cat, dog, goat, sheep, and cattle but has not been observed in the pig [322]. In the rabbit, achromotrichia and alopecia are a more sensitive index of copper deficiency in the rabbit than is anemia [323]. A marked loss of pigmentation in cattle hair as a result of copper deficiency has been reported in Japan [324]. The mechanism involving copper in the pigmentation process is unknown. A breakdown in the conversion of tyrosine to melanin is the most likely explanation as this conversion is catalyzed by the copper-containing polyphenol oxidases [325].

Copper and Keratinization. A reduction in the quantity and quality of wool from copper-deficient Australian sheep has been observed [302,303,326, 327]. Copper supplementation of such sheep increases the weight of wool produced [190]. The deterioration in the process of keratinization, signified by a crimping defect, appears to be a specific effect of copper deficiency. In copper deficiency there are fewer disulfide groups and the alignment or orientation of the long-chain keratin fibrillae in the fiber may be changed [328]. In addition, the polypeptide chains of keratin have more N-terminal glycine and alanine than normal wool [329].

Copper and Fertility. In female rats, copper deficiency results in reproductive disorders, due to fetal death and resorption [330,331]. The estrus cycles remain unaffected and conception is not inhibited. Hens fed a severely Cu-deficient diet showed a marked drop of egg production and hatchability. The mortality is probably due to defects in red blood cell and in connective tissue formation [332] during early embryonic development.

In several areas, low fertility in cattle has been associated with copper deficiency [333-336]. Depressed or delayed estrus is common in dairy cows in copper-deficient areas.

Zipper et al. [337] reported that a small length of copper wire placed in the lower segment of rabbit uterus inhibited pregnancy. The presence of metal loops inserted into the testes of maturing rats inhibited spermato-

genesis [338]. The addition of metallic copper to an intrauterine device
significantly enhanced its contraceptive effectiveness in humans [339-341].

Copper and Cardiovascular Disorders. Bennetts and co-workers [333-335]
first noticed cardiac lesions in western Australian cattle suffering from
"falling disease." In this disease there is an atrophy of the myocardium
with replacement fibrosis with dense collagenous tissue. Death results due
to cardiac failure after mild exercise or excitement. Sheep, horses, and
pigs are rarely affected. In chicks [298,342-344], pigs [345-347], guinea
pigs [313], and rats [348] on copper-deficient diets, ruptures of the coronary and pulmonary arteries have been observed. In these species, the tensile strength of the aorta was markedly reduced and the myocardium was abnormally friable. A derangement of the elastic membranes of the aorta was
evident. The elastin content of deficient pigs [349] and chicks [350] is
decreased. Desmosine and isodesmosine, which are key cross-linking groups
of elastin [351] are decreased in the elastin of copper-deficient animals
[352-353]. Both substances, which are derived from lysine, need an ϵ-amino
group to be removed and oxidized [354], possibly to an aldehyde (a reaction
catalyzed by amino oxidases, which are copper-containing enzymes [355-357]).
The amino oxidase of the plasma of Cu-deficient pigs [358] and ewes and
lambs [359] is lower than those of animals on normal diets.

Copper and Scouring (Diarrhea) of Cattle. In cattle in the severely
copper-deficient areas of Australia, intermittent diarrhea occurs [333-335].
In parts of Holland [360,361], a similar disease occurs, where it is known
as scouring disease. In Zealand, a disease of cattle feeding on peatland
has been named "peat scours" [305]. A similar condition in cattle occurs
in England [362]. The disease is prevented or cured by copper therapy.
Diarrhea is not a common manifestation of copper deficiency in other species [306].

Copper and Wilson's Disease. Hepatolenticular degeneration (Wilson's
disease) is an inherited autosomal recessive disorder, described first by
Wilson in his monograph of 1912 [363]. In this disease the liver, basal
ganglia of the brain, cornea, and kidneys are most severely affected.
Chronic degeneration of the basal nuclei is associated with degeneration
of the hepatic parenchyma, which leads to eventual cirrhosis. The disease
is inexorably progressive and ultimately fatal. The most consistent salient
feature has been severe diminution or occasional absence of serum ceruloplasmin.

Two major hypotheses have been advanced to account for the pathological findings of Wilson's disease.

1. The abnormal gene suppresses the synthesis of normal ceruloplasmin [364-367]. As a consequence of ceruloplasmin deficiency, copper absorption from the gut is accelerated. Copper is then deposited in excessive quantities in the tissues. Structural damage and functional impairment ensue in the organs involved, particularly the liver, basal ganglia, and renal tubules.

2. An abnormal protein, presumably determined by the mutant gene, has an enhanced affinity for copper. This, in turn, deprives ceruloplasmin of its copper, blocking its formation, hence the deficiency [368,369].

The first hypothesis does not provide a mechanism. The second mechanism has not been proven, as no special abnormal proteins have been discovered. The biochemical defect may be related to a decreased cytochrome oxidase activity. Individuals with Wilson's disease have extremely low levels of cytochrome oxidase in their leucocytes, comparable to the low levels of ceruloplasmin in their sera [370]. Carrier individuals display intermediate levels of cytochrome oxidase in the leucocytes and ceruloplasmin in the serum.

Torsion dystony is somewhat similar to Wilson's disease and is also a copper metabolic defect [371]. This clinical and pathological condition is also called dystonia lenticularis.

Copper and Menkes Kinky Hair Syndrome (Trichopoliodystrophy). Menkes syndrome is a progressive brain disease of male infants, which usually causes death before 3 years of age and which is characterized by severely retarded growth and development, "kinky hair" (pili torti) hypothermia, arterial tortuosity, scorbutic bone changes, and cerebral gliosis with cystic degeneration [372]. Menkes syndrome is associated with profound hypocupremia, hypoceruloplasminemia, and diminished concentrations in hair [373-376]. Alterations of the free sulfhydryl groups of hair may result in its tendency to twist [373]. Changes in the elastic fibers of arterial walls and scorbutic bone deformities [373,374] may be related to copper deficiency. There is also a defect in intestinal copper absorption which could be caused either by a disturbance of the intracellular handling of copper in the duodenal mucosa or by impairment of copper transport across the serosal cell membrane [375]. Parenteral administration of copper may possibly be therapeutically beneficial [373-375]. Potential screening of infants for Menkes syndrome and Wilson's disease by analyses of serum copper may become a major application of clinical pathology laboratories [377].

Copper and Hodgkin's Disease. Measurements of serum copper are valuable as a laboratory adjunct to monitoring relapse in patients with Hodgkin's lymphoma [378,379]. There is a close correlation between the concentration of serum copper and the clinical activity of the lymphoma. The increased serum concentration of copper is the result of hyperceruloplasminemia, which occurs as a manifestation of the "acute phase reaction." Fluctuations in serum concentration may help to guide the physician in anticipating the clinical response to treatment in patients with Hodgkin's disease.

Copper and Psoriasis. In general, patients with psoriasis tended to have higher serum copper levels [380-382]. Kekki et al. [381] attributed the increase of copper levels to the nonceruloplasmin-bound fraction. Koskelo et al. [383] reported normal ceruloplasmin serum levels in uncomplicated psoriasis, but found elevated ceruloplasmin levels in patients with psoriasis and roentgenologically confirmed arthritis.

Copper and Prostaglandin Synthesis. The presence of Cu^{2+} in homogenates of sheep vesicular tissue stimulates the conversion of arachidonic acid to prostaglandin $F_{2\alpha}$. Simultaneously, prostaglandin E_2 production is decreased [384]. This effect is caused by a selective inactivation of prostaglandin E_2 synthetase which occurs naturally, but which is accelerated by Cu^{2+}.

FLUORINE

Chemistry of Fluorine

Fluorine is a gaseous element found in Group VIIA of the periodic table. Fluorine's abundance in the earth's crust is 0.03%. Fluorine is found chiefly as the mineral fluorite or fluorspar (CaF_2), as cryolite (Na_3AlF_6), and as fluorapatite [$CaF_2 \cdot 3Ca_3(PO_4)_2$]. There is only one stable and naturally occurring nuclear species of fluorine, ^{19}F, but short-lived radioactive isotopes with mass numbers 17, 18, 20, and 21 have been prepared. The most common oxidation state of fluorine is 1-.

Large-scale production of fluorine is accomplished by the electrolysis of fused potassium hydrogen fluoride (KHF_2) in a copper apparatus with graphite electrodes. One important use of fluorine is the addition of 1 ppm to drinking water to prevent tooth decay. Fluorinated compounds stabilize lubricating oil over a wide temperature range; Freon-12 (CCl_2F_2) is used as a refrigerant; sodium fluoracetate (compound 1080) is a rat poison; fluoro-DDT is an insecticide; and Teflon (tetrafluoroethylene) resin, a plastic, withstands aqua regia and endures relatively high temperatures. Hydrogen fluoride (HF) attacks silicates readily and is used for etching glass.

The highly reactive fluorine combines readily with nearly all the other elements and even with the noble gases krypton and xenon. It reacts with all metals, forming a large number of single, double, and complex salts, and also with most of the nonmetals. Because of its small size, it forms many stable complexes with positive ions, e.g., silicon hexafluoridates (SiF_6^2), aluminum hexafluoridates (AlF_6^{3-}), and many others.

Essentiality of Fluorine

Two groups of investigators [385,386] have found no differences in the weight and growth of groups of animals on fluoride-deficient diets and fluoride-supplemented diets. Evans and Phillips [387] found that a mineralized milk diet containing 1.6 ppm F (dry basis) was adequate for the growth, health, and fertility of rats through five generations. Lawrenz [388] fed rats on a lower fluoride (0.47 ppm) diet for a period of 207 days. Some evidence of fluorine depletion was observed.

McClendon and Gershon-Cohen [389] fed weanling rats for 66 days with a basal diet prepared from materials grown in water culture and claimed to be "fluorine free." The rats averaged 51 g live weight and had 10 carious molars per animal, compared with an average of 128 g live weight and 0.5 carious molar per animal, compared with an average of 128 g live weight and 0.5 carious molar per animal in rats fed a supplemented fluorine diet. Schwarz and Milne [390] reported that fluorine stimulates the growth of rats fed a highly purified amino acid diet. However, the control rats grew suboptimally and the weight differences between the deficient and the control animals were small. Clearly, more research is necessary before it can be stated that fluorine is essential for growth.

At present [390], a requirement of 1-2 ppm of diet appears to be beneficial. Foods high in fluorine include seafoods (5-10 ppm) [391] and tea (100 ppm) [392]. Cereal and other grains contain 1 to 3 ppm, and cow's milk contains 1 to 2 ppm (dry basis) [393]. When water is artificially fluoridated, the consumption of 1200 to 1500 ml/day of water containing 1 ppm F provides 1.2-1.5 mg F, which is more than is normally ingested in normal North American diets which contribute about 0.3-0.5 mg F daily [394,395], approximately 80% of which is absorbed [396,397].

Metabolism of Fluorine

Soluble fluorides are rapidly and almost completely absorbed from the gastrointestinal tract. Radiofluoride (^{18}F) has been detected in the blood of sheep 5 min after a dose was placed in the stomach, the peak being reached in 3 hr [398]. In humans given small oral doses of soluble fluoride, blood maxima are observed within 1 hr, and 20-30% appeared in the urine in 3-4 hr [399,400]. Insoluble forms of fluoride are almost as well absorbed as the soluble compounds. The fluorine of calcium fluoride was 96% absorbed and that of cryolite was 93% absorbed [401].

Fluoride readily crosses cell membranes including that of the red cells. The fluoride concentration of the plasma is normally twice that of the red cells, with less than 5% bound to plasma solutes under physiological conditions [401]. The disappearance curve of ^{18}F from the blood is triphasic in nature [399,400]. The first phase presumably represents mixing of the fluoride with the body water; the second, uptake by the skeleton; and the third, excretion in the urine. Most of the absorbed fluoride which escapes retention by the bones and teeth is excreted rapidly in the urine. Organically bound fluorine may also be important. In human blood serum, fluorine travels electrophoretically in the area of the albumin peak. The fluorine-containing compound is not a protein but a weak, lipid-soluble organic acid [402,403]. In eggs, fluorine has been reported to be associated primarily with the lipid portion of the yolk [404].

Other biological effects include stimulating growth in tissue culture, activating citrulline synthesis by liver and enzymatic decomposition of nitromethane; fluoride also activates adenyl cyclase (mediator of hormone effects) [405].

Health Effects of Fluorine

Fluorine and Dental Caries. A relationship between dental caries and increasing fluoride concentration was first shown by Dean [406]. In a study of 7257 children, 12-14 years old, caries decreased in permanent teeth as the fluoride concentration of the drinking water increased above 1.3 ppm. An inverse relationship has also been observed in many countries between fluoride naturally present in water and dental caries [407-409]. The water supplies of hundreds of communities have been treated with sodium fluoride or fluosilicate at 0.8 to 1.2 ppm. Comparisons between these communities [410,411] and adjacent communities without fluoridation showed the value of artificially fluoridating water supplies. Topical applications of fluorides have achieved some success [412-414]. In Switzerland, salt has shown considerable promise as a fluoride vehicle [415,416]. Fluoride fortification of cereals may also have some promise, judging by limited European experience [415,417].

Fluorine, Osteoporosis, and Aortic Calcification. Osteoporosis is a disease of the elderly characterized by a decrease in bone density often accompanied by collapsed vertebrae. Individuals suffering from osteoporosis have had improvement when treated with large amounts of fluoride [418-422]. Leone et al. [423] have found substantially less osteoporosis in a high-fluoride area of Texas (8 ppm in water) than a low-fluoride area (0.09 ppm in the water) in Massachusetts. Similar results were obtained by Bernstein et al. [424] in a comparative study of a high- and low-fluoride area of North Dakota.

Leone et al. [425] have compared the mortality of a high- and low-fluoride area of Texas. The low-fluoride area had a much greater incidence of heart attacks. Calcification of the aorta was much greater in the low-fluoride area. The levels of fluoride that prevented osteoporosis and aortic calcification is above that considered safe for children.

Fluorine, Hematocrits, and Fertility. During the stress of pregnancy, feeding diets low in fluoride may result in decreased hematocrits in mice [426]. Also, a decrease in fertility apparently occurs [427]. The number of litters produced by first and second generation was reduced, but litter size was not affected. The condition was prevented by the addition of 50 µg fluorine/ml drinking water. Although this amount is toxic for man, it is not an unusual amount to be fed to rodents. Certainly more research is needed in this regard.

MANGANESE

Chemistry

Manganese, whose atomic number is 25 and atomic weight is 54.938, is located in Group VIIA of the periodic table, horizontally between chromium and iron. Manganese exists in three, and possibly four, allotrophic modifications. Alpha and beta manganese are hard, brittle metals that will scratch glass. Gamma manganese is flexible and soft and can be bent and easily cut. It changes to the alpha form at ordinary temperatures. Manganese makes up about 0.10% of the earth's crust. The main ores are pyrolusite (MnO_2), psilomelane [$BaMnMn_8O_{16}(OH)_4$], wad, hydrous Mn oxides, manganite ($Mn_2O_3 \cdot H_2O$), hausmannite (Mn_3O_4), braunite ($3Mn_2O_3 \cdot MnSiO_3$), rhodochrosite ($MnCO_3$), and rhodonite ($MnSiO_3$).

The element can exist in its compounds in the valence states of 1, 2, 3, 4, 6, and 7. The most stable compounds are those of valence 2, 6, and 7. The dioxide MnO_2 is also quite stable. The lower oxides, MnO and Mn_2O_3, are basic; the higher oxides, acidic. Manganese liberates hydrogen slowly from water at room temperature and readily from acids. Manganese metal oxidizes superficially in air and rusts in moist air. Boiling concentrated solutions of potassium or sodium hydroxide have no action on manganese.

More than 95% of the manganese is used in the form of ferroalloys by the metal industries, chiefly for steel manufacture. It is used in ferromanganese, manganese, iron, carbon, and silicon steel. Manganese is also used in dry cells, in batteries, and in glassmaking to counteract the green color from iron. It also supplies pink and black coloring in glassmaking. Manganese is added to soils to combat chlorosis of crops. The powerful oxidizing properties of potassium permanganate are utilized for disinfecting, deodorizing, and decolorizing, and this compound is an important analytic reagent.

Essentiality of Manganese

Manganese was first shown to be required by plants and microorganisms by McHarque [428] in 1923. In 1931, Hart and associates [429,430] found manganese to be necessary for growth in mice and for normal ovarian activity in mice and rats. Orent and McCollum [431] showed that manganese is required to prevent testicular degeneration in male rats and for ovarian function in female rats. Five years later, two diseases of poultry, perosis or "slipped tendon" [432,433] and nutritional chondrodystrophy [434], were caused by inadequate intakes of manganese.

Young rats require about 2 mg/day [435] or 40 ppm of dry diet and rabbits require 1-4 mg/day [436]. About 11-14 ppm was found satisfactory for the growth of pigs [437].

About 25 ppm Mn seems to meet the full requirements of cattle. The minimum requirements for chickens and turkeys are about 40-54 ppm [438, 439].

Nuts, cereals, and dried fruits have the greatest manganese concentration [440] and average concentrations range from 20 to 23 ppm, whereas poultry products, fish, and seafoods are as low as 0.2 to 0.5 ppm. Schroeder et al. [441] have found similar results. Tea and cloves were found to be exceptionally rich in manganese. Adults consuming a typical Dutch diet consumed an average of 2.3 Mn/day [442], which is similar to the 2.4 mg Mn daily calculated by Schroeder et al. [441] for adults on an institutional diet in the United States. The mean manganese intake of nine American college women was reported as 3.7 mg daily [443], which is lower than the 6.4-7.5 mg measured for two adults by Tipton et al. [444]. A vegetarian diet contained an average of 7 mg Mn [445]. Adults on an English diet consumed an average of 7 mg Mn daily of which 3.3 mg came from tea [446].

Metabolism of Manganese

Greenberg [447,448] found that only 3-4% of orally administered radiomanganese is absorbed by rats. The absorbed manganese quickly appeared in the bile and was excreted in the feces. Bile flow is the main route of manganese excretion and constitutes the main regulatory mechanism. Excretion also occurs via the pancreatic juice [449]. Excretion of manganese also takes place into the duodenum and jejunum and to a lesser extent into the terminal ileum [450]. Very little manganese is excreted in the urine [451,452].

Injected radiomanganese disappears rapidly from the bloodstream [453-454]. Radiomanganese enters into the capillaries, the mitochondria, and the nuclear fraction [453]. In general, a high proportion of the body manganese must be in a highly dynamic mobile state.

Pyruvate carboxylase is the only known manganese-containing metalloprotein with a fixed amount of the metal per molecule of protein [455]. However, liver arginase has been claimed to contain manganese as an essential component [456,457]. A firmly bound manganese compound, which is nondialyzable, nonexchangeable, and not available for chelation with EDTA, occurs in human and rabbit erythrocytes and may be a manganese-porphyrin compound [458]. In human blood serum, manganese occurs almost totally bound to a β1-globulin [459-461]. Complexes of manganese and other bivalent cations with RNA and DNA have been identified [462].

In the mammalian liver most of the manganese is present in the arginase extract, indicating that in this organ the metal exists largely in combination with protein [457]. Fore and Morgan [463] have shown that about 20% of the manganese of liver and kidney is loosely held.

Hemoglobin levels are not affected by lack of manganese [464,465]. In growth, inhibition results partly from reduced food consumption and partly from an impaired utilization of the ingested food [466].

Health Effects of Manganese

Manganese and Bone Growth. Skeletal abnormalities, ranging from gross
and crippling deformities to mild rarefaction of bone occur in all species.
The following deformities, according to species, have been observed: in
mice, rats, and rabbits, retarded bone growth with shortening and bowing of
the forelegs [464,467,468]; in pigs, lameness, enlarged hock joints and
crooked and shortened legs [469,470]; in cattle, leg deformities with "over-
knuckling" [471]; in sheep, joint pains with poor locomotion and balance
[472]; in goats, tareal joint excrescences and ataxia [473]; the disease
perosis or "slipped tendon" [432,433] in chicks, poults, and ducklings; and
in chick embryos, nutritional chondrodystrophy [474].

Leach and Muenster [475] discovered that radiosulfate uptake is lowered
in the cartilage of the Mn-deficient chick and that the total concentration
of hexosamines and hexuronic acid is reduced in this tissue. Everson and
associates [476-478] demonstrated a significant reduction in the concentration of acid mucopolysaccharides (AMPS) in the rib and epiphyseal cartilage
in newborn guinea pigs. A severe reduction of cartilage chondroitin sulfate
content is associated with manganese deficiency [479]. The critical sites
of manganese function in chondroitin sulfate synthesis have been identified
by Leach et al. [480]. These are the two enzyme systems: (a) polymerase
enzyme, which is responsible for the polymerization of uridine diphosphate
(UDP)-N-acetyl galactosamine to UDP-glucuronic acid to form the polysaccharide, and (b) galactotransferase, an enzyme which incorporates galactose
from UDP-galactose into the galactose-galactose-xylose trisaccharide which
serves as the linkage between the polysaccharide and the protein associated
with it.

Manganese and Reproductive Function. Defective ovulation, testicular
degeneration, and infant mortality were reported in the earliest studies
showing the essentiality of manganese in the diet of rats [429-431]. The
mortality was thought to be due to deficient lactation, but the young grew
normally when placed with Mn-deficient mothers [481]. Shils and McCollum
[468] showed Mn-deficient rats experience no loss of ability to suckle
normal young and no lack of normal interest. Manganese deficiency can be
reflected by ataxia or stillbirth in the young or irregular estrous cycles
or lack of interest in mating by the adults. Impairment of reproductive
function occurs in poultry, who show lowered egg production and decreased
hatchability even in the absence of signs of perosis and chondrodystrophy
[438,482].

The omission of manganese from the maternal diet of guinea pigs results
in a decrease of litter size and an increase in the percentage of young de-
livered prematurely or born dead [483]. Cows [484,485] and goats [473]
exhibit delayed estrus and conception on low-Mn rations. Similar results
were found with pigs [486,487].

In the Mn-deficient male rat and rabbit, the sterility and absence of
libido is associated with seminal tubular degeneration and complete lack of
spermatozoa [464,466], indicating that manganese may be specifically involved in spermatogenesis.

Manganese and Neonatal Ataxia. Ataxia in the offspring of Mn-deficient
animals was first observed in the chick by Caskey and Norris [488]. Manganese administration did not cure the ataxia. Shils and McCollum [468] and
others [483,489,490] have reported ataxia, incoordination, and poor equilibrium in many of the young from Mn-deficient rats and guinea pigs.

Histological examination of the brain and spinal cord has not disclosed
any lesions which could account for the ataxia [468,490-492]. Acetylcholin-
esterase and a number of other enzymes in the brains of rats and guinea pigs
were not significantly different when comparing Mn-sufficient to Mn-deficient
animals [468,483]. Cerebrospinal fluid pressures do not differ significantly
in normal and deficient young [493]. Greater brain excitability and convul-
sability was observed in these animals [494].

A structural defect in the inner ear has emerged as a possible causative
factor of ataxia in Mn-deficient rats and guinea pigs [489,495,496]. The
ataxic symptoms arose from impaired vestibular function, itself an effect
of lack of manganese upon cartilage mucopolysaccharide synthesis and hence,
bone development of the skull, particularly of the otoliths. Some Mn-deficient guinea pigs also exhibit abnormal curvatures of the semicircular canals
and misshapen ampullae [496]. Defective motion and posture characteristics
of the Mn-deficient young may result from faulty otolith development during
fetal life. An otolith defect has also been observed in Mn-deficient mink
[497].

Manganese and Carbohydrate Metabolism. Manganese may play a part in
gluconeogenesis through its presence in the metalloenzyme pyruvate decar-
boxylase. Aplasia or marked hypoplasia of guinea pig pancreas occurred in
Mn-deficient animals [498,499], and decreased the number of pancreatic
islets, with less intensely granulated beta cells and more alpha cells.
An Mn-deficient guinea pig shows a decreased capacity to utilize glucose

and exhibits a diabetic-like curve in response to glucose loading. Manganese supplementation completely reversed the reduced glucose utilization.

Manganese administration to diabetic subjects has a hypoglycemic effect [500,501], and both pancreatectomy and diabetes have been correlated with decreased levels in blood and tissues [502,503]. Decreased concentrations of stainable mucopolysaccharides occur in the skin of young rats born to diabetic mothers [504]. Insulin may regulate the utilization of glucose in the synthesis of mucopolysaccharides [505]. Perhaps impairment of glucose utilization in the Mn-deficient guinea pig is related to the connective tissue defect that occurs in these animals.

Manganese and Lipid Metabolism. An interaction between manganese and choline in skeletal development was observed several years ago [506-508]. Liver and bone fat are reduced in manganese- and choline-supplemented rats, and back fat is reduced in pigs [487]. Manganese stimulates the hepatic synthesis of cholesterol and fatty acids in rats [509]. Manganous ion is a necessary cofactor for the conversion of mevalonic acid to squalene by mevalonic kenase [510]. A phosphorylated derivative of mevalonic acid is an intermediate in this reaction and requires manganese for its synthesis [511].

Bell and Hurley [512] have observed a reduction in the nonspecific choline esterase activity, cytochrome, oxidase, and choline lipid staining of manganese-deficient mouse epidermis. It has been suggested [513] that liver ultrastructure resulting from a deficiency of manganese or from choline may be similar.

IRON

Chemistry of Iron

Iron, whose atomic number is 26 and which has an atomic weight of 55.847, is classified in Group VIIIB of the periodic table. About 5% of the earth's crust is iron. Iron is tetramorphous. The deltal form exists above 1400° C and is weakly paramagnetic. Below 1400° C there is a transition to gamma iron which is also weakly paramagnetic. At 895° C there is a transition to beta iron which is stable to 766° C, where alpha iron is obtained. In the alpha form, iron is a soft, ductile, gray-white metal of high tensile strength. Its chief ores are hematite (Fe_2O_3), brown ore, which is hydrated iron oxide ($Fe_2O_3 \cdot nH_2O$) such as limonite, magnetite (Fe_3O_4), and siderite ($FeCO_3$).

The most important oxidation states of iron are 2+ or 3+. The 4+ state is realized in perferrite (FeO_3^{2-}), and the 6+ state is realized in ferrate (FeO_4^{2-}). In contact with nonoxidizing acids, iron dissolves by reducing hydrogen ion to hydrogen gas, forming ferrous ion. Oxidizing agents produce ferrous ion if the metal is in excess and ferric if the oxidizing agent is in excess. Upon immersion in concentrated nitric acid, iron does not dissolve but is made passive and will not dissolve in dilute acids. Under usual atmospheric conditions iron rusts to form hydrated ferric oxides. Both ferrous and ferric iron form complex ions, such as the ferrocyanide ion [$Fe(Cn)_6^{4-}$] and the ferricyanide ion [$Fe(Cn)_6^{3-}$]. Prussian blue, an important pigment, is ferric ferrocyanide ($Fe[Fe(CN)_6]_3$).

Iron is the most useful metal of material civilization; it has made possible plants, tools, machinery, and many other products of the Industrial Revolution. Iron's principal use is to alloy it with carbon; a moderate amount produces steel, an excess produces cast iron. Special alloys with other metals such as manganese or chromium result in manganese steel or chromium steel.

Essentiality of Iron

Keilin established that iron, through its presence in the hemoprotein enzymes, the cytochromes, is vitally concerned in the oxidative mechanism of all living cells [514]. Subsequently, iron-containing flavoprotein enzymes were discovered [515,516], and it became clear that iron is intimately involved in oxygen utilization by the tissue as well as in oxygen transport as part of the hemoglobin molecule. Lack of dietary iron was shown to inhibit some of the iron-dependent enzymic processes in the animal, in addition to its effect in limiting hemoglobin formation [517-520].

Human iron deficiency is characterized clinically by listlessness and fatigue, palpitation on exertion, sore tongue on occasion, angular dysphagia, and koilonychia [521]. In children, anorexia, depressed growth, and decreased resistance to infection are commonly observed. In iron-deficient anemia, abnormalities of the gastrointestinal tract, including achlorhydria and superficial gastritis, have been observed [522,523]. Iron-deficiency anemia is much more common in women than in men because women of fertile age are subject to additional iron losses in menstruation, pregnancy, and lactation. The incidence of iron deficiency in women has been reported as 20-25% in different Swedish [524] and English [525] studies. In U.S. studies with pregnant women, iron-deficiency anemia ranging from 15% [526]

to 58% [527] have been observed. The principal cause of anemia in adult
men and postmenopausal women is chronic bleeding due to infections, malig-
nancy, bleeding ulcers, and hookworm infestation. Economic disadvantage
[528,529], infection, vegetarian-type diets [530], and excessive sweating
can also lead to iron-deficiency anemia.

During the suckling period, both young animals and humans can become
iron deficient [531,532]. In U.S. infants, an incidence of iron-deficiency
anemia from as low as 8% to as high as 64% [533,534] has been reported.
Iron-deficiency anemia occurs most frequently between 4 and 24 months of
age. There is a regular need for supplementation with medicinal iron or
with iron-fortified foods [533-535].

Piglets denied access to sources of iron other than sow's milk develop
anemia within 2 to 4 weeks of birth. The disease is a typical iron deficiency [536-538]. Pigs seem to be particularly sensitive to iron-deficiency
anemia because of their high growth rate and its relatively poor endowment
with iron at birth. Lambs and calves fed a whole-milk diet develop a mild
anemia [539]. Heavy infestation of grazing animals with helmith intestinal
parasites results in an iron-deficiency type of anemia in lambs and calves
[540,541].

The richest sources of iron are the organ meats (liver, kidney, and
heart), egg yolk, dried legumes, cocoa, cane molasses, shellfish, and pars-
ley [542]. Poor sources include milk and milk products, white sugar, white
flour and bread (unenriched), polished rice, sago, potatoes, and most fresh
fruit. Foods of intermediate iron content are the muscle meats, fish, and
poultry, nuts, green vegetables, and whole-meal flour and bread. Iron
utensils such as cast iron skillets or Dutch ovens contribute significantly
to the iron content of cooked food [543]. Foods having an acid reaction
such as spaghetti sauce or apple butter removed the greatest amounts of
iron from the iron skillet. Substitution of aluminum and stainless steel
in the manufacture of cooking equipment has reduced iron intake.

Cider and wine made in Europe or the United States may have 2 to 16
mg of iron or more per liter [544]. The iron in city water supplies is
usually low, but amounts greater than 5 mg/l may be found in the water from
some deep wells or bore holes [543].

Average U.S. diets supply 14-20 mg Fe per man daily [545]. Australian
diets supplied 20-22 mg Fe per adult male daily [546]. A poor Indian diet
provides only 9 mg of total iron daily [547]. A convenient figure to remember is that the diets of people who live in the so-called Western countries

contain about 5 to 7 mg of iron per 1000 calories [548]. The United States recommended daily allowance is 15 mg daily for children under 1 year, 10 mg daily for children ages 1-3, 18 mg for adults and children 4 or more years of age, and 18 mg for pregnant or lactating women [549].

Metabolism of Iron

In monogastric species, absorption of iron takes place mainly in the duodenum [550-552] in the ferrous form [553,554]. Iron occurs in foods in inorganic form, in combination with protein, in heme compounds as constituents of hemoglobin and myoglobin, or other organic complexes. Heme iron is absorbed directly into the mucosal cells of the intestine. Both inorganic iron and iron bound to protein need to be reduced to the ferrous state and released from conjugation for effective absorption. Gastric juice and other digestive secretions help accomplish these transformations. About 5-10% of the iron in food is absorbed depending on the food source. Iron-deficient subjects absorb 10-20% of the iron. The amount of absorption depends on the bioavailability of the iron of each food [543].

Amino acids such as histidine or lysine assist in iron absorption [555,556]. Ascorbic acid and cysteine may also assist in reducing and releasing food iron [557,558]. Ascorbic acid reduces ferric to ferrous ion in vitro, and the efficiency of iron absorption is increased when large doses of ascorbic acid are administered with iron salts [559-561]. On the other hand, when phytate is added to diets, iron absorption can be significantly reduced in man [559, 562-563].

The efficiency of iron absorption changes in various disease states. Increased absorption occurs in aplastic anemia, hemolytic anemia, pernicious anemia, pyridoxine deficiency, hemochromatosis, and transfusional siderosis [564-566]. Increased iron absorption is also related to increased erythropoiesis [567,568], hypoxia [569], depletion of body iron stores [570,571], and increased iron turnover [572]. Iron absorption is decreased in transfusional polycythemia [567] and has been related to tissue iron overload [573].

Much of the absorbed iron is continuously circuited throughout the body, of which the cycle plasma-erythroid marrow-red cell-senescent red cell-plasma is quantitatively the most important. Other subsidiary metabolic circuits exist, including the cycles plasma-ferritin and hemosiderin-plasma, and plasma-myoglobin and iron-containing enzymes-plasma. The iron of plasma is apparently the link between cycles and facilitates ready exchange among them.

Iron is stored in tissues as ferritin and hemosiderin. The iron of plasma is bound to transferrin which is a β_1-globulin with a molecular weight of about 86,000 and has two iron-binding sites. There are more iron-binding sites than atoms of iron present in normal plasma, so that no free iron is present. When all the binding sites are filled, this represents the total amount bound or the total iron-binding capacity (TIBC). Normal human total iron is 63-202 µg/100 ml, and 250-416 µg/100 ml is the normal value for TIBC.

In young iron-deficient rats, cytochrome c may be reduced to as little as half of normal concentrations in the skeletal muscles, heart, liver, kidney, and intestinal mucosa [574-577] with a smaller reduction in the brain [574]. Catalase activity appears to be little affected [578,579]. Succinic dehydrogenase activity is reduced in the cardiac muscle of iron-deficient rats [580,581] and chicks [520]. Variable degrees of hemeprotein depletion in different tissues in response to iron deprivation are not understood, but may be related to organ function, growth rate, and cell turnover [575, 576].

Health Effects of Iron

Diseases Related to Increase in Serum or Plasma Iron. Increases in serum or plasma iron are brought about by several conditions: increased red cell destruction (hemolytic anemia, decreased survival of red cells), in cases of decreased utilization (decreased blood formation as in lead poisoning or pyridoxine deficiency), in situations in which release of iron occurs (release of ferritin in necrotic hepatitis), in states where iron storage is defective (as in pernicious anemia), in conditions in which there is an increased rate of absorption (e.g., homochromatosis, hemosiderosis).

Diseases Related to Decreases in Serum or Plasma Iron. Decreases in serum or plasma iron are generally due to a deficiency in the total amount of iron present in the body which may be caused by a lack of sufficient intake or absorption of iron (chronic blood loss or nephrosis) or by an increased demand on the body stores (pregnancy). Diminished iron levels may also be caused by a decreased release of iron from body stores (reticoendothelial system) as seen in infections or turpentine abscesses.

Diseases Related to Changes in the Total Iron-Binding Capacity. Increases in the total iron-binding capacity of serum may be caused by an increased production of the iron-binding protein transferrin, as found in the various states of chronic iron deficiency, or it may be caused by an increased release of ferritin, as in hepatocellular necrosis. Decreases in the total iron-binding capacity may be caused by a deficiency in ferritin, as found in cirrhosis and homochromatosis, or as a result of an excessive loss of protein (transferrin), as occurs in nephrosis.

MOLYBDENUM

Chemistry of Molybdenum

Molybdenum is classified in Group VIB of the periodic table and is therefore related to chromium and tungsten. It has an atomic number of 42 and a molecular weight of 95.94. It makes up about 0.0015% of the earth's crust. There are seven natural stable isotopes with mass numbers of 92, 94, 95, 96, 97, 98, and 100. The only important ore is molybdenite (MoS_2); however some powellite [calcium tungstomolybdate, $Ca(Mo_3,W)O_4$] and deposits containing wulfenite (lead molybdate, $PbMoO_4$) have also been worked.

The main valences are 2+, 3+, 4+, 5+, and 6+. The most important compound is the trioxide (MoO_3), from which most of the known compounds can be prepared. Molybdenum is resistant to hydrochloric, sulfuric, phosphoric, and hydrofluoric acids under many conditions of concentration and temperature. It is attacked by oxidizing acids, molten oxidizing salts, and fused alkalis. It is rapidly oxidized in air at temperatures above $500°$ C.

Metallic molybdenum has been widely used in electronic tubes for anodes, grids, and support members. It is also used in steels and high-speed tools. Molybdic oxide has found use as a catalyst and in molybdated dyes and pigments.

Essentiality of Molybdenum

Bortels [582] showed molybdenum is an essential nutrient for the growth of Azotobacter. Molybdenum was later found to be necessary for all nitrogen-fixing organisms and for Aspergillus niger [583]. By 1939, Arnon and Stout [584] had shown that molybdenum is required by higher plants independent of nitrogen fixation.

The first indication that molybdenum was essential for animal nutrition came in 1953 when it was shown that the flavoprotein enzyme xanthine oxidase is a molybdenum-containing metalloenzyme which requires molybdenum for its activity [585-587]. Using purified diets, it was shown that molybdenum is essential in the diet of lambs, chicks, and turkey poults [588-590]. Molybdenum deficiency has never been reported either in man or in other farm animals.

Tipton et al. [591] found the mean dietary intake of two adults to be close to 100 µg Mo/day. In another study carried out on 24 girls, 7-9 years old [592], the average intake was 75 µg Mo/day. Most of the dietary molybdenum appeared in the urine.

The molybdenum content of foods varies greatly. Legumes, cereal grains, leafy vegetables, liver, and kidney are among the richest sources of molybdenum, with fruits, root and stem vegetables, muscle meats, and dairy products among the poorest [593-595]. Leguminous seeds vary from 0.2 to 4.7 ppm Mo, and cereal grains vary from 0.12 to 1.14 ppm [595]. Wheat, flour, and bread ranged from 0.30 to 0.66 ppm Mo. Determinations of the response in the intestinal xanthine oxidase levels of rats fed low-Mo diets indicate that 50-100% of the total Mo in various foods is available for this purpose [595].

Metabolism of Molybdenum

Studies with both stable and radioactive molybdenum (^{99}Mo) indicate that molybdenum is readily and rapidly absorbed from most diets. The hexavalent water-soluble forms, such as ammonium molybdate, and the molybdenum of high-Mo herbage are particularly well absorbed by cattle [596]. Insoluble compounds such as MoO_3 and $CaMoO_4$, but not MoS_2, are well absorbed by rabbits and guinea pigs when fed in large doses [597]. Administered ^{99}Mo reached a peak in the blood of swine in 2-4 hr, whereas the average time in cattle was 96 hr. Over 75% of both orally and intravenously administered ^{99}Mo was excreted in the urine of swine in 120 hr. Fecal excretion was the main route in cattle. Only 15% was excreted in the urine in 168 hr by the intravenously dosed cattle [598]. Urine was the major route of excretion in pigs [599], rats [600], and man [601], employing ^{99}Mo.

Sulfate ion has an influence on molybdenum retention. In rats [602], in cattle [603], and in sheep [604-606] there is a reduction of molybdenum retention when these animals are on a high-sulfate diet. Dick [604] has postulated that inorganic sulfate impedes or blocks reabsorption of molybdenum through the kidney tubule.

Xanthine oxidase or xanthine dehydrogenase in animals and the nitrate reductase of plants are the only known molybdenum-containing metalloproteins. The only known biochemical function of molybdenum in animals, other than a copper interaction, is related to the activity of xanthine oxidase. The purified enzyme isolated from cow's milk is a reddish-brown protein with a molecular weight of 275,000 [607], containing 8 atoms of iron, 2 molecules

of flavine adenine dinucleotide (FAD), and usually 1.3 to 1.5 atoms of Mo
per molecule of protein [608,609]. The molybdenum is firmly bound to the
protein and cannot be removed without destroying the xanthine oxidase activity [610].

Molybdenum is associated with NADH dehydrogenase [611] and may have a
role in the terminal NADH oxidation in beef heart [612]. A molybdohemepro-
tein, sulfite oxidase has been isolated from bovine liver [613]. This enzyme catalyzes the oxidation of sulfite to sulfate. Seelig [614] has proposed a role of a copper-molybdenum interaction in iron-deficiency and iron-
storage diseases.

Health Effects of Molybdenum

Molybdenum and Dental Caries. Claims have been made based upon epidemiological studies carried out in Hungary [615,616] and New Zealand [617,
618] that molybdenum exerts a beneficial effect on the incidence and severity
of dental caries and that it might enhance the well-established effect of
fluoride.

In two of the earliest experiments [619,620] with rats, a reduction in
caries was observed when molybdenum was supplied during tooth formation.
Other experiments with rats who were fed a cariogenic diet [595,621-623] and
were given supplemental molybdenum at levels up to 50 ppm failed to demonstrate any significant effect. Buttner [621,622] found that addition of 25
to 50 ppm Mo and 50 ppm F to the water was more effective than 50 ppm F
alone. In similar experiments Malthus et al. [623] found no significant
differences. Fluoride uptake by intact human enamel is not increased by
Mo salts added to solutions of NaF, and neither fluoride retention in bones
of rats [617,618,620] nor the fluoride content of the saliva [624] is increased when ^{99}Mo and ^{18}F are given together by stomach tube, compared to
animals receiving ^{18}F alone. Obviously, further work is needed before molybdenum can be assigned a preventative or an ameliorative role in dental
caries.

Molybdenum and Anemia. Bala and Liftshits [625] have reported that
the mean molybdenum content of the whole blood of healthy subjects was 1.47
± 0.12 µg/100 ml, evenly distributed between erythrocytes and the plasma.
In leukemia patients, the molybdenum level was significantly increased in
the whole blood and in the erythrocytes but not in the plasma. In all the
types of anemia studied, the molybdenum content of the whole blood and
erythrocytes was reduced and there was also a substantial decrease in plasma

molybdenum in iron-deficiency and cancer anemia. After posthemorrhagic
anemia, the molybdenum content of the blood decreased solely as a result of
a decrease in the number of erythrocytes. In other anemias, erythrocyte
saturation with molybdenum is greatly reduced. This reduction in erythrocyte molybdenum is the result of a molybdenum decrease in the nonhemoglobin
protein fraction of the cells. It is possible that in iron-deficiency
anemia there is a concurrent molybdenum deficiency arising from a metabolic
disturbance linked with iron.

Molybdenum and Renal Calculi. A high incidence of renal xanthine calculi in sheep, especially in castrated male sheep, was recognized in the
Moutere Hills of New Zealand [626]. The livers of the sheep also have subnormal levels of molybdenum. Because other pastures of the world are low
in molybdenum and these calculi are not present, other factors may also be
important in xanthine calculus formation.

NICKEL

Chemistry

Nickel is classified in Group VIII of the periodic table. Its atomic
number is 28 and its atomic weight is 58.71. Stable isotopes of 58, 60,
61, 62, and 64 have been reported. Nickel constitutes about 0.016% of the
earth's crust and constitutes about 0.02% of igneous rocks. The most important sources of the metal are the mixed sulfide ores containing pentlandite
[(Fe, Ni)S], nickel-bearing pyrrhotite (Fe_5S_6 to $Fe_{16}S_{17}$), and nickel-bearing
chalcopyrite ($CuFeS_2$). Oxide ores range from hydrous magnesium silicates,
e.g., garnierite (Ni, Mg)$SiO_3 \cdot nH_2O$(varies), to nickel-bearing iron oxide
(laterite).

The main valence state of nickel is 2+, although 1+ and 4+ states do
exist in specialized situations. These latter ions are not stable in aqueous
solution. Nickel reacts slowly with strong acids under ordinary conditions
to liberate hydrogen and form Ni^{2+}. Nickel salts are slightly acid and
yield a precipitate of hydrous nickel oxide when the pH of dilute solutions
is raised above 6.7. The metal is uniquely resistant to the action of alkalies and is frequently used for containers to handle concentrated solutions
of sodium hydroxide. Most nickel salts form double compounds with other
salts and coordination complexes with ammonia. Nickel also forms coordination complexes with alkali cyanides similar to those of palladium and platinum.

Nickel compounds are used in electroplating, in ground-coat enamels, in storage batteries of the Edison type, and in nickel-alloy cooking utensils. More than 2,000,000 lb of the metal are used in catalytic applications each year. Nickel catalysts are used for hydrogenating fats and oils, in synthesis of organic chemicals and pharmaceuticals, in petroleum chemistry, and in gaseous fuel production. Nickel is used in nickel-chromium steels and in nickel silver and nickel steel.

Essentiality of Nickel

Nielsen et al. [627-630] have found that feeding a diet containing less than 40 ppb nickel resulted in an apparent nickel-deficiency syndrome in chicks. When compared to control chicks given 3-5 ppm nickel, the deficient chicks showed (a) pigmentation changes in the shank skin, (b) thicker legs with slightly swollen hocks, (c) dermatitis of the shank skin, (d) less friable liver, which may be related to the fat content, and (e) an enhanced accumulation of a tracer dose of ^{63}Ni in bone, liver, and aorta.

In a second experiment [631] the abnormalities were diminished or inconsistent in regard to leg structure or dermatitis. The other gross sign, a decrease in friability of the liver in deficient chicks, was observed in the second experiment. Sunderman et al. [632] have also attempted to repeat the first experiment. While observing no gross effects, they did observe ultrastructural changes in the liver. These included dilation of the perimitochondrial rough endoplasmic reticulum in 15 to 20% of the hepatocytes. In general, no significant weight differences were observed between the experimental and the control group.

In nickel-deficient rats several indexes of metabolism were consistently found [630]. These included decreased oxygen uptake by liver homogenates in the presence of α-glycerophosphate, an increase in liver lipids, a decrease in the liver phospholipids, and no apparent change in liver cholesterol.

Seven first-generation, nickel-deficient female rats which were mated had a significant fetal loss at birth (15%) compared with no perinatal mortality in the newborn pups of the six controls [630]. The nickel-deficient pups [631] had a rougher coat and were less active. Electronic monitoring of matched litters of second- and third-generation deficient and control sucklings showed that the nickel-deficient rats were more lethargic.

Nickel is widespread in its occurrence and is distributed widely in foods. Estimates of the daily human intake are from about 0.24 to 1.0 mg

Ni/day [633-640]. Vegetable material contains much more nickel than material from animal origin. Estimates of from 0.15 to 0.35 ppm Ni have been made for fruits, tubers, and grains [635,641]. Some items high in nickel were tea (7.6 ppm), buckwheat seed (6.4 ppm), herring, and oysters (6.0 ppm on a dry-weight basis) [635,641-644]. Low levels of nickel were observed in muscle meats, eggs, and milk.

Metabolism of Nickel

Studies [636,645] have indicated that normal dogs excrete 90% of ingested nickel in the feces and 10% in the urine. In man, urine nickel has been studied by several investigators. The average μg Ni/l has been found to be 20, 10, and 18 [646-648], respectively. Rats [649,650] have also been shown to absorb nickel poorly and to excrete it mainly in the feces. In two studies [639,651], the average daily fecal nickel concentration was 258 μg.

Studies with radioactive nickel (^{63}Ni) indicate that the compound is widely distributed in low concentrations in the tissues and rapidly eliminated. In rats given ^{63}Ni as nickel chloride [652], 61% of a single injection of ^{63}Ni was excreted via the urine within 72 hr, and 5.9% appeared in the feces. After 72 hr, only the kidney contained significant amounts of ^{63}Ni. Mean levels of nickel reported for human blood plasma were 0.04 [653], 0.03 [654], 0.02 [655], and 0.06 μg Ni/g blood [656]. The average level in red cells is similar to that reported in plasma, 0.053 μg Ni/g [656].

Nickel activates several enzyme systems including arginase [657], acetyl coenzyme A synthetase [658], carboxylase [659], trypsin [660], and phosphoglucomutase [661]. Another in vitro effect of nickel is the enhancement of the adhesiveness of polymorphonuclear leukocytes [662-664]. Nickel stabilizes RNA [665] and DNA [666] against thermal denaturation and is very effective in the preservation of tobacco mosaic virus RNA infectivity [667, 668]. Nickel may have a role in the compact structure of ribosomes against thermal denaturation [669-671] in that nickel will restore the sedimentation characteristics of Escherichia coli ribosomes which have been subjected to EDTA denaturation. Nickel may help maintain the configuration of the protein molecules of crystalline complexes of ribonuclease [672].

Significant concentrations of nickel are present in DNA [673,674] and RNA [643,662,668] from phylogenetically diverse sources. Nickel and other metals which are present may help stabilize the structure of nucleic acids.

A metalloprotein in human serum is rich in nickel [675]. The protein is an α-1 macroglobulin. It has been isolated from rabbit serum and has been designated "nickeloplasmin" [676]. It has an estimated molecular weight of 7.0×10^5 and contains 0.9 g atoms of nickel/mol.

Indirect evidence that suggests that nickel and other metals may play a role in pigmentation in several species of animals, fish, birds, and insects has been obtained by Kikkawa and co-workers [677,678].

Health Effects of Nickel

Concentrations of serum nickel become increased in patients following acute myocardial infarction, stroke, burns, and septicemia [679-681]. Diminished mean concentrations of serum nickel are found in patients with hepatic cirrhosis and with chronic renal insufficiency [679,680]. Measurements of nickel in serum, urine, feces, and hair are used as measures of environmental and occupational exposure to nickel [651,682,683].

SELENIUM

Chemistry of Selenium

Selenium is found in Group VIA of the periodic table between sulfur and tellurium. It has three important allotropic modifications: monoclinic (red) selenium, which has two crystalline forms; metallic (gray) selenium, which also exists in two forms; and amorphous selenium, which has three forms, vitreous, red amorphous, and colloidal selenium. Its abundance in the earth's crust is 0.000009%. There are no important ores of selenium, and it is usually recovered as a by-product of the refining of the sulfide ores of other metals, such as copper. Selenium has six stable isotopes with mass numbers 74, 76, 77, 78, 80, and 82.

The most important oxidation states of selenium are 2-, 2+, 4+, and 6+. Some of the known selenium compounds are H_2Se, metallic selenides, SeO_2, H_2SeO_3, SeF_4, Se_2Cl_2, and H_2SEO_4 (selenic acid). Selenic acid possesses the unusual property of dissolving gold. The most notable selenium compound is the oxychloride ($SeOCl_2$), a yellowish corrosive liquid which attacks most metals and is a good solvent for sulfur, selenium, tellurium rubber, bakelite, gums, resins, celluloid, gelatin, glue, asphalt, and other materials. Selenium also forms a large number of organic compounds that are analogous to those of sulfur.

The greatest amounts of selenium are used for the manufacture of the photoelectric cell. Some selenium is used for xerography and the electronics

industry also makes use of the element in selenium rectifiers. Selenium is
used in ceramics and in the rubber industry. A small amount corrects the
green color of glass, and a large amount gives the ruby color to glass, so
important in taillights and signals. Red enamelware contains selenium. In
the rubber industry, selenium is used along with sulfur and tellurium to
increase the tensile strength, abrasion resistance, and life of rubber.
Selenium is used as a catalyst and in flameproofing electric cable.

Essentiality of Selenium

Schwarz [684] found that rats fed a torula yeast diet develop a fatal
liver necrosis which could be prevented by brewer's yeast, despite the absence of sufficient cystine or vitamin E to account for its protective action. This led Schwarz [684] to postulate the presence of a third anti-
liver-necrosis factor, designated "Factor 3." Selenite supplements were
shown to protect against liver necrosis in the same manner as Factor 3 itself [685].

Subsequent selenium therapy was found to be effective in the treatment
of various myopathies including white muscle disease (WMD) in lambs, calves,
and foals [686-690] and hepatosis dietetica in pigs [691,692]. Selenium-
supplemented sheep had improved growth as well as fertility and reduced
postnatal losses in certain areas [687,688,693]. Neither the resorption
sterility in rats [694] nor the encephalomalacia in chicks [695] that arises
on vitamin E-deficient diets responds to selenium.

Unequivocal evidence that selenium is essential for growth independent
of vitamin E was not obtained until Thompson and Scott [696] fed purified
crystalline amino acid diets containing less than 0.005 ppm Se to chicks.
With variable amounts of vitamin E, growth was inferior to that obtained
with selenium and no added vitamin E. McCoy and Weswig [697] and Wu et al.
[698] reported similar data with rats. Selenium was also found to be essential for the growth of quail [699].

Selenium levels are greatest in meat, especially kidney and liver.
Vegetable and fruit products are quite low in selenium. Barley, wheat, and
rice have intermediate selenium levels [700,701]. The human requirement is
not known.

A dietary intake of 0.1 ppm provides an adequate intake by grazing
sheep and cattle [702]. A minimum requirement of 0.06 ppm Se for the prevention of WMD in lambs was reported by Oldfield et al. [703]. Gardiner
and Gorman [704] have shown that white muscle disease can occur in lambs
grazing Australian pastures estimated to contain 0.05 ppm Se. A torula

yeast diet containing 0.056 ppm Se and 100 IU vitamin E/lb could not maintain maximum growth in chicks unless it was supplemented with 0.04 ppm as
sodium selenite [705]. The selenium requirement in turkey poults ranged
from 0.18 to 0.28 ppm depending on vitamin E levels [696]. The importance
of vitamin E in chick selenium requirements is illustrated by the experiments
of Scott et al. [706]. Selenium requirements for using purified diets ranged
from 100 ppm vitamin E and 0.01 ppm selenium to 10 ppm vitamin E and 0.05 ppm
Se.

Metabolism of Selenium

Studies with ^{75}Se at physiological levels indicate that the duodenum
is the main site of absorption of selenium in sheep or pigs [707]. The
total net absorption represented approximately 35% of the ingested isotope
in sheep and 85% in pigs. Monogastric animals have a higher intestinal absorption of selenium than ruminants [708,709]. Radioselenium is more efficiently retained from Se-deficient than from Se-supplemented diets by chicks
[710], rats [711,712], and sheep [713,714].

Absorbed selenium is at first carried mainly in the plasma [715], apparently in association with the plasma proteins [716]. From the plasma,
selenium enters all the tissues, including the bones, the hair, and the
erythrocytes [709,715,717,718]. The intracellular distribution of ^{75}Se was
uniform among the particulates and soluble fraction in liver, whereas nearly
75% of the activity in kidney cortex was found in the nuclear fraction [714].
Of the subcellular fractions, the microsomes appear to be the initial site
for incorporating selenium into protein [719].

Selenium is believed to replace sulfur in certain amino acids to form
selenocystine or selenomethionine which are incorporated into protein [720,
721]. On the other hand, Cummings and Martin [722] have offered evidence
that the selenium associated with cystine or methionine is merely selenite
bound to the sulfur compounds.

Selenium is transmissible through the placenta to the fetus. This has
been observed in the mouse [723], rat [724], dog [725,726], and sheep [713,
714]. Selenium administration to the mother during pregnancy prevents WMD
in lambs and calves.

Purification of ovine erythrocyte glutathione peroxidase chromatographed
on Sephadex G150 showed a coincidence of protein concentration, glutathione
peroxidase activity, and selenium content [727], indicating glutathione
peroxidase to be a selenium-containing enzyme. Dietary supplementation of

selenium increases glutathione peroxidase activity of rat erythrocytes [727]. Glutathione peroxidase in conjunction with reduced glutathione (GSH) causes the breakdown of hydrogen peroxide to water. GSH and glutathione peroxidase are important in maintaining membrane integrity in the face of "oxidant stress" imposed by various drugs such as primaquine, sulfanilamide, etc. GSH and glutathione peroxidase protect the cell by their role in peroxide decomposition and possibly by maintaining protein-SH groups through SH-SS interchange.

Additional selenoproteins in animal tissues have also become evident, such as the muscle protein studied by Whanger et al. [728], which appears to have the properties of a cytochrome. Another selenoprotein has been found in plasma [729]. A role for Se in the microsomal system of liver has been proposed by Diplock [730], and a role in catalyzing cytochrome c reduction by glutathione has been postulated [731]. Selenium may also be concerned in the biosynthesis of ubiquinone (coenzyme Q) [732-734].

Health Effects of Selenium

Selenium and Muscular Dystrophy. Nutritional muscular dystrophy is a degenerative disease of the striated muscles which occurs, without a neural involvement, in a wide range of animal species. The disease has been observed in lambs, calves, foals, rabbits, and even marsupials. White muscle disease rarely occurs in mature animals. In lambs, it is most common between 3 and 6 weeks of age. The deep muscles overlying the cervical vertebrae are particularly affected with the typical chalky white striations. Animals may also have severe heart involvement. Bilateral symmetrical distribution of the skeletal muscle lesions is characteristic of muscular dystrophy or white muscle disease in lambs. WMD in lambs is characterized further by subnormal levels of selenium in blood and tissues and by abnormally high levels of serum glutamic oxalacetic transaminase (SGOT) and of lactic dehydrogenase (LDH) [735-737]. Only partial control of congenital muscular dystrophy can be secured with tocopherol [687,688,690,693,738] administration. Because of its economic significance, WMD in lambs has received the most attention, but similar degenerative changes occur in foals [693], pigs [739], and chicks [705]. In all these species, the disease can be prevented by selenium supplementation.

Exudative Diathesis in Chicks. Exudative diathesis was first observed in chicks consuming vitamin E-free diets containing cod-liver oil [740]. Edema first appears on the breast, wing, and neck and later has the appearance of massive cutaneous hemorrhages, arising from abnormal permeability

of the capillary walls and accumulation of fluid throughout the body. A
greenish-blue discoloration occurs under the ventral skin. Plasma proteins
are low in the blood of affected chicks, and an anemia develops which may
be related to the hemorrhages that occur [741].

Chicks are most commonly affected at 3-6 weeks of age. α-tocopherol
and ethoxyquin reduce the incidence and severity of the disease. The addition of selenium is completely effective in preventing the disease and the
chicks grow better than when supplemented with tocopherol alone [742-744].
White muscle disease affecting the breast muscles often develops along with
the exudative diathesis, and a congenital myopathy characterized by the
hatching of dead chicks or chicks dying 3-4 days later is another Se-respon-
sive condition in this species [743]. Encephalomalacia does not respond to
selenium supplements but only to the addition of vitamin E to the diets.

Hepatosis Dietetica in Pigs. When young pigs are fed diets low in
vitamin E or selenium, mortality is high and deaths occur suddenly. Severe
necrotic liver lesions are apparent, usually with some degree of myocardial
and skeletal muscle degeneration. There is deposition of ceroid pigment in
adipose tissue, which gives a yellowish-brown color to the body fat [691-
693,739,745]. Selenium supplements are completely effective in preventing
the mortality and liver lesions, but selenium may not be as effective as
vitamin E in preventing the skeletal muscle degeneration or pigment deposition which occurs in this disease [692,739].

Selenium-Responsive Unthriftiness in Sheep and Cattle. In New Zealand
a serious condition known as "ill-thrift" occurs in lambs at pasture and
can occur in beef and dairy cattle of all ages [693,745]. Ill-thrift can
be prevented by selenium treatment, with striking increases in growth and
wool yield in some instances [693,703,745-748]. In lambs neither vitamin
E nor the antioxidant ethoxyquin has any effect on unthriftiness [749].

Peridontal Disease of Ewes. Peridontal disease in ewes occurs at 3-5
years of age and is characterized by loosening and shedding of permanent
molars or incisors in conjunction with gingival hyperplasia, resorption,
and replacement fibrosis of alveolar bone, alveolar infection, and bony
exostoses on the adjacent part of the mandible or maxilla [750,751]. The
disease virtually disappeared on affected properties after selenium dosing.

Selenium and Fertility in Animals. In parts of California, annual
losses occur due to the birth of premature, weak, or dead calves. These
losses were shown to be completely prevented by injecting cows, 50-60 days

before calving, with a sodium selenite-vitamin E mixture [752]. Similar results were obtained with selenium alone [753] in New Zealand.

Selenium deficiency results in reduced hatchability of fertile eggs and reduced viability of newly hatched Japanese quail [754]. Rats fed a low-Se, torula yeast diet with adequate vitamin E have poor hair growth and reduced fertility [697]. Immotile sperms, with separation of heads from tails, were found in five of the eight males. Rats fed Se-deficient diets also had degenerative changes of the epididymis as well as impaired testicular function [698]. One ppm Se as Na_2SeO_3 restored hair coat, growth, and reproductive capabilities of the rats.

Selenium and Cancer. Sodium selenide as well as several other antioxidants prevented skin tumor formation in mice [755,756]. Sodium selenite-supplemented torula yeast diets also significantly decreased skin tumor formation in mice [756]. In addition, there is an inverse relationship between the soil content of selenium and human cancer mortality in several countries [757,758]. In some unpublished work we have observed a significant inverse correlation coefficient between the blood content of selenium and the age-adjusted human cancer mortality in 19 cities.

When the mortality from several types of cancer are compared in the high- and low-selenium areas, there are much lower death rates from the types of cancer in organs which might come into contact with selenium than in the organs which do not come into contact directly with selenium. There is a much lower death rate from cancer of the digestive organs in the high-selenium areas [757,758].

Selenium as well as other antioxidants may be stabilizing or breaking down malonaldehyde, a product of peroxidative breakdown of unsaturated fatty acids. Malonaldehyde is a carcinogen [759,760] which is present in foods such as beans and chicken. In some unpublished work we have observed as much as 4 mg/100 g of chicken. Malonaldehyde is also present in human feces indicating the entire gastrointestinal tract has come into contact with a carcinogen.

Selenium in the form of sodium selenite as well as other antioxidants reduced carcinogen-induced chromosome breakage when compared to the controls [761,762]. Selenium blood levels are lower in patients with gastrointestinal cancer or liver metastases [763].

Clayton and Baumann [764] found that the inclusion of 5 ppm of selenium in a purified diet reduced the incidence of liver tumors in rats induced by

N^1-methyl-p-dimethylaminoazobenzene. Dietary selenium has also reduced N-2-
fluorenyl-acetamide-induced cancer in vitamin E-supplemented depleted rats
[765]. The subject of selenium and cancer has been reviewed by Shapiro
[766]. Dietary Se at levels above that generally accepted as nutritionally
adequate (0.1 ppm) enhances the primary immune response in mice as measured
by the plaque-forming cell test and by hemagglutination [767].

Selenium and Heart Disease. Patients taking selenium-tocopherol cap-
sules (Tolsem) have shown reduced incidence of anginal pain in 22 of 24
cases [768]. Similar results in other trials by Ingvoldstad [769] have been
summarized.

Rats fed selenium-deficient diets develop abnormal electrocardiograms
[770]. Selenium-deficient lambs also have abnormal electrocardiograms accompanied by blood pressure changes and histopathology [771]. In piglets
born of selenium- and vitamin E-deprived sows, progressive vascular damage
was observed. Connective tissue lesions of the heart were noted. This
change appears to characterize mulberry heart disease of swine and may result in the sudden death of the animal.

Cadmium has been observed to cause hypertension in rats and is also
present in high concentration in kidney and urine of hypertensive patients
[772,773]. The cadmium pressor effect caused by 2.5 and 10 ppm of cadmium
in the drinking water can be reversed by 3 ppm selenium in the drinking
water [774].

In a recent epidemiological study, it was shown that the age-specific
death rates per 100,000 for cardiovascular-renal cerebrovascular, coronary,
and hypertensive heart disease were all significantly lower ($P < 0.001$) in
the very high selenium area than in the low-selenium area [775]. For the
most part, there was an inverse gradation in mortality and selenium bioavailability. Comparisons between nine types of heart mortality in 17 cities
showed significantly lower death rates in regard to arteriosclerotic and
hypertensive heart disease for both males and females.

Nonwhite mortality rates were markedly greater for cerebrovascular
hypertensive heart disease [775]. The nonwhite are located in inner city
areas where there is a greater chance of airborne cadmium pollution which
has been previously correlated with arteriosclerotic and hypertensive heart
diseases.

A positive correlation has been observed between age-adjusted arteriosclerotic heart disease and colon cancer [776] which has also previously

been shown to be inversely related to selenium, indicating possible similarities in the mechanisms of the two diseases.

SILICON

Chemistry of Silicon

Silicon is the second most abundant of the elements in the earth's
crust (27.72%), surpassed in quantity only by oxygen. Silicon occurs mainly
in the silicate form. The general formulas are SiO_2 or SiO_3 or multiples
thereof. Several isotopes with mass numbers 28, 29, and 30 are known. Silicon is found in Group IVA of the periodic table, between carbon and germanium. Silicon is a metalloid (exhibits both metallic and nonmetallic properties) and a semiconductor. Silicon is gray-black, crystalline, lustrous,
brittle, and exceedingly hard.

Silicon is reactive at high temperatures, combining directly with most
elements to form silicides, such as magnesium silicide (Mg_2Si) and silicon
compounds, such as silicon dioxide (SiO_2), silicon fluoride (SiF_4), and
silicon carbide (SiC). Silicon dissolves in hot sodium hydroxide with the
evolution of hydrogen.

$$Si + 4NaOH \rightarrow Na_4SiO_4 + 2H_2$$

Silicon forms two well-defined oxyacids: orthosilicic acid (H_4SiO_4) and
metasilicic acid (H_2SiO_3). They exist only in solution and decompose irre-
versibly into silicon dioxide if the water is evaporated. Oxidation states
of silicon are 4-, 2+, and 4+.

The silicates are the foundation material for various ceramic industries.
These industries include glass, vitreous enamels, portland cement, abrasives,
building brick, paving brick, tile, earthenware (pottery, sewer pipe), and
whiteware (china, decorative porcelain). Silicon carbide is one of the
hardest materials ever made and is useful in grinding wheels and in abrasive
paper and cloth products. Silicates are important constituents of glass.
By fusion with two or more oxides, commonly sodium oxide Na_2O and lime CaO,
both introduced as carbonate, silica forms the silica glass. Silicone polymers are a group of synthetic polymers composed of silicon, carbon, hydrogen,
and oxygen. They are noted for their ability to withstand comparatively
high temperatures without decomposing. Silicon added to steel improves the
magnetic (electrical) characteristics of steel.

Essentiality of Silicon

Carlisle [777,778] first reported that silicon is necessary for an early
stage of bone calcification in rats and chicks. The first clear evidence
that silicon is essential for animals was reported in 1972 [779,780]. Chicks
fed a silicon-deficient diet had depressed growth, along with pallor of the
legs, comb, skin, and mucous membranes. Subcutaneous tissue had a muddy to
yellowish color in contrast to the white-pinkish subcutaneous tissue of the
silicon-adequate control animals. The comb of deficient chicks was severely
attenuated and they had no wattles. Feathering was retarded. Silicon may be
involved in some aspect of bone calcification because leg bones had a thinner
cortex and were shorter and of smaller circumference than the controls. Fe-
murs and tibias fractured more easily, cranial bones were flatter, and beaks
were more flexible. Silicon deficiency also results in depressed growth and
skull deformations [781]. Skeletal alterations [782] involve the cartilage
matrix. In the silicon-deficient chick metatarsus and tibial epiphyses,
epiphyseal plates and spongiosae, there is a significant decrease in hexosamines.

The chick requirement for silicon as sodium silicate is in the range
of 100 to 200 µg/g [783]. Other forms may be more available than the silicate. Foods high in silicon include unrefined grains such as unpolished
rice. Beer is a saturated solution of silicon containing approximately
1200 µg/g. Dietary items of animal origin, except skin (i.e., chicken),
are relatively low in silicon.

Metabolism of Silicon

Silicon may have a role in mucopolysaccharide metabolism. Silicon is
a constituent of certain glycosaminoglycans and polyuronides where it is
apparently bound to the polysaccharide matrix [784]. There are 330 to 554
µg of bound silicon/g of purified hyaluronic acid from the umbilical cord,
chondroitin 4-sulfate, dermatan sulfate, and heparan sulfate. Lesser amounts
of 57 to 191 µg/g were found in chondroitin 6-sulfate, heparin, and keratan
sulfate-2 from cartilage. Vitreous humor hyaluronic acid and cornes keratan
sulfate-1 were silicon free.

Schwarz has suggested that silicon is present as a silanolate, i.e.,
an ether (or ester-like derivative of silicic acid). He postulated that
silicon has a structural role in the glycosaminoglycans and polyuronides.
Silicon may link portions of either the same polysaccharides to each other,
acid mucopolysaccharides to each other, or acid mucopolysaccharides to

proteins. Silicon may function as a biological cross-linking agent and may contribute to the structure and resilience of connective tissue.

Health Effects of Silicon

Silicon and Aging. Embryonic or rapidly growing tissue has a far greater mucopolysaccharide content than adult or aging tissue. Silicon is known to be a component of the mucopolysaccharides [782]. The silicon content of the aorta, skin, and thymus is found to decline significantly with age in contrast with other analyzed tissues which showed little or no change.

Leslie et al. [785] also found a decrease in silicon content of rat skin with age. In contrast, other tissues, such as brain, liver, spleen, lung, and femur, showed an increase.

Similarly in human skin, the silicon content of the dermis diminishes with age [786,787]. The silicon content of the aorta decreases considerably with age [788], and arterial wall silicon decreases with the development of atherosclerosis [789]. Silicon absorption changes in the blood and intestinal tissues of rats in relation to age, sex, and various endocrine glands [790]. The decline of hormonal activity in senescence could well account for the modifications in silicon observed in aged animals.

Silicon Urolithiasis. Although silica is readily eliminated, under some conditions a part of it is deposited in the kidney, bladder, or urethra to form calculi or uroliths. Small calculi are excreted harmlessly, but sometimes they become so large that they block the passage of urine and the death of the animal ansues. Silica urolithiasis is a serious problem in grazing wethers in western Australia [791] and in grazing steers in the western regions of Canada [792,793] and the northwestern regions of the United States [794,795].

Attempts to form siliceous calculi by adding silicates to the diet [777,793] or by restricting water consumption [796] have been unsuccessful even when the urine level was two to three times the 70-80 μg/ml level at which silicon normally precipitates in bovine urine [797]. The mechanism by which the calculi are formed is unknown.

TIN

Chemistry of Tin

Tin is a soft, ductile, metallic element whose atomic number is 50, and whose atomic weight is 118.69. It is classified in Group IV of the

periodic table. Tin is present in the igneous rocks of the earth's crust
to the extent of about 0.001%. Cassiterite (SnO_2), the only tin-bearing
mineral of commercial importance, occurs in low-grade alluvial and lode
deposits.

The valence number of tin is 2+ and 4+. There are 10 naturally occurring isotopes. Tin can also exist in two allotropic forms: white tin (β)
and gray tin (α).

Halogen acids dissolve tin, particularly when hot and concentrated.
Both hot sulfuric and cold, dilute nitric acid will dissolve tin. Hot
nitric acid converts the tin to metastannic acid (hydrated tin oxide).
Dilute solutions of weak alkalies, such as ammonium hydroxide or sodium
carbonate, have little effect on tin. Strong alkalies, such as sodium or
potassium hydroxide, dissolve tin with the formation of stannates.

Tin is used for electroplating food containers, in solders, in bronze,
in aluminum tin, and for improving the metallic properties of various alloys.

Essentiality of Tin

Trace amounts of tin occur in many tissues and dietary items, but until
recently the element has been considered an "environmental contaminant" instead of an essential dietary factor. Stimulatory activities in plants have
been reported [798,799].

In 1970, it was reported that tin is essential for the growth of rats
maintained on purified amino acid diets in a trace element-controlled environment [800]. Rats required 1 µg tin as stannic sulfate per gram of
experimental diet for optimal growth. Trimethyl tin hydroxide, dibutyl tin
maleate, stannic sulfate, and potassium stannate enhanced growth at dose
levels supplying 100 µg% (1 ppm) of tin to the diet. When supplied in the
form of stannic sulfate, 50, 100, and 200 µg% of tin increased growth by
24, 53, and 59%, respectively (Table 2). These levels of tin are similar
to those normally present in foods, feeds, and tissues.

Metabolism of Tin

Kehoe et al. [801] have carried out a thorough spectrochemical study
of human tissues and fluids. They found tin in 80% of the samples. Distribution of tin was even, but no tin has been found in the brain [801,802].
Kehoe reported 0.1 ppm in muscle, 0.2 ppm in kidney, heart, spleen, and intestines, and 0.8 ppm Sn in fresh bone. Tin [802] tended to accumulate in
the lungs with advancing age, but not in the liver, kidney, aorta, or

TABLE 2. Growth Effect of Tin Compounds in Rats in Trace Element-Controlled Environment.[a] (Duration of Experiments 26-29 Days)

Compounds	Dose (μg Sn/100 g)	No. of Animals	Average Daily Weight Gain (g) $\bar{x}$ (± SE)	Increase (%)	P Value
Basal A					
Control	--	5	1.89 ± 0.06	--	--
Trimethyl tin hydroxide, $(CH_3)_3SnOH$	100	4	2.22 ± 0.09	18	0.02
Dibutyl tin maleate, $(C_4H_9)_2Sn(OOCCH=)_2$	100	5	2.16 ± 0.14	14	0.1
Basal B					
Control	--	7	1.27 ± 0.11	--	--
Stannic sulfate, $Sn(SO_4)_2 \cdot 2H_2O$	100	7	1.67 ± 0.07	31	0.01
Potassium stannate, $K_2SnO_3 \cdot 3H_2O$[b]	100	8	1.55 ± 0.10	22	0.1
Control	--	5[c]	1.10 ± 0.05	--	--
Stannic sulfate, $Sn(SO_4)_2 \cdot 2H_2O$	50	8	1.37 ± 0.10	24	0.02
Stannic sulfate	100	8	1.68 ± 0.10	53	<0.001
Stannic sulfate	200	8	1.75 ± 0.10	59	<0.001

[a] Reprinted from Ref. 800 by courtesy of Academic Press.
[b] Better formulated as $K_2[Sn(OH)_6]$.
[c] Two control animals died in the course of the experiment. One animal was eliminated because it was outside of the normal error.

intestines. Groups from Europe, Africa, and Asia had lower mean and median values for kidney, liver, and lung than the Americans.

Kehoe et al. reported the mean daily intake by a normal adult American to be 17 mg. This intake is several times greater than the 1.5 and 2.5 mg/day obtained by Tipton et al. [803] and the 3.5 mg/day calculated by Schroeder et al. [802]. Schroeder and co-workers [802] estimated that a 2400-kcal diet composed largely of fresh meats, grain products and vegetables which are low in tin content would supply 1 mg/day. But a diet including a substantial proportion of canned vegetables and fish could supply as much as 38 mg/day.

Large amounts of tin can accumulate in foods in contact with tinplate [804], particularly when nonlacquered. The introduction of lacquered cans and the crimping of the tops, thus allowing little direct contact of the food with solder, reduces the source of tin for modern civilized man. The lower daily intakes of tin reported by Schroeder [802] and Tipton [803] may be due to the modern improvements in canning, compared to a few decades earlier when Kehoe et al. [801] obtained their high estimates of daily tin intakes.

Evidence indicates that tin is poorly absorbed and is excreted mainly in the feces. The amounts excreted daily in the urine have been estimated to be 23.4 µg [805], 16 µg [801], and 8-11 µg/day for two adults [803]. Fecal excretion approximated the total amount of tin ingested with the food [802].

Health Effects of Tin

Tin has a number of chemical properties that offer possibilities for a biological function. Tetravalent tin has a strong tendency to form coordination complexes with four, five, six, and possibly eight ligands. Thus, tin [800] may contribute to the tertiary structure of proteins or other components of biological importance. Tin [800] may participate in oxidation-reduction reactions in biological systems because the $Sn^{2+} \rightleftarrows Sn^{4+}$ potential of 0.13 volts is within the physiological range near the oxidation-reduction potential of flavine enzymes. Tin also forms covalent bonds with carbon and a large number of organotin compounds are known. Some of these serve as catalysts in polymerization, transesterification, olefin condensation, and other reactions.

A colloidal mixture of 99 $\underline{m}$ Tc-Sn has been used for liver scanning [806] and for brain [807] and skeletal [808] scintigraphy.

VANADIUM

Chemistry

Vanadium is widely distributed in various minerals, coal, and petroleum. Although it is estimated to comprise between 0.02 and 0.03% of the earth's crust, ores of commercial value occur in only a few places. The principal commercial ores are partonite, roscoelite, vanadinite, and carnotite.

Vanadium has the atomic number 23 and an atomic weight of 50.94. It is the first member of subgroup V of the periodic table, which also includes niobium and tantalum in order of increasing atomic weight. Like its congeners in the subgroup, vanadium may be described as seminoble. When heated with oxygen, nitrogen, carbon, and sulfur, it forms the oxides V_2O_3, VO, VO_2, and V_2O_5, the nitride VN, the carbides VC and V_4C_3, and the sulfides VS_2 and V_2S_5. Subgroup V forms compounds with a maximum oxidation state of 5. The other oxidation states possessed by vanadium in its compounds are 2, 3, or 4. Vanadium dissolves in nitric acid but not hydrochloric or sulfuric acid. The basicity of the hydrogen-oxygen compounds of vanadium varies with the oxidation state. In the two lower oxidation states, 2 and 3, these compounds are basic; in oxidation states 4 and 5, they are amphoteric.

Vanadium is added to constructional steels to improve elastic properties, toughness, and yield-to-tensile strength ratios. Vanadium foil is used to bond steel and titanium in cladding pure titanium metal to steel.

Essentiality of Vanadium

Vanadium has been demonstrated to be an essential requirement in two microorganisms: the mold Aspergillus niger [809] and the green alga Scenedesmus obiquus, where it may be concerned with photosynthesis [810]. A need for vanadium has also been demonstrated for a thermophilic yeast, Candida sloofi, when grown at high enough temperatures [811]. Growth effects in higher plants have been related to the capacity of vanadium to substitute for molybdenum as a catalyst of nitrogen fixation in Azotobacter and other bacteria [812-814]. In regard to mammalian metabolism, vanadium enhances the development of wing and tail feathers in chicks raised under carefully controlled conditions on a casein-based diet; however, the growth rates of these chicks were not affected [815]. Using a highly purified amino acid diet, Schwarz has demonstrated that vanadium added to the diet enhances growth by over 40% [816] (Table 3). It appears that the physiologically essential levels of vanadium lie at or below 0.1 ppm of dry matter. The

TABLE 3. Growth Response of Rats to Varying Levels of Vanadium Supplements (Sodium Orthovanadate, Na_3VO_4). Pooled Results of Five Successive Experiments Are Shown for Each Dose. Total Increase Is Given as the Percentage Gain over a 21- to 28-Day Period[a]

Dose ($\mu g/100$ g of diet)	Unsupplemented Controls		Supplemented Animals		Total Increase (%)	P
	Rats[b] (no.)	Average Daily Weight Gain (g) (± 5E)	Rats (no.)	Average Daily Weight Gain (g) (± 5E)		
1	7	1.05 ± 0.08	7	1.27 ± 0.10	21	N.S.[c]
5	16	1.04 ± 0.08	16	1.38 ± 0.08	33	< 0.01
10	6	1.02 ± 0.14	7	1.38 ± 0.07	35	< 0.05
25	14	0.87 ± 0.10	14	1.21 ± 0.09	41	< 0.02
50	6	1.02 ± 0.14	7	1.49 ± 0.12	46	< 0.02

[a] Klaus Schwarz and D. B. Milne, Science, 174, 426-428 (1971). (Copyright 1971 by the American Association for the Advancement of Science.)

[b] A total of 37 rats served as controls in five successive experiments.

[c] N.S., not significant.

rat requirement is approximately as much vanadium as is needed in the media for Aspergillus niger and Scenedesmus obliquus to support growth; the effective concentration in these media was in the order of 10^{-8}, equivalent to 0.1 ppm of dry weight in the medium. The amount of vanadium required by the rat is also quite close to that calculated as the daily vanadium intake for man. A rat weighing 75 g needs 1 to 2 μg of vanadium per day (25 $\mu g/100$ g of diet) for an optimal growth response, while a human with an average weight of 75 kg has been estimated to consume 2 mg of vanadium daily [816]. The total amount in man's body is estimated to be 17 to 43 mg [817]. In Schwarz's rat experiment, the vanadyl acetate [$VO(CH_3COO^-)_2$] and the vanadyl sulfate ($VOSO_4$) had significant growth effects while sodium metavanadate ($NaVO_3 \cdot 4H_2O$) and the sodium pyrovanadate ($Na_4V_2O_7$) had little or no growth effect (Table 4). Nielsen has estimated that a vanadium intake of approximately 100 ng/g for chicks is probably adequate with an experimental diet composed of 26% protein, 6% fat, and 57% carbohydrate with a balance of minerals, vitamins, and nonnutritive fiber. Depressed growth occurs for chicks at 30 to 35 ng vanadium/g. Strasia [819] found that rats fed less than 100 ng vanadium/g exhibited reduced body growth and a significantly increased blood packed-cell volume when compared with controls receiving at least 0.5 μg vanadium/g. He also noted an increase in blood and bone iron in deficient rats.

TABLE 4. Effect of Different Vanadium Salts on Growth of Rats in an "Ultra-clean" Environment[a]

Dose (µg/100 g of diet)	Rats (no.)	Average Increase (%)	P[b]
Sodium metavanadate, $NaVO_3 \cdot 4H_2O$			
5	8	8	N.S.
5	8	18	N.S.
Sodium pyrovanadate, $Na_4V_2O_7$			
5	8	-8	N.S.
10	8	9	N.S.
Vanadyl sulfate, $VOSO_4$			
1	8	4	N.S.
5	7	27	< 0.05
Vanadyl acetate, $VO(CH_3COO^-)_2$			
5	7	16	N.S.
10	8	21	< 0.05
25	8	18	< 0.10

[a]Klaus Schwarz and D. B. Milne, Science, 174, 426-428 (1971). (Copyright 1971 by the American Association for the Advancement of Science.)
[b]N.S., not significant.

The major determinant of vanadium intake is the type of fat in the diet. A diet high in unsaturated fatty acids from vegetable sources results in higher vanadium intakes than one containing saturated fats from animal sources. Up to 43 ppm were found in soybean oil and in corn, olive, linseed, and peanut oils. Such high concentrations were not found in castor and codliver oil or in lard or butter. Beef, pork, deer, and chicken fats were relatively high in this element. Söremark [820], using neutron activation analysis, found less than 0.1 ng vanadium/g in peas, carrots, beets, and pears, compared to 52 ng/g in radishes. Milk generally contains less than 0.1 ng/g (fresh basis), and liver, fish, and meat contain up to 10 ng per g. A large number of vanadium food analyses have been summarized by Schlettwein-Gsell [821].

In a study of blood from male donors from 19 U.S. cities, Allaway and co-workers [822] found over 90% of the samples contained less than 1 µg V per 100 ml of whole blood. The highest concentration was 2 µg/100 ml. These concentrations are lower than those reported by Butt et al. [823] and

by Schroeder [817]. Schroeder reported 23 μg V/100 ml blood in the serum
of elderly controls.

Vanadium Metabolism

Vanadium salts at intakes beyond physiological levels are poorly absorbed from the gastrointestinal tract and appear in the feces. Between
0.1 and 1.0% of the vanadium in 100 mg of the soluble diammonium oxytartaro-
vanadate was absorbed from the human gut [824] in one study. In another
study, 60% of absorbed vanadium was excreted in the urine in the first 24
hr [825]. Small amounts of vanadium (0-8 μg/day) are normally excreted in
the urine of man [817,826]. Söreberg and Ullberg [827] found the greatest
amount of ^{48}V in the bones and teeth of mice, and Hathcock et al. [828]
found the greatest retention in the bones and kidneys of chicks. Hopkins
and Tilton [829] found that liver, kidneys, spleen, and testes accumulated
^{48}V up to 4 hr after injection and retained most of this activity up to 96
hr. During this period, the amount of ^{48}V in the liver subcellular supernatant fraction decreased from 57 to 11%, whereas the mitochondrial and
nuclear fractions increased from 14 to 40%. It was suggested that the
marked liver retention of ^{48}V was due to its movement into the mitochondrial
and nuclear fractions.

Although the function of vanadium in intermediary metabolism is unknown,
it catalyzes the in vitro oxidation of phospholipids by mammalian liver
protein fractions [830]. Vanadium is highly active as a catalyst in the
nonenzymatic oxidation of catecholamines, dihydroxyphenylalanine, and 5-
hydroxyindoles [831]. Vanadium and iron atoms are present in ribonucleic
acid from yeast [832].

Health Effects of Vanadium

Vanadium and Cholesterol, Triglyceride, and Glucose Metabolism. Vanadium reduces the in vivo cholesterol level in plasma in the aorta in rabbits
and in healthy human subjects as well [824,833-836]. This inhibition was
accompanied by decreased plasma phospholipids. Mean serum cholesterol levels
in workmen exposed to industrial sources of vanadium were found to be slightly
but significantly lower (205 mg/100 ml) than that of controls (228 mg/100 ml).
In older human patients and in patients with hypercholesterololemia or
ischemic heart disease, vanadium does not lower serum cholesterol [817,837-
840]. Curran and Burch [837] observed a stimulation of cholesterol biosynthesis by vanadium in 500- to 600-g rats.

Its antiatherosclerotic action in younger subjects appears to be due to interference with cholesterol synthesis by inhibiting utilization of mevalonic acid [824] and also acceleration of cholesterol catabolism [833]. Vanadium inhibits synthesis of cholesterol from acetate as well but not from squalene [840]. The microsomal enzyme system referred to as squalene synthetase is a site of vanadium inhibition, because vanadium inhibits the conversion of labeled farnesyl pyrophosphate to squalene [841]. A possible explanation of the age-related effect of vanadium on cholesterol biosynthesis in the rat [837] is that in the young animal, vanadium may decrease cholesterol synthesis both by enhancing acetoacetyl-CoA deacylase, thus reducing the acetoacetyl pool, and by its inhibition of squalene synthesis. The older animals may not be affected because there is no effect or an actual increase in the acetoacetyl CoA pool due to an inhibition of acetoacetyl-CoA deacylase with consequent increased cholesterol synthesis. Vanadium counteracts the stimulation of cholesterol synthesis induced by manganese, and manganese nullifies both the stimulatory effect of vanadium on hepatic phospholipid oxidation and its depressant action on cholesterol synthesis [842, 843]. Vanadium-deficient chicks had decreased plasma levels of cholesterol at 28 days of age, but at 49 their plasma cholesterol concentrations were greater than those of the control animals. With a diet based on peanut meal-sucrose-lard containing 30 to 35 ng vanadium/g, similarly decreased plasma cholesterol levels were found as early as 14 days of deficiency, whereas after only 28 days, significantly increased plasma cholesterol levels occurred [818]. Recent data indicate that plasma triglyceride levels are also significantly increased in vanadium-deficient chicks [844,845]. Although Bernheim et al. [846] showed no effect of vanadium on glucose substrate, reinvestigation with the intact animal using sensitive radiotracer techniques showed that glucose utilization was significantly increased 1 to 3 hr after vanadium administration. This may explain why triglyceride levels are lower with vanadium as glucose is a precursor of glycerol in the glycolytic scheme of carbohydrate metabolism.

Vanadium, Other Trace Elements, and Cardiovascular Disease. It may be of interest to note that hard waters, whose consumption is statistically associated with a lower incidence of cardiovascular disease in many areas of the world, contain vanadium whereas soft waters do not [847]. Furthermore, Schroeder [848] found a significant negative correlation between the vanadium content of municipal waters and atherosclerotic heart death rates.

In addition to the possible correlation between vanadium content of municipal waters and atherosclerotic heart disease, there is evidence that trace elements may play a general role in preventing cardiovascular diseases. A very interesting example is the statistical association found by several investigators in different countries between the softness of drinking water and the incidence of cardiovascular diseases. Reports from England, Ireland, Japan, Sweden, and the United States show that death rates from ischemic heart disease and from other cardiovascular diseases are higher in areas supplied with soft water than in areas served by hard water [848-861].

In soft-water areas at necropsy, the prevalence of myocardial scars, of atheroma, and of stenosis of the lumen has also been found to be higher in soft-water areas [854]. These findings suggest that the lack of certain minerals in drinking water is perhaps detrimental to cardiovascular health or, alternatively, that the presence of specific minerals such as vanadium or other minerals in the water may protect against the disease [848].

Vanadium and Dental Caries. The occurrence of vanadium in human enamel and dentin suggests that it may exchange in the apatite tooth substance [862,863]. Microradioautography indicates that $^{48}V_2O_5$ injected subcutaneously into mice is highly concentrated in the areas of rapid mineralization in tooth dentin and bone [827]. Vanadium is also incorporated into the tooth structure of rats and retained in the molars up to 90 days after injection [864]. Rygh [865-867] has reported that the addition of vanadium and of strontium to specially purified diets promoted mineralization of the bones and teeth and reduced the number of carious teeth in rats and guinea pigs. Geyer [868] observed a high degree of protection against caries in hamsters fed a cariogenic diet when vanadium was administered as V_2O_5, either orally or parenterally. Kruger [869] observed that administering vanadium intraperitoneally to rats during tooth development was effective in reducing dental caries.

Other studies failed to show beneficial effects of vanadium. Ten ppm of vanadium actually increased caries when young hamsters were given a cariogenic diet [870]. In three other studies with rats, administration of varying levels of vanadium in the drinking water was unsuccessful in decreasing caries incidence [871-874].

An inverse relationship between vanadium levels in the water supply and caries incidence in children born and reared in various localities has been reported [874]. The number of children included in some cases was small, and Hadjimarkos has pointed out [875,876] that the drinking water does not constitute an important source of vanadium to man. Because Wyoming is a high selenium area, the effects attributed to vanadium on dental caries may actually be confounded with the cariogenic effect of selenium reported by Hadjimarkos.

Vanadium and Bone Development. Vanadium deficiency also has adverse effects on chick bone development [877]. Histologically, the vanadium-deficient chick tibia shows severe disorganization of the cells of the epiphysis. The cells appear compressed and their nuclei flattened. These abnormalities result in a shortened, thickened leg structure. The uptake and distribution of $^{35}SO_4^{2-}$ and hexosamine concentrations in the epiphysis are similar to those of the controls. Therefore, it seems that mucopoly-saccharide metabolism is not affected by vanadium deficiency. On the other hand, Summers and Moran [878] observed no significant differences in blood phosphorus or bone ash levels in young chicks when their diet was supple-mented with vanadium.

Vanadium and Reproduction. In rats, reproductive performance is im-paired by vanadium deprivation [844,845]. When five fourth-generation female rats were mated, there were significantly fewer live births and significantly more deaths of neonatal pups than with vanadium-sufficient controls. Vana-dium salts or chelating agents have induced glycoprotein mating factors in diploid yeast of Hansenula wingei [879].

Vanadium and Other Health Effects. The complete inhibition of growth of Mycobacterium tuberculosis can be achieved by including 5 μg of m-vandate ion in the medium. This inhibition can be reversed by addition of manganous or chromate ion [880]. Dietary administration of small quantities of vana-dium markedly reduces pulmonary tuberculosis lesions in rabbits and produces a minimal but significant depression of disease in mice infected with a mouse-adapted strain of human tubercle bacillus [881,882]. In general, in animals with generalized tuberculosis [882] the level of vanadium and other trace elements in the lungs and liver was found to be decreased. The amount of vanadium is also sharply reduced in the liver of subjects who died of tuberculosis. The similarity of data obtained in animals and man suggests a medical application of vanadium in a complex therapy of tuberculosis.

ZINC

Chemistry of Zinc

Zinc is found in Group IIB of the periodic table. Its abundance in the earth's crust is 0.022%. Zinc is obtained primarily from zinc blende (sphalerite) and marmatite, which are zinc sulfide ores. Sphalerite is

the source of 90% of the metallic zinc produced today. Other zinc ores
are smithsonite or calamine, a zinc carbonate ore; willemite, a zinc silicate ore; zincite, a zinc oxide ore; and franklinite, an oxide of zinc,
iron, and manganese. The main isotopes are 64, 66, 67, 68, and 70. Zinc
occurs in the 2+ state.

The ion Zn^{2+} is colorless and exists in a hydrated form in neutral and
acidic aqueous solutions; but the hydroxide is precipitated in alkaline solution. With excess base, the hydroxide redissolves to form zincate ion,
ZnO_2^{2-}. The zinc ion forms many complex ions in aqueous solutions such as
$Zn(NH_3)_4^{2+}$ and $Zn(CN)_4^{2-}$ as well as others.

The largest single world use for zinc is the protection of steel against
atmospheric corrosion. Another important use is in the die-casting process.
Combination of the zinc and steel helps the alloy to solidify almost instan-
taneously. Alloyed with copper, zinc forms the important group of alloys
known as the brasses. Zinc oxide is used widely in paint. The rubber industry uses a considerable quantity of zinc oxide. Zinc oxide helps provide
motor car tires with high thermal conductivity and heat capacity, good adhes-
ive characteristics, and resistance to deterioration by sunlight. Some
compounds find use as antiseptics. Other useful compounds of zinc are zinc
peroxide, zinc chloride, zinc sulfide, zinc sulfate, and zinc carbonate.

Essentiality of Zinc

About 100 years ago, Raulin [883] showed that zinc was essential in
the nutrition of Aspergillus niger. In 1926, zinc was found to be essential
for the higher forms of plant life [884,885]. Indications of a function for
zinc came from the work of Birckner [886]. In 1934, Todd and associates
[887], using semipurified diets, found zinc to be essential for the rat.
In 1954, Tucker and Salmon [888] reported that zinc cures and prevents
parakeratosis in pigs. O'Dell and co-workers [889,890] showed that zinc
is required for growth, feathering, and skeletal development in poultry.
Prasad and co-workers [891-893] related this element to the occurrence of
dwarfism and hypogonadism in Middle Eastern boys. Zinc deficiency can occur
in cattle under natural conditions [894-896].

The zinc requirement for rats is about 11-18 ppm depending on the protein source [897,898], but Swenerton and Hurley [899] have found 60 ppm inadequate and 100 ppm adequate in preventing long-term testicular changes.
Pigs require 45-46 ppm to prevent parakeratosis [900,901]. The minimum
dietary zinc level for growth and health in chicks appears to be 35-40 ppm

on soybean protein diets [889,890,902-904] and 25-30 ppm on casein or egg
white diets [902,905]. Lambs grew all right on 15-18 ppm [906,907], but
testicular development and spermatogenesis was best at 32 ppm [907]. Calves
require 8 to 9 ppm for growth [906,908], although 10-14 ppm is necessary to
maintain normal plasma zinc levels.

Adult human diets supply from 5 to 22 mg Zn/day in one study [909,910],
but most mixed diets supply from 12 to 15 mg/day [911]. Tribble and Scoular
[912] found the average zinc intake of college women aged 17-27 years to be
12 mg/day, of which 6.6 mg/day was retained. Engel et al. [913] observed
daily zinc intakes ranging from 4.6 to 9.3 mg/day and suggested that 6 mg
Zn/day is adequate for the normal needs of preadolescent girls. The United
States recommended daily allowance is 5 mg for infants, 8 mg for children
up to age 4, 15 mg for adults and children 4 or more years of age, and 15
mg for pregnant or lactating women [914].

Foods vary greatly in zinc content. White sugar, pome and citrus
fruits are among the lowest in zinc (less than 1 ppm). Wheat germ and bran
(40-120 ppm) and oysters, which may contain over 1000 ppm Zn, are among the
richest sources of this element [911]. Disodium EDTA and calcium sodium EDTA
are used in some canned food to reduce deterioration from heavy metals and
and may affect zinc availability. A lesser use of galvanized iron pipes
and containers may also be of significance. There is evidence of regional
differences in plasma zinc levels in human adults in the United States [915].
The high phytate content of rural Iranian bread may be a possible cause of
human zinc deficiency reported in that country [916]. High levels of histidine have alleviated parakeratosis in zinc-deficient swine [917].

Metabolism of Zinc

In liver and mammary cells, zinc is present in the nuclear, mitochondrial, and supernatant fractions, with the highest concentrations in the
supernatant and the microsomes [918,919]. Experiments with radiozinc injections in mice indicate about one-sixth of the ^{65}Zn in these tissues is
firmly bound to protein and cannot be removed by EDTA or by long dialysis
[918]. This fraction probably consists of the zinc bound to nucleic acids
or of zinc metalloproteins. The remainder, which is dialyzable or removable
by EDTA, is bound to the imadazole or sulfhydryl groups of proteins [920].

As early as 1939, zinc was found to be a constituent of the enzyme
carbonic anhydrase [921]. Subsequently, many other zinc-containing metalloenzymes were discovered, including pancreatic carboxypeptidase, alkaline

phosphatase, alcohol, malic, lactic, and glutamic dehydrogenases, and tryp-
tophan desmolase [922,923].   Zinc was found to act as a co-factor in a
variety of enzyme systems including arginase [922].   Zinc metalloenzymes
and enzymes requiring zinc are listed in Table 5.   Zinc is involved in a
wide range of metabolic activities and is vitally concerned with RNA and
protein synthesis and metabolism in plants [924], microorganisms [925], and
higher animals [926-928].

TABLE 5. Zinc Metalloenzymes and Metalloproteins

Enzyme	Source
Alcohol dehydrogenase	Yeast; equine and human liver
Lactate dehydrogenase	Rabbit muscle
D-lactate-cytochrome c reductase	Yeast
Glyceraldehyde-3-phosphate dehydrogenase	Bovine and porcine muscle; yeast
Glutamate dehydrogenase	Bovine liver
Aldolase	Yeast; Aspergillus niger, E. coli
Carbonic anhydrase	Bovine, simian, human, and porcine erythrocytes; rat prostate, shark, parsley
Alkaline phosphatase	E. coli, porcine kidney, human placenta and leukocytes
Procarboxypeptidase A and B	Bovine, porcine, and Pacific spiny dogfish pancreas
Carboxypeptidase A and B	Bovine, porcine, and Pacific spiny dogfish pancreas
Neutral protease	Bacillus subtilis, B. megatherium, Aeromonas proteolyticum, Serratia
Thermolysin	Bacillus thermoproteolyticus
Leucine aminopeptidase	Porcine kidney
Pyruvate carboxylase	Yeast
Phosphomannose isomerase	Yeast
AMP-aminohydrolase	Rabbit muscle
Dipeptidase	Porcine kidney, mouse ascites, tumor cells
Aspartate transcarboxylase	E. coli
DNA-polymerase	E. coli, sea urchin
Proteinase	Cottonmouth (water moccasin)
α-Macroglobulin	Human serum
Corneal collagenase	Mammalian tissue

TABLE 5 (Continued)

Enzyme	Source
ALA-dehydralase	Mammalian tissue
Proteins containing both zinc and cadmium	
Metallothionein	Equine kidney and liver; human kidney and liver; rabbit liver
Metalloenzymes containing both calcium and zinc	
Amylase	B. subtilis
Metalloenzymes containing both zinc and manganese	
Superoxide dismutase	E. coli

Impaired in vivo synthesis of DNA in the liver of two Zn-deficient rats compared to the controls has been observed in several studies [926, 927,929]. The incorporation of ^{32}P into rat liver nucleotides [930] and of tritiated thymidine into the DNA of liver, testis, kidney, and spleen [927,931] is depressed. Thymidine kinase, which is required for DNA synthesis, is decreased in zinc-deficient tissues [932]. The oxidation of ^{14}C-labeled lysine and leucine is increased [933] in zinc deficiency. Decreased RNA liver concentration and decreased thymus DNA concentration also occur in Zn-deficient baby pigs [934], and both RNA and DNA are decreased in zinc-deficient rats, possibly due to an increase of RNAase or DNAase [935]. Decreased RNA polymerase has been observed in zinc-deficient rats [936]. Zinc may also be important for reverse transcriptase activity [937].

The proteolytic activity of the pancreas is reduced in the Zn-deficient rat [938,939]. This observation led to the discovery that pancreatic carboxypeptidase is a zinc metalloenzyme [940]. Zinc may also play a part in the normal production or action of insulin in vivo. A serious impairment of blood glucose utilization in Zn-deficient rats has been observed [941, 942]. Deficient rats also revealed a greatly increased resistance to insulin coma. Zinc may be necessary for normal insulin secretion. Serum insulin is sharply reduced in zinc-deficient rats [943]. Glucose uptake by adipose tissue is increased by zinc and by insulin [943,944]. Decreased glucose uptake may explain the high-fasting, free-fatty-acid levels in the blood and the virtual absence of adipose tissue in animals with advanced zinc deficiency.

Health Effects of Zinc

Zinc and Keratogenesis. Rats and mice with zinc deficiency developed gross epithelial lesions and alopecia. Histological studies revealed a condition of parakeratosis, i.e., a hyperatinization of the epithelial cells of the skin [945]. In more severe zinc deficiency in rats, scaling and cracking of the paws with deep fissures, coarseness, and loss of hair, and dermatitis [922] occurs. In pigs, parakeratosis occurs around the eyes and mouth and on the scrotum and lower parts of the legs [946]. Similar patterns are seen in zinc-deficient ruminants [907,947]. Zinc deficiency is evident in sheep through changes in the wool and horns [906,907] and changes in hoof structure and wool growth. The wool fibers lose their crimp and become thin and loose and readily shed.

In the Zn-deficient chick [889,890], turkey poult [948], and pheasant [949], feathering is poor and abnormal and dermatitis is usual. Feathering but not dermatitis is severely affected [950,951]. The epidermal changes seen in zinc-deficient animals may be related to vitamin A deficiency. Zinc is necessary to maintain a normal concentration of rat plasma vitamin A [952]. Zinc is necessary for normal mobilization of vitamin A from the liver.

Zinc and Bone Growth. Bowing of the hind legs and stiffness of the joints in Zn-deficient calves [953,954] is rapidly reversible by zinc feeding. Skeletal malformations in the fetuses from Zn-deficient rats [955] have been observed. Skeletal abnormalities have been observed in baby pigs [956] and in growing birds. In chicks, poults, pheasants, and quail [904, 940-943] the long bones are shortened and thickened in proportion to the degree of zinc deficiency [957]. Changes and disproportions occur in other bones, giving rise to a perosis histologically similar to that of manganese deficiency [889,890,904]. Although the exact mechanism of action of zinc in bone formation is not known, decreased osteoblastic activity in the bony collar of the long bones has been noted [889,890,904]. The action of zinc on bones may also be related to a reduction of food intake in zinc-deficient animals [887,906].

Zinc and Wound Healing. Pories and Strain and associates [958,959] observed an accelerated rate of wound healing in rats accidentally fed zinc. Patients suffering from major burns have subnormal hair zinc levels [959]. Wound healing is impaired in Zn-deficient calves [946] and rats [960]. The mode of action of zinc in tissue repair is unknown. Zinc is preferentially

concentrated in healing tissues in rats, both in skin and muscle wounds
[961], and in bone fractures [962], suggesting a heightened zinc requirement
for tissue synthesis during the healing process. Zinc-deficient animals
show a decreased rate of wound healing [963]. Several investigators have
reported no effect of supplemental zinc on wound healing in rats [964,965].
It is likely that the zinc status of the animals was low or deficient in
the effective experiments.

In zinc-deficient animals, collagen synthesis is markedly reduced.
Impaired wound healing and growth retardation as a result of zinc deficiency
may be related directly to lack of collagen formation [966].

Adrenal corticosteroids are known to help reduce tissue inflammation
and injury. A relationship might exist between zinc levels and adrenal-
corticosteroid levels [967]. Patients with untreated adrenal cortical insufficiency exhibit serum concentrations of zinc and copper significantly
higher than the controls.

Zinc and Reproduction. Atrophic seminiferous tubules were first observed in zinc-deficient male rats [945]. Zinc deficiency also retarded
development of the testes, epididymes, and prostate and pituitary glands
with atrophy of the testicular germinal epithelium. The availability of
sufficient zinc for incorporation of high concentrations into sperm during
the final stages of maturation seems to be essential for the maintenance
of spermatogenesis and for the survival of the germinal epithelium [907,
968,969].

Hypogonadism, with suppression in the development of the secondary
sexual characteristics, is conspicuous of zinc deficiency of young men in
parts of Iran and Egypt [892,893]. Hypogonadism also occurs in Zn-deficient bull calves [970,971], kids [972], and ram lambs [907]. Zinc levels
of human spermatozoa are high [973]. In female rats, zinc deficiency caused
a severe disruption of estrus [955]. In rats maintained on a marginally
Zn-deficient diet (9 ppm) throughout the period from weaning to maturity
and then mated, estrous cycles were not disrupted and mating took place
normally. If these diets were continued throughout pregnancy, less than
half had living young at term [955]. Severe zinc deficiency imposed upon
normal adult female rats from the first day of gestation markedly affected
the behavior of the female both before and after parturition, and 75% of
the young died within 2 hr of birth [974]. Decreased hatchability of eggs
and chick embryos with grossly impaired development and high mortality was
observed in Zn-deficient hens [975,976]. Suboptimal zinc levels fed to
sows reduced litter size [977]. Others have also observed zinc deficiency

during pregnancy causes a high incidence of abortions [978,979] and malformations in the rat. Teratogenic effects [980] have been observed by feeding
EDTA to rats during pregnancy. Pups of lactating zinc-deficient mothers
are also zinc deficient [981].

    Zinc and Atherosclerosis. Pories et al. [982] have studied 13 patients
with advanced vascular disease who were given zinc sulfate orally up to 29
months. Twelve of these 13 showed marked clinical improvement; nine returned
to normal activity. About half of the patients of Henzel and associates
[983] also improved. Hair and plasma zinc levels are usually significantly
subnormal in patients with atherosclerosis and myocardial infarctions [982,
984,985], and the aortic wall has an extremely active turnover of ^{65}Zn [986]
which becomes more active when the arterial wall is injured. Atherosclerosis
may be an expression of inadequate arterial repair [982], which like wound
healing in skin, muscle, and bone is related to zinc levels.

    Zinc serum levels fall sharply to acute myocardial infarction within
a day of onset [987] and then rose to normal values within 7 to 10 days.
An imbalance between copper and zinc has been hypothesized as contributing
to the risk of coronary heart disease [988].

    Zinc and Cancer. Subnormal plasma zinc levels have been reported in
patients with malignant tumors [989-991]. Marked changes in leukocyte zinc
occur in patients with chronic leukemia. Zinc concentration in the peripheral leukocytes is greatly reduced and cannot be raised by zinc injections.
In clinical remission, a rise to normal levels occurs [992]. The zinc content of the leukocytes also decreases in patients with a variety of neoplastic diseases, and this difference has been suggested as a diagnostic
test for cancer [993]. Zinc plays a role in the transformation of lymphocytes by phytohemagglutinin [994,995].

    Poswillo and Cohen [996] have reported the inhibition of chemical
carcinogenesis in the hamster cheek pouch by dietary zinc deficiency.
DeWys et al. [997] reported the inhibition of Walker 256 carcinosarcoma by
dietary zinc deficiency. Similar results were reported by McQuilty et al.
[998]. Because zinc is necessary for growth of normal tissue, zinc may
also be necessary for tumor growth. Zinc deficiency depressed the growth
of P 388 leukemia in weanling mice after the third posttransplantation day
[999]. Growth of a transplantable hepatoma induced by 3^1-methyl-4-dimethyl-
aminoazobenzene was significantly reduced in rats maintained on a low-zinc
diet [1000]. Zinc levels are higher in certain types of human cancer tissue
[1001].

EDTA inhibits the synthesis of DNA by chick embryo cells in tissue culture, and this inhibition can only be reversed by zinc [1002]. In contrast, EDTA did not significantly inhibit DNA synthesis in Hela and L cells [1003], ascites tumor cells [1004], or in chick embryo cells transformed by Rous sarcoma virus [1002].

Zinc — Infections, Anemia, and Cirrhosis. Subnormal plasma zinc levels have been reported in patients in chronic and acute infections [991], in untreated pernicious anemia [1005-1008], and in post-alcoholic cirrhosis of the liver and other liver diseases [1009-1012]. The lower plasma zinc levels may indicate abnormalities in zinc metabolism, but their possible mechanisms are not understood. Because it is lowered in so many diseases, measurements of zinc in plasma or urine may have limited importance in clinical diagnosis or prognosis [1013].

Zinc and Hypogeusia. Several adult patients with low serum zinc developed decreased taste acuity (hypogeusia). Oral zinc supplementation relieved this problem [1014,1015].

Zinc — Chronic Leg Ulcers and Bedsores. Oral zinc sulfate therapy has promoted the healing of chronic venous leg ulcerations that had failed to respond to conventional medical therapy [1016-1019]. Two investigators have observed a therapeutic response to oral doses of zinc sulfate in subjects with bedsores [1020,1021].

Zinc — Epilepsy, Retardation of Brain Growth, and Acromegaly. If copper or zinc are injected intraventricularly, severe epileptic seizures are induced in animals [1022]. Lower doses of zinc produce yawning and stretching behavior. In further studies, plasma levels of zinc and copper were measured in 30 treated epileptic patients and 32 age- and sex-matched control subjects. There was no difference in copper levels, but zinc concentration was significantly decreased in the patients. Zinc deficiency in suckling rats during critical periods for brain growth retards brain maturation [1023]. In untreated acromegaly, zinc levels are significantly lower than in the controls [1024].

Zinc — Dialysis and Colds. Zinc serum levels are decreased in the plasma of dialysis patients [1025]. Magnesium and copper levels were increased. Zinc ions at biochemical levels inhibit the replication of rhinoviruses, a subgroup of the picoraviruses, some of which can cause the common cold [1026].

REFERENCES

1. K. Schwarz and W. Mertz, Arch. Biochem. Biophys., 72, 515 (1957).

2. K. Schwarz and W. Mertz, Arch. Biochem. Biophys., 85, 292 (1959).

3. E. E. Roginski and W. Mertz, J. Nutr., 93, 249 (1967).

4. D. Perlman, J. Bacteriol., 49, 167 (1945).

5. W. Mertz, Physiol. Rev., 49, 163 (1969).

6. R. A. Levine, D. H. P. Streeten, and R. J. Doisy, Metab. Clin. Exp., 17, 114 (1968).

7. H. A. Schroeder, J. J. Balassa, and I. H. Tipton, J. Chron. Dis., 15, 941 (1962).

8. W. H. Glinsmann and W. Mertz, Metab. Clin. Exp., 15, 510 (1966).

9. R. A. Levine, D. H. Streeten, and R. J. Doisy, Metab. Clin. Exp., 17, 114 (1968).

10. I. H. Tipton, P. L. Stewart, and P. G. Martin, Health Phys., 12, 1683 (1966).

11. M. M. Braideck and F. H. Emery, J. Amer. Water Works Ass., 27, 557 (1935).

12. J. P. Carter, A. Kattab, K. A. Abd-Al-Hadi, J. T. Davis, A. E. Gholmy, and V. N. Patwardhan, Amer. J. Clin. Nutr., 21, 195 (1968).

13. L. L. Hopkins, Jr., O. Ransome-Kuti, and A. S. Majaj, Amer. J. Clin. Nutr., 21, 203 (1968).

14. W. Mertz and E. E. Roginski, in Newer Trace Elements in Nutrition (W. Mertz and W. E. Cornatzer, eds.), Marcel Dekker, New York, 1971, p. 123.

15. E. W. Toepfer, W. Mertz, E. E. Roginski, and M. M. Polansky, J. Agr. Food Chem., 21, 69 (1973).

16. G. D. Christian, E. C. Knoblock, W. L. Purdy, and W. Mertz, Biochem. Biophys. Acta, 66, 420 (1963).

17. R. M. Donaldson and R. F. Barreras, J. Lab. Clin. Med., 68, 484 (1966).

18. W. Mertz, E. E. Roginski, and R. Reba, Amer. J. Physiol., 209, 489 (1965).

19. W. J. Visek, I. B. Whitney, U. S. G. Kuhn, and C. L. Comar, Proc. Soc. Exp. Biol. Med., 84, 610 (1963).

20. L. W. Conn, H. L. Webster, and A. H. Johnston, Amer. J. Hyg., 15, 760 (1932).

21. E. A. Kane, W. C. Jacobson, and L. A. Moore, J. Nutr., 44, 583 (1950).

22. E. A. Kane, W. C. Jacobson, and L. A. Moore, J. Nutr., 47, 263 (1952).

23. B. A. Kottk and M. T. Subbiah, J. Lab. Clin. Med., 78, 811 (1971).

24. M. T. Fisher, P. R. Atkins, and G. F. Joplin, Clin. Chim. Acta, 41, 109 (1972).

25. R. D. Mackenzie, R. Anwar, R. U. Byerrum, and C. A. Hoppert, Arch. Biochem. Biophys., 79, 200 (1959).

26. S. J. Gray and K. Sterling, J. Clin. Invest., 29, 1604 (1950).

27. L. L. Hopkins, Jr., and K. Schwarz, Biochim. Biophys. Acta, 90, 484 (1964).

28. K. A. Aas and F. H. Gardner, J. Clin. Invest., 37, 1257 (1958).

29. M. Cooper and C. A. Owen, J. Lab. Clin. Med., 47, 65 (1956).

30. S. C. Shih, W. N. Tauxe, and V. F. Fairbanks, Amer. J. Clin. Pathol., 55, 431 (1971).

31. A. L. Pawlak, H. Karon, L. Torlinski, and S. Dzieciuchowicz, Clin. Chim. Acta, 35, 395 (1971).

32. I. O. Szymanski, G. S. Lipson, and C. R. Valeri, Transfusion, 13, 13 (1973).

33. P. D. Berk and T. F. Blaschke, Ann. Intern. Med., 77, 527 (1972).

34. L. L. Hopkins, Jr., Amer. J. Physiol., 209, 731 (1965).

35. T. F. Mancuro and W. C. Hueper, Ind. Med. Surg., 20, 358 (1951).

36. P. V. Vittorio and E. W. Wright, Can. J. Biochem. Physiol., 41, 1349 (1963).

37. C. Edwards, K. B. Olson, G. Heggen, and J. Glenn, Proc. Soc. Exp. Biol. Med., 107, 94 (1961).

38. W. E. C. Wacker and B. L. Vallee, J. Biol. Chem., 234, 3257 (1959).

39. W. E. C. Wacker, M. P. Gordon, and J. W. Huff, Biochemistry, 2, 716 (1963).

40. C. C. Chatterjee, R. K. Roy, N. Sasmal, S. K. Banerjee, and P. K. Majumder, J. Nutr., 103, 509 (1973).

41. W. H. Glinsmann, F. J. Feldman, and W. Mertz, Science, 152, 1243 (1966).

42. W. Mertz, E. E. Roginski, F. J. Feldman, and D. E. Thurman, J. Nutr., 99, 363 (1969).

43. E. E. Roginski, F. J. Feldman, and W. Mertz, Fed. Proc., 27, 482 (1968).

44. A. Milosha, Nauk. Zap. Stanislav. Derzh. Med. Inst., 3, 85 (1959).

45. L. A. Pribluda, Dokl. Akad. Beloruss. SSR, 7, 135 (1963).

46. H. J. Votava, C. J. Hahn, and G. W. Evans, Biochem. Biophys. Res. Commun., 55, 312 (1973).

47. K. Schwarz and W. Mertz, Fed. Proc., 20 (Suppl. 2), 111 (1961).

48. I. W. F. Davidson and W. L. Blackwell, Proc. Soc. Exp. Biol. Med., 127, 66 (1968).

49. W. Mertz, E. E. Roginski, and K. Schwarz, J. Biol. Chem., 236, 318 (1961).

50. H. A. Schroeder, J. Nutr., 88, 439 (1966).

51. L. Sherman, J. A. Glennon, W. J. Brech, G. H. Klomberg, and E. S. Gordon, Metab. Clin. Exp., 17, 439 (1968).

52. H. A. Schroeder, Amer. J. Clin. Nutr., 21, 230 (1968).

53. L. L. Hopkins, Jr. and M. G. Price, Proc. Western Hemisphere Nutr. Congr., Puerto Rico, Vol. II, 40 (1968).

54. I. W. F. Davidson and R. L. Burt, Amer. J. Obstet. Gynecol., 116, 601 (1973).

55. A. G. Mowat and J. D. Baum, New Engl. J. Med., 284, 621 (1971).

56. J. D. Baum, A. G. Mowat, and J. A. Kirk, J. Lab. Clin. Med., 77, 501 (1971).

57. K. M. Hambridge, Amer. J. Clin. Nutr., 27, 505 (1974).

58. K. M. Hambridge, B. Martinez, J. A. Jones, C. E. Boyle, W. E. Hathaway, and D. O'Brien, Pediatr. Res., 6, 133 (1972).

59. J. M. Morgan, Metab., 21, 313 (1972).

60. H. A. Schroeder and J. J. Balassa, Amer. J. Physiol., 209, 433 (1965).

61. H. A. Schroeder, W. H. Vinton, Jr., and J. J. Balassa, Proc. Soc. Exp. Biol. Med., 109, 859 (1962).

62. H. A. Schroeder, J. Nutr., 97, 237 (1969).

63. H. W. Staub, G. Reussner, and R. Thiessen, Jr., Science, 166, 746 (1969).

64. S. Goldenberg and H. T. Blumenthal, in Diabetes Mellitus, Diagnosis and Treatment, Amer. Diabetes Ass., New York, 1964, p. 177.

65. W. Mertz, E. E. Roginski, and H. A. Schroeder, J. Nutr., 86, 107 (1965).

66. G. L. Curran, J. Biol. Chem., 210, 765 (1954).

67. E. E. Roginski and W. Mertz, Fed. Proc., 26, 301 (1967).

68. E. E. Roginski and W. Mertz, J. Nutr., 97, 525 (1969).

69. L. L. Hopkins, Jr. and A. S. Majaj, Proceedings Seventh International Congress Nutrition, Vol. 5, Pergamon, New York, 1967, p. 721.

70. L. L. Hopkins, Jr., O. Ransome-Kuti, and A. S. Majaj, Amer. J. Clin. Nutr., 21, 203 (1968).

71. C. T. Gurson and G. Saner, Amer. J. Clin. Nutr., 24, 1313 (1971).

72. J. P. Carter, A. Kattab, K. Abd-El-Hadi, J. T. Davis, A. L. Gholmy, and V. N. Patwardhan, Amer. J. Clin. Nutr., 21, 195 (1968).

73. K. M. Hambridge and J. D. Baum, Amer. J. Clin. Nutr., 25, 376 (1972).

74. I. H. Tipton, in Metal Binding in Medicine, Lippincott, Philadelphia, 1960, p. 27.

75. K. M. Hambridge and J. D. Baum, Clin. Res., 19, 220 (1971).

76. K. M. Hambridge and D. O. Rodgerson, Amer. J. Obstet. Gynecol., 103, 320 (1969).

77. K. M. Hambridge, D. O. Rodgerson, and D. O'Brien, Diabetes, 17, 517 (1968).

78. W. Mertz and E. E. Roginski, J. Nutr., 97, 531 (1969).

79. H. A. Schroeder, J. J. Balassa, and W. H. Vinton, Jr., J. Nutr., 83, 239 (1964).

80. H. A. Schroeder, J. J. Balassa, and W. H. Vinton, Jr., J. Nutr., 86, 51 (1965).

81. H. A. Schroeder, W. H. Vinton, Jr., and J. J. Balassa, J. Nutr., 80, 39 (1963).

82. H. A. Schroeder, W. H. Vinton, Jr., and J. J. Balassa, J. Nutr., 80, 48 (1963).

83. C. T. Gurson and G. Saner, Amer. J. Clin. Nutr., 27, 988 (1973).

84. J. L. Scott, R. McMillan, J. V. Marino, and J. G. Davidson, Blood, 41, 155 (1973).

85. K. Aho, P. Virkola, and O. P. Heinonen, Acta Endocrinol., 68, 196 (1971).

86. D. Sharma and J. Tuomi, Acta Vet. Scand., 14, 651 (1973).

87. N. Vidon, B. Crozatier, and J. J. Bernier, Arch. Fr. Mal. App. Dig., 62, 201 (1973).

88. B. C. Aston, N. Z. J. Agr., 28, 38 (1924).

89. B. C. Aston, N. Z. J. Agr., 28, 301 (1924).

90. B. C. Aston, N. Z. J. Agr., 29, 14 (1924).

91. B. C. Aston, N. Z. J. Agr., 29, 84 (1924).

92. E. J. Underwood and J. F. Filmer, Aust. Vet. J., 11, 84 (1935).

93. E. J. Underwood and R. J. Harvey, Aust. Vet. J., 14, 183 (1938).

94. E. L. Rickes, N. G. Brink, F. R. Koniusky, T. R. Wood, and K. Folkers, Science, 108, 134 (1948).

95. E. L. Smith, Nature (London), 162, 144 (1948).

96. S. E. Smith, B. A. Koch, and K. L. Turk, J. Nutr., 44, 455 (1951).

97. E. G. Hallsworth, S. B. Wilson, and E. A. Greenwood, Nature (London), 187, 79 (1960).

98. H. M. Reisenhauer, Nature (London), 186, 375 (1960).

99. P. G. Ozanne, E. A. Greenwood, and T. C. Shaw, Aust. J. Agr. Res., 14, 39 (1963).

100. J. K. Powrie, Aust. J. Soil, 23, 198 (1960).

101. I. H. Tipton, P. L. Stewart, and P. G. Martin, Health Phys., 12, 1683 (1966).

102. H. A. Schroeder, A. P. Nason, and I. H. Tipton, J. Chronic Dis., 20, 869 (1967).

103. G. Hurwitz and R. C. Beeson, Food Res., 9, 348 (1944).

104. N. D. Sylvester and L. H. Lampitt, J. Soc. Chem. Ind. (London), 59, 57 (1940).

105. H. R. Marston, S. H. Allen, and R. M. Smith, Nature (London), 190, 1085 (1961).

106. E. D. Andrews, N. Z. J. Agr. Res., 8, 788 (1965).

107. J. F. Filmer and E. J. Underwood, Aust. Vet. J., 10, 84 (1934).

108. J. F. Filmer and E. J. Underwood, Aust. Vet. J., 13, 57 (1937).

109. H. R. Marston, Physiol. Rev., 32, 66 (1952).

110. M. Somers and J. M. Gawthorne, Aust. J. Exp. Biol. Med. Sci., 47, 227 (1969).

111. K. J. McNaught, N. Z. J. Sci. Technol., Sect. A, 20, 14 (1938).

112. J. Stewart, Brit. Commonwealth Offic. Sci. Conf., 1949, Australia, 1951, p. 281.

113. H. J. Lee and H. R. Marston, Aust. J. Agr. Res., 20, 1109 (1969).

114. H. J. Lee, Aust. Vet. J., 26, 152 (1950).

115. C. L. Comar, G. K. Davis and R. F. Taylor, Arch. Biochem., 9, 149 (1946).

116. C. L. Comar and G. K. Davis, Arch. Biochem., 12, 257 (1947).

117. R. W. Engel, N. O. Price, and R. F. Miller, J. Nutr., 92, 197 (1967).

118. W. S. Beck, M. Flavin, and S. Ochoa, J. Biol. Chem., 229, 997 (1957).

119. W. S. Beck and S. Ochoa, J. Biol. Chem., 232, 931 (1958).

120. S. Gurnani, S. P. Misty, and B. C. Johnson, Biochim. Biophys. Acta, 38, 187 (1960).

121. R. M. Smith and K. J. Monty, Biochem. Biophys. Res. Commun., 1, 105 (1959).

122. M. C. Dawbarn, H. Forsyth, and D. Kilpatrick, Aust. J. Exp. Biol. Med. Sci., 41, 1 (1963).

123. R. M. Smith, W. S. Osborne-White, and G. R. Russell, Biochem. J., 112, 703 (1969).

124. I. Chanarin, M. C. Bennett, and V. Berry, J. Clin. Pathol., 15, 269 (1962).

125. A. L. Luhby, J. M. Cooperman, and D. N. Teller, Proc. Soc. Exp. Biol. Med., 101, 350 (1959).

126. M. Silverman and A. J. Pitney, J. Biol. Chem., 233, 1179 (1958).

127. E. L. R. Stokstad, R. E. Webb, and E. Shah, J. Nutr., 88, 225 (1966).

128. M. R. Spivey-Fox and W. J. Ludwig, Proc. Soc. Exp. Biol. Med., 108, 703 (1961).

129. J. M. Gawthorne, Aust. J. Biol. Sci., 21, 789 (1968).

130. J. B. Buchanan, Medicine (Baltimore), 43, 697 (1964).

131. V. Herbert and R. Zalusky, J. Clin. Invest., 41, 1263 (1962).

132. V. Herbert, Semin. Nucl. Med., 2, 220 (1972).

133. M. F. Cottrall, D. G. Wells, N. G. Trott, and N. E. G. Richardson, Blood, 38, 604 (1971).

134. R. F. Schilling, J. Lab. Clin. Med., 42, 860 (1953).

135. J. H. Katz, J. DiMase, and R. M. Donaldson, Jr., J. Lab. Clin. Med., 61, 266 (1953).

136. B. K. Armstrong and H. J. Woodlif, J. Clin. Pathol., 23, 569 (1970).

137. P. A. McIntyre and H. N. Wagner, Jr., J. Lab. Clin. Med., 68, 966 (1966).

138. R. W. Heinle, A. D. Welch, V. Scharf, G. C. Meacham, and W. H. Prusoff, Trans. Ass. Amer. Physicians, 65, 214 (1952).

139. G. B. J. Glass, Physiol. Rev., 43, 529 (1963).

140. P. G. Reizenstein, E. P. Cronkite, and S. H. Cohn, Blood, 18, 45 (1961).

141. K. S. Lau, C. Gottlieb, L. R. Wasserman, and V. Herbert, Blood, 26, 202 (1965).

142. L. Wide and A. Killander, Scand. J. Clin. Lab. Invest., 27, 151 (1971).

143. I. L. Schloesser and R. F. Schilling, Amer. J. Clin. Nutr., 12, 70 (1963).

144. S. J. Winawer, R. R. Streiff, and N. Zamcheck, Gastroenterology, 53, 130 (1967).

145. J. D. Hines, Amer. J. Clin. Nutr., 19, 260 (1966).

146. M. Pollycove, L. Apt, and M. J. Colbert, N. Engl. J. Med., 255, 164 (1956).

147. R. J. Harrison, C. C. Booth, and D. L. Mollin, Lancet, 1, 727 (1956).

148. P. M. Conner and M. C. Pirola, Med. J. Aust., 2, 451 (1963).

149. B. C. Lampkin and E. F. Saunders, J. Pediatr., 75, 1053 (1969).

150. B. Ungar, A. Stocks, F. Martin, S. Whittingham, and I. R. Mackay, Lancet, 2, 415 (1968).

151. J. Meecham and E. W. Jones, Lancet, 1, 535 (1967).

152. S. Ardeman, I. Chanarin, B. Krafchik, and W. Singer, Quart. J. Med., 35, 421 (1966).

153. M. G. Whiteside, D. L. Mollin, N. F. Coghill, A. W. Williams, and B. Anderson, Gut, 5, 385 (1964).

154. S. Whittingham, I. R. Mackay, B. Ungar, and J. D. Mathews, Lancet, 1, 951 (1969).

155. G. Perman, R. Gullberg, P. G. Reizenstein, B. Snellman, and L. G. Allgen, Acta Med. Scand., 168, 117 (1960).

156. P. A. McIntyre, M. V. Sachs, J. R. Krevans, and C. L. Conley, Arch. Intern. Med., 98, 541 (1956).

157. V. Herbert and W. B. Castle, J. Clin. Invest., 40, 1978 (1961).

158. W. Veeger, J. Abels, N. Hellemans, and H. O. Nieweg, N. Engl. J. Med., 267, 1341 (1962).

159. W. T. Cooke, Ann. R. Coll. Surg., 17, 137 (1955).

160. T. M. Bayless, M. S. Wheby, and V. L. Swanson, Amer. J. Clin. Nutr., 21, 1030 (1968).

161. J. J. Stewart, D. J. Pollock, A. V. Hoffbrand, D. L. Mollin, and C. C. Booth, Quart. J. Med., 36, 425 (1967).

162. R. B. Scott, R. B. Kammer, W. F. Burger, and F. G. Middleton, Ann. Intern. Med., 69, 111 (1968).

163. M. Katz, S. K. Lee, and B. A. Cooper, N. Engl. J. Med., 287, 425 (1972).

164. S. Schimoda, D. R. Saunders, and C. E. Rubin, Gastroenterology, 55, 705 (1968).

165. H. Y. Shum, B. J. O'Neill, and A. M. Streeter, Lancet, 1, 1303 (1971).

166. R. Grasbeck, R. Gordin, I. Kantero, and B. Kuhlback, Acta Med. Scand., 167, 289 (1960).

167. O. Imerslund, Acta Paediatr. Scand., 49 (Suppl. 119), 1 (1960).

168. I. L. Mackenzie, R. M. Donaldson, J. S. Trier, and V. I. Mathan, N. Engl. J. Med., 286, 1021 (1972).

169. N. HaKami, P. E. Neiman, and G. P. Canellos, N. Engl. J. Med., 285, 1163 (1971).

170. O. Heinivaara and I. P. Palva, Acta Med. Scand., 175, 469 (1964).

171. O. Heinivaara and I. P. Pavla, Acta Med. Scand., 177, 337 (1965).

172. O. Heinivaara, I. P. Pavla, M. Siorala, and R. Pelkonen, Ann. Med. Intern. Fenn., 53, 75 (1964).

173. P. P. Toskes and J. J. Deren, Gastroenterology, 62, 1232 (1972).

174. D. I. Webb, R. B. Chodos, C. Q. Mahar, and W. W. Faloon, N. Engl. J. Med., 279, 845 (1968).

175. J. Lindenbaum and C. S. Lieber, Nature, 224, 806 (1969).

176. G. H. Tomkin, D. R. Hadden, J. A. Weaver, and D. A. D. Montgomery, Brit. Med. J., 2, 685 (1971).

177. E. D. Jacobson, R. B. Chodos, and W. W. Faloon, Amer. J. Med., 28, 524 (1960).

178. L. W. Sullivan, The Megablastic Anemias, in Hematology: Principles and Practice (C. E. Mengel, E. Frei III, and R. Nachman, eds.), Yearbook Medical Publishers, Chicago, 1972, pp. 95-131.

179. V. Herbert, Blood, 32, 305 (1968).

180. H. S. Gilbert, S. Krauss, B. Pasternack, V. Herbert, and L. R. Wasserman, Ann. Intern. Med., 71, 719 (1969).

181. B. M. Freeman and D. R. Langslow, Comp. Biochem. Physiol., 46A, 427 (1973).

182. M. Telib and F. H. Schmidt, Endokrinol., 61, 395 (1973).

183. R. J. Smith, Blood, 42, 893 (1973).

184. M. O. Schultze, C. A. Elvehjem, and E. B. Hart, J. Biol. Chem., 106, 735 (1934).

185. C. F. Mills and G. Murray, J. Sci. Food Agr., 9, 547 (1960).

186. J. M. Evvard, V. E. Nelson, and W. E. Sewell, Proc. Iowa Acad. Sci., 35, 211 (1928).

187. Agricultural Research Council, Nutr. Requir. Farm Livestock No. 3 (1967).

188. E. J. Underwood, in Trace Elements in Human and Animal Nutrition (E. J. Underwood, ed.), Academic, New York, 1971, p. 96.

189. A. T. Dick, Aust. J. Agr. Res., 5, 511 (1954).

190. H. R. Marston and H. J. Lee, J. Agr. Sci., 38, 229 (1948).

191. H. R. Marston, H. J. Lee, and I. W. McDonald, J. Agr. Sci., 38, 216 (1948).

192. H. R. Marston, H. J. Lee, and I. W. McDonald, J. Agr. Sci., 38, 222 (1948).

193. A. G. Spais, Rec. Med. Vet., 135, 161 (1959).

194. A. G. Spais, T. K. Lazaridis, and A. G. Agiannidis, Res. Vet. Sci.,
     9, 337 (1968).

195. R. Allcroft and W. H. Parker, Brit. J. Nutr., 3, 205 (1949).

196. G. Lewis and R. Allcroft, Proceedings of the Fifth International
     Congress on Nutrition, Washington, D. C., 1960.

197. R. Allcroft, Vet. Rec., 64, 17 (1952).

198. R. Allcroft and G. Lewis, J. Sci. Food Agr., 8 (Suppl.), 96 (1957).

199. A. H. Hunter, A. Eden, and H. H. Green, J. Comp. Pathol., 55, 19
     (1945).

200. J. R. M. Innes and G. D. Shearer, J. Comp. Pathol., 53, 1 (1940).

201. G. D. Shearer, J. R. M. Innes, and E. I. McDougal, Vet. J., 96, 309
     (1940).

202. G. D. Shearer and E. I. McDougal, J. Agr. Sci., 34, 207 (1944).

203. W. V. Camargo, H. J. Lee, and D. W. Dewey, Proc. Aust. Soc. Anim.
     Prod., 4, 12 (1962).

204. I. J. Cunningham, N. Z. Vet. J., 7, 15 (1959).

205. G. R. Moule, A. K. Sutherland, and J. M. Harvey, Queensl. J. Agr.
     Sci., 18, 93 (1959).

206. A. K. Sutherland, G. R. Moule, and J. M. Harvey, Aust. Vet. J., 31,
     141 (1955).

207. R. G. Hemingway, A. MacPherson, and N. S. Ritchie, Proc. First Int.
     Symp., Trace Element Metab. Anim., 1969, p. 264 (1970).

208. F. I. Scoular, J. Nutr., 16, 437 (1938).

209. R. W. Engel, N. O. Price, and R. F. Miller, J. Nutr., 92, 197 (1967).

210. G. E. Cartwright, in Symposium on Copper Metabolism (W. D. McElroy
     and B. Glass, eds.), Johns Hopkins Press, Baltimore, 1950, p. 274.

211. R. M. Leverton and E. S. Binkley, J. Nutr., 27, 43 (1944).

212. I. H. Tipton, P. L. Stewart, and P. G. Martin, Health Phys., 12, 1683
     (1966).

213. H. A. Schroeder, A. P. Nason, I. H. Tipton, and J. J. Balassa, J.
     Chronic Dis., 19, 1007 (1966).

214. S. L. Thompsett, Biochem. J., 34, 961 (1940).

215. R. Belz, Voeding, 6, 236 (1960).

216. L. S. P. Davidson, H. W. Fullerton, J. W. Howie, J. M. Croll, J. B.
     Orr, and W. M. Godden, Brit. Med. J., 2, 685 (1933).

217. H. N. De, Indian J. Med. Res., 37, 301 (1941).

218. E. G. Zook and J. Lehmann, J. Ass. Offic. Agr. Chem., 48, 850 (1965).

219. W. Mertz, J. Amer. Diet. Ass., 64, 163 (1974).

220. C. W. Lindow, C. A. Elvehjem, and W. H. Peterson, J. Biol. Chem., 82,
     465 (1929).

221. R. A. McCance and E. M. Widdowson, in The Chemical Composition of
     Foods, Chem. Publ. Co., New York, 1947.

222. C. P. Czerniejewski, C. W. Shank, W. G. Bechtel, and W. B. Brodley, Cereal Chem., 41, 65 (1964).

223. A. Sacks, V. E. Levine, F. C. Hill, and R. C. Hill, Arch. Intern. Med., 71, 489 (1943).

224. J. P. Bowland, R. Braude, A. G. Chamberlain, R. F. Glascock, and K. G. Mitchell, Brit. J. Nutr., 15, 59 (1961).

225. B. Starcher, J. Nutr., 97, 321 (1969).

226. D. R. VanCampen and E. A. Mitchell, J. Nutr., 86, 120 (1965).

227. C. L. Comar, in Symposium on Copper Metabolism (W. D. McElroy and B. Glass, eds.), Johns Hopkins Press, Baltimore, 1950, p. 191.

228. G. E. Cartwright and M. M. Wintrobe, Amer. J. Clin. Nutr., 14, 224 (1964).

229. G. E. Cartwright and M. M. Wintrobe, Amer. J. Clin. Nutr., 15, 94 (1964).

230. M. O. Schultze, C. A. Elvehjem, and E. B. Hart, J. Biol. Chem., 115, 453 (1936).

231. M. O. Schultze, C. A. Elvehjem, and E. B. Hart, J. Biol. Chem., 116, 93 (1936).

232. M. O. Schultze, C. A. Elvehjem, and E. B. Hart, J. Biol. Chem., 116, 107 (1936).

233. J. W. Lassiter and M. C. Bell, J. Anim. Sci., 19, 754 (1960).

234. D. H. Cox and L. H. Harris, J. Nutr., 70, 514 (1960).

235. D. R. Grant-Frost and E. J. Underwood, Aust. J. Exp. Biol. Med. Sci., 36, 339 (1958).

236. A. C. Magee and G. Matrone, J. Nutr., 72, 233 (1960).

237. D. R. VanCampen, J. Nutr., 88, 125 (1966).

238. A. T. Dick, Soil Sci., 81, 229 (1956).

239. A. T. Dick and L. B. Bull, Aust. Vet. J., 21, 70 (1945).

240. C. H. Hill, G. Matrone, W. L. Payne, and C. W. Barber, J. Nutr., 80, 227 (1963).

241. G. Matrone, Proc. First Int. Symp. Trace Element Metab. Anim., 1969, p. 354 (1970).

242. P. N. Davis, L. C. Norris, and F. H. Kratzer, J. Nutr., 77, 217 (1962).

243. W. W. Carlton and W. Henderson, J. Nutr., 85, 67 (1965).

244. C. E. Hunt and W. W. Carlton, J. Nutr., 87, 385 (1965).

245. J. A. Bush, J. P. Mahoney, C. J. Gubler, G. E. Cartwright and M. M. Wintrobe, J. Lab. Clin. Med., 47, 898 (1956).

246. G. Gregoriadis and T. L. Sourkes, Can. J. Biochem., 45, 1841 (1967).

247. H. Porter, Proc. First Int. Symp. Trace Element Metab. Anim., 1969, p. 237 (1970).

248. H. Porter, W. Weiner, and M. Barker, Biochem. Biophys. Acta, 52, 419 (1961).

249. G. E. Herman and E. Kun, Exp. Cell Res., 22, 257 (1961).

250. R. E. Theirs and B. L. Vallee, J. Biol. Chem., 226, 911 (1957).

251. D. B. Milne and P. H. Weswig, J. Nutr., 95, 429 (1968).

252. H. Markowitz, C. J. Gubler, J. P. Mahoney, G. E. Cartwright, and M. M. Wintrobe, J. Clin. Invest., 34, 1498 (1955).

253. I. Sternlieb, A. G. Morell, and I. H. Scheinberg, Trans. Ass. Amer. Phys., 75, 228 (1962).

254. A. H. VanRavesteyn, Acta Med. Scand., 118, 163 (1944).

255. J. P. Mahoney, J. A. Bush, C. J. Gubler, W. H. Moretz, G. E. Cartwright, and M. M. Wintrobe, J. Clin. Invest., 46, 702 (1955).

256. D. Gitlin and C. A. Janeway, Nature (London), 185, 693 (1960).

257. D. Gitlin, W. A. Hughes, and C. A. Janeway, Nature (London), 185, 151 (1960).

258. A. B. Beck, Aust. J. Agr. Res., 12, 743 (1961).

259. C. D. Klaassen, Proc. Soc. Exp. Biol. Med., 144, 8 (1973).

260. A. P. Giorgio, G. E. Cartwright, and M. M. Wintrobe, Amer. J. Clin. Pathol., 41, 22 (1964).

261. G. E. Cartwright, C. J. Gubler, and M. M. Wintrobe, J. Clin. Invest., 33, 685 (1954).

262. P. E. Chen, Chin. Med. J., 75, 917 (1957).

263. T. S. Hamilton and H. H. Mitchell, J. Biol. Chem., 178, 345 (1949).

264. A. E. Moffitt, Biochem. Pharmacol., 22, 1463 (1973).

265. A. B. Beck, Aust. J. Exp. Biol. Med. Sci., 19, 145 (1941).

266. A. B. Beck, Aust. J. Exp. Biol. Med. Sci., 19, 249 (1941).

267. M. E. Lahey, C. J. Gubler, M. S. Chase, G. E. Cartwright, and M. M. Wintrobe, Blood, 7, 1053 (1952).

268. S. E. Smith and M. Medlicott, Amer. J. Physiol., 141, 354 (1944).

269. S. E. Smith, M. Medlicott, and G. H. Ellis, Amer. J. Physiol., 142, 179 (1944).

270. H. W. Bennetts and A. B. Beck, Aust. J. Common. Counc. Sci. Ind. Res. Bull., 147 (1942).

271. I. J. Cunningham, N. Z. J. Sci. Technol., Sec. A, 27, 372 (1946).

272. I. J. Cunningham, N. Z. J. Sci. Technol., Sec. A, 27, 381 (1946).

273. E. I. McDougall, J. Agr. Sci., 37, 329 (1947).

274. G. Matrone, Fed. Proc., 19, 659 (1960).

275. J. H. Baxter and J. J. VanWyk, Bull. Johns Hopkins Hosp., 93, 1 (1953).

276. J. H. Baxter, J. J. VanWyk, and R. H. Follis, Jr., Bull. Johns Hopkins Hosp., 93, 25 (1953).

277. J. J. VanWyk, J. H. Baxter, J. H. Akeroyd, and A. G. Motulsky, Bull. Johns Hopkins Hosp., 93, 51 (1953).

278. S. E. Smith and G. H. Ellis, Arch. Biochem., 15, 81 (1947).

279. J. A. Bush, W. N. Jensen, J. W. Athens, H. Ashenbrucker, G. E. Cartwright, and M. M. Wintrobe, J. Exp. Med., 103, 701 (1956).

280. C. H. Gallagher, J. D. Judah, and K. R. Rees, Proc. Roy. Soc., London, Sec. B, 145, 134 (1956).

281. C. H. Gallagher, J. D. Judah, and K. R. Rees, Proc. Roy. Soc., London, Sec. B, 145, 195 (1956).

282. G. R. Lee, G. E. Cartwright, and M. M. Wintrobe, Proc. Soc. Exp. Biol. Med., 127, 977 (1968).

283. R. L. Anderson and S. B. Tove, Nature (London), 182, 315 (1958).

284. M. S. Chase, C. J. Gubler, G. E. Cartwright, and M. M. Wintrobe, J. Biol. Chem., 199, 757 (1952).

285. M. S. Chase, C. J. Gubler, G. E. Cartwright, and M. M. Wintrobe, Proc. Soc. Exp. Biol. Med., 80, 749 (1952).

286. C. J. Gubler, M. E. Lahey, M. S. Chase, G. E. Cartwright, and M. M. Wintrobe, Blood, 7, 1075 (1952).

287. G. R. Lee, S. Nacht, J. N. Lukens, and G. E. Cartwright, J. Clin. Invest., 47, 2058 (1968).

288. A. Cordano, J. M. Baertl, and G. G. Graham, Pediatrics, 34, 324 (1964).

289. A. Cordano, R. P. Placko, and G. G. Graham, Blood, 28, 280 (1966).

290. R. A. Al-Rashid and J. Spangler, N. Engl. J. Med., 285, 841 (1971).

291. J. T. Karpel and V. H. Peden, J. Pediatr., 80, 32 (1972).

292. G. G. Graham and A. Cordano, Johns Hopkins Med. J., 124, 139 (1969).

293. W. M. Dunlap, G. W. James, and D. M. Hume, Ann. Int. Med., 80, 470 (1974).

294. R. W. Vilter, R. C. Bozian, E. V. Hess, D. C. Zellner, and H. C. Petering, N. Engl. J. Med., 291, 1881 (1974).

295. M. M. Wintrobe, G. E. Cartwright, and C. J. Gubler, J. Nutr., 50, 395 (1953).

296. C. E. Hunt, W. W. Carlton, and P. M. Newberne, Fed. Proc., 25, 432 (1966).

297. C. H. Gallagher, Aust. Vet. J., 33, 311 (1957).

298. B. L. O'Dell, B. C. Hardwick, G. Reynolds, and J. E. Savage, Proc. Soc. Exp. Biol. Med., 108, 402 (1961).

299. R. B. Rucker, H. E. Parker, and J. C. Rogler, J. Nutr., 98, 57 (1969).

300. R. H. Follis, Jr., J. A. Bush, G. E. Cartwright, and M. M. Wintrobe, Bull. Johns Hopkins Hosp., 97, 405 (1955).

301. H. S. Teague and L. E. Carpenter, J. Nutr., 43, 389 (1951).

302. H. W. Bennetts, Aust. Vet. J., 8, 137 (1932).

303. H. W. Bennetts, Aust. Vet. J., 8, 183 (1932).

304. K. Guggenheim, E. Tal, and U. Zor, Brit. J. Nutr., 18, 529 (1964).

305. I. J. Cunningham, in Symposium on Copper Metabolism (W. D. McElroy and B. Glass, eds.), Johns Hopkins Press, Baltimore, 1950, p. 246.

306. G. K. Davis, in Symposium on Copper Metabolism (W. D. McElroy and B. Glass, eds.), Johns Hopkins Press, Baltimore, 1950, p. 216.

307. P. Bornstein, A. H. Kang, and K. A. Piez, Proc. Nat. Acad. Sci. U. S., 55, 417 (1966).

308. J. J. Harding, Advan. Protein Chem., 20, 109 (1965).

309. H. W. Bennetts and F. E. Chapman, Aust. Vet. J., 13, 138 (1937).

310. R. S. Hedger, D. A. Howard, and M. L. Burdin, Vet. Rec., 76, 493 (1964).

311. E. C. Owen, R. Proudfoot, J. M. Robertson, R. M. Barlow, E. J. Butler, and B. S. W. Smith, J. Comp. Pathol., 75, 241 (1965).

312. K. C. A. Schultz, P. K. VanderMerwe, P. J. Rensburg, and J. S. Swart, Onderstepoort J. Vet. Res., 25, 35 (1961).

313. G. J. Everson, M. C. Tsai, and T. Wang, J. Nutr., 93, 533 (1967).

314. J. M. Joyce, N. Z. Vet. J., 3, 157 (1955).

315. W. J. Wilkie, Aust. Vet. J., 35, 203 (1959).

316. W. W. Carlton and W. A. Kelly, J. Nutr., 97, 42 (1969).

317. B. F. Fell, C. F. Mills, and R. Boyne, Res. Vet. Sci., 6, 10 (1965).

318. M. O. Schultze, J. Biol. Chem., 129, 729 (1939).

319. M. O. Schultze, J. Biol. Chem., 138, 219 (1941).

320. C. J. Gubler, G. E. Cartwright, and M. M. Wintrobe, J. Biol. Chem., 224, 533 (1957).

321. E. W. Hurst, Aust. J. Exp. Biol. Med. Sci., 20, 297 (1942).

322. E. J. Linderwood, in Trace Elements in Human and Animal Nutrition, Academic, New York, 1971, p. 87.

323. S. E. Smith and G. H. Ellis, Arch. Biochem., 15, 81 (1947).

324. S. Uesaka, R. Kawashima, A. Iritani, K. Namikawa, N. Nakanishi, and T. Nishimo, Bull. Res. Inst. Food Sci., Kyoto Univ., 24 (1960).

325. H. S. Raper, Physiol. Rev., 8, 245 (1928).

326. H. J. Lee, J. Agr. Sci., 47, 218 (1956).

327. H. R. Marston, R. G. Thomas, D. Murnane, E. W. Lines, I. W. McDonald, H. O. Moore, and L. B. Bull, Aust. Common. Counc. Sci. Ind. Res. Bull., 113 (1938).

328. H. R. Marston, in Proceedings of the Symposium on Fibrous Proteins, Society of Dyers and Colourists, Leeds, 1946.

329. R. W. Burley and W. T. deKoch, Arch. Biochem. Biophys., 68, 21 (1957).

330. B. Dutt and C. F. Mills, J. Comp. Pathol., 70, 120 (1960).

331. G. A. Hall and J. McC. Howell, Brit. J. Nutr., 23, 41 (1969).

332. C. F. Simpson, J. E. Jones, and R. H. Harms, J. Nutr., 91, 283 (1967).

333. H. W. Bennetts and H. T. B. Hall, Aust. Vet. J., 15, 52 (1939).

334. H. W. Bennetts, R. Harley, and S. T. Evans, Aust. Vet. J., 18, 50 (1942).

335. H. W. Bennetts, A. B. Beck, and R. Harley, Aust. Vet. J., 24, 237 (1948).

336. E. E. VanKoetsveld, Diergeneesk., Jaarb., 83, 229 (1958).

337. J. A. Zipper, M. Medel, and R. Prager, J. Obstet. Gynecol., 105, 529 (1969).

338. V. Zbuzkova and F. A. Kincl, Acta Endocrinol., 66, 379 (1971).

339. J. A. Zipper, H. J. Tatum, M. Medel, L. Pastene, and M. Rivera, Nobel Symposium, 15, 199 (1971).

340. L. Fortier, Y. Lefebvre, M. Larose, R. Lanctot, Amer. J. Obstet. Gynecol., 115, 291 (1973).

341. M. Elstein and K. Ferrer, Brit. Med. J., 1, 507 (1972).

342. W. W. Carlton and W. Henderson, J. Nutr., 81, 200 (1963).

343. C. F. Simpson and R. H. Harms, Exp. Mol. Pathol., 3, 390 (1964).

344. C. E. Hunt, J. Landesman, and P. M. Newberne, Brit. J. Nutr., 24, 607 (1970).

345. W. H. Carnes, G. S. Shields, G. E. Cartwright, and M. M. Wintrobe, Fed. Proc., 20, 118 (1961).

346. W. F. Coulson and W. H. Carnes, Amer. J. Pathol., 43, 945 (1963).

347. G. S. Shields, W. F. Coulson, D. A. Kimball, W. H. Carnes, G. E. Cartwright, and M. M. Wintrobe, Fed. Proc., 20, 118 (1961).

348. W. A. Kelly, J. W. Kesterson, and W. W. Carlton, Exp. Mol. Pathol., 20, 40 (1974).

349. N. Weismann, G. S. Shields, and W. H. Carnes, J. Biol. Chem., 238, 3115 (1963).

350. B. Starcher, C. H. Hill, and G. Matrone, J. Nutr., 82, 318 (1964).

351. S. Partridge, D. F. Elsden, J. Thomas, A. Dorfman, A. Telser, and P. L. Ho, Biochem. J., 93, 308 (1964).

352. E. J. Miller, E. R. Martin, C. E. Mecca, and K. A. Piez, J. Biol. Chem., 240, 3623 (1965).

353. B. L. O'Dell, D. W. Bird, D. F. Ruggles, and J. E. Savage, J. Nutr., 88, 9 (1966).

354. C. H. Hill, B. Starcher, and C. Kim, Fed. Proc., 26, 129 (1968).

355. F. Buffoni and H. Blaschko, Proc. Roy. Soc., London, Ser. B, 161, 153 (1964).

356. J. M. Hill and P. G. Mann, Biochem. J., 85, 198 (1962).

357. H. Yamada and K. T. Yasunobu, J. Biol. Chem., 237, 1511 (1962).

358. H. Blaschko, F. Buffoni, N. Weissmann, W. H. Carnes, and W. F. Coulson, Biochem. J., 96, 48 (1965).

359. C. F. Mills, A. C. Dalgarno, and R. B. Williams, Biochem. Biophys. Res. Commun., 24, 537 (1966).

360. B. Sjollema, Biochem. Z., 267, 151 (1933).

361. B. Sjollema, Biochem. Z., 295, 372 (1938).

362. R. Allcroft and W. H. Parker, Brit. J. Nutr., 3, 205 (1949).

363. S. A. K. Wilson, Brain, 34, 295 (1912).

364. A. G. Bearn, Amer. J. Med., 15, 442 (1953).

365. I. H. Scheinberg and D. Gitlin, Science, 116, 484 (1952).

366. G. E. Cartwright, R. E. Hodges, C. J. Gubler, J. P. Mahoney, K. Daum, M. M. Wintrobe, and W. B. Bean, J. Clin. Invest., 33, 1487 (1954).

367. C. J. Earl, M. J. Moulton, and B. Selverstone, Amer. J. Med., 17, 205 (1954).

368. F. L. Iber, T. C. Chalmers, and L. L. Uzman, Metabolism, 6, 388 (1957).

369. L. L. Uzman, F. L. Iber, and T. C. Chalmers, Amer. J. Med. Sci., 231, 511 (1956).

370. M. H. K. Shokeir and D. C. Shreffler, Proc. Nat. Acad. Sci. U.S., 62, 867 (1969).

371. Y. Herishanu and E. Loewinger, Eur. Neurol., 8, 251 (1972).

372. J. H. Menkes, Pediatrics, 50, 181 (1972).

373. D. M. Danks, B. J. Stevens, P. E. Campbell, J. M. Gillespie, J. Walker-Smith, J. Blomfield, and B. Turner, Lancet, 1, 1100 (1972).

374. D. M. Danks, P. E. Campbell, B. J. Stevens, V. Mayne, and E. Cartwright, Pediatrics, 50, 188 (1972).

375. D. M. Danks, E. Cartwright, B. J. Stevens, and R. R. W. Townley, Science, 179, 1140 (1973).

376. S. Singh and M. J. Bresnan, Amer. J. Dis. Child., 125, 572 (1973).

377. F. W. Sunderman, Jr., Human Pathol., 4, 549 (1974).

378. M. Hrgovcic, C. F. Tessmer, T. M. Minckler, B. Mosier, and G. H. Taylor, Cancer, 21, 743 (1968).

379. R. L. Warren, A. M. Jelliffe, J. V. Watson, and C. B. Hobbs, Clin. Radiol., 20, 247 (1969).

380. G. Lipkin, F. Herrmann, and L. Mandol, J. Invest. Derm., 39, 593 (1962).

381. M. Kekki, P. Koskelo, and A. Lassus, J. Invest. Derm., 47, 159 (1966).

382. M. M. Molokhia and B. Portnoy, Brit. J. Derm., 83, 376 (1970).

383. P. Koskelo, M. Kekki, M. Virkkunen, A. Lassus, and R. Somer, Acta Rheum. Scand., 12, 261 (1966).

384. I. S. Maddox, Biochem. Biophys. Acta, 306, 74 (1973).

385. G. R. Sharpless and E. V. McCollum, J. Nutr., 6, 163 (1933).

386. A. R. Doberenz, A. A. Kurnick, E. B. Kurtz, A. R. Kemmerer, and B. L. Reid, Proc. Soc. Exp. Biol. Med., 117, 689 (1964).

387. R. J. Evans and P. H. Phillips, J. Nutr., 18, 353 (1939).

388. H. H. Mitchell and M. Edman, Nutr. Abstr. Rev., 21, 787 (1952).

389. F. J. McClendon and J. Gershon-Cohen, J. Agr. Food Chem., 1, 464 (1953).

390. K. Schwarz and D. B. Milne, Bioinorg. Chem., 1, 331 (1972).

391. F. J. McClure and R. C. Likins, J. Dent. Res., 30, 172 (1951).

392. M. F. Harrison, Brit. J. Nutr., 3, 162 (1949).

393. F. H. Nielsen and H. H. Sandstead, Amer. J. Clin. Nutr., 27, 515 (1974).

394. W. Machle, E. W. Scott, and J. Treon, Amer. J. Hyg., 29, 139 (1939).

395. F. J. McClure, Amer. J. Dis. Child., 66, 362 (1942).

396. J. Cholak, J. Occup. Med., <u>1</u>, 501 (1959).

397. W. Machle, E. W. Scott, and E. J. Largent, J. Ind. Hyg. Toxicol., <u>24</u>, 199 (1942).

398. A. W. Pierce, Nutr. Abstr. Rev., <u>9</u>, 253 (1939-1940).

399. C. H. Carlson, W. D. Armstrong, and L. Singer, Amer. J. Physiol., <u>199</u>, 187 (1960).

400. C. H. Carlson, W. D. Armstrong, and L. Singer, Proc. Soc. Exp. Biol. Med., <u>104</u>, 235 (1960).

401. E. J. Largent and F. F. Heyroth, J. Ind. Hyg. Toxicol., <u>31</u>, 134 (1949).

402. J. T. Rotruck, W. G. Hoekstra, A. L. Pope, H. Ganther, A. B. Swanson, and D. G. Hafeman, Fed. Proc., <u>31</u>, 691 (1972).

403. J. A. Weatherell, in Handbook of Experimental Pharmacology, Vol. 20, Springer Verlag, New York, 1966, p. 141.

404. J. Pinsent, Biochem. J., <u>57</u>, 10 (1954).

405. K. Schwarz, Fed. Proc., <u>33</u>, 1748 (1974).

406. H. T. Dean, in Fluorine and Dental Health, Amer. Ass. Advan. Sci., Washington, D. C., 1942, pp. 6-11 and 23-31.

407. J. R. Forrest, G. J. Parfitt, and E. R. Bransby, Mon. Bull. Min. Health Pub. Health Lab. Serv., <u>10</u>, 104 (1951).

408. F. S. McKay, Amer. J. Pub. Health, <u>38</u>, 828 (1948).

409. A. L. Russell and E. Elvove, Pub. Health Rep., <u>66</u>, 1389 (1951).

410. F. A. Arnold, Jr., Amer. J. Pub. Health, <u>47</u>, 539 (1957).

411. M. N. Naylor, Health Educ. J., <u>28</u>, 136 (1969).

412. R. Harris, Aust. Dent. J., <u>4</u>, 257 (1959).

413. J. W. Knutson and D. W. Armstrong, Pub. Health Rep., <u>58</u>, 1701 (1943); <u>60</u>, 1085 (1945); <u>61</u>, 1683 (1946); <u>62</u>, 425 (1947).

414. W. A. Jordan, J. R. Snyder, and V. Wilson, Pub. Health Rep., <u>73</u>, 1010 (1958).

415. M. Marthaler, Schweiz. Bull. Eidg. Gesundheitsamtes, Part B, <u>2</u> (1962).

416. H. J. Wespi, Schweiz. Bull. Eidg. Gesundheitsamtes, Part B, <u>2</u> (1962).

417. R. Ege, Tandlaegebladet, <u>65</u>, 445 (1961).

418. M. I. Aeschlimann, J. A. Grant, and J. F. Grigler, Jr., Metab. Clin. Exp., <u>15</u>, 905 (1966).

419. R. M. Cass, J. D. Croft, P. Perkins, W. Nye, C. Waterhouse, and R. Terry, Arch. Intern. Med., <u>118</u>, 111 (1966).

420. P. Cohen and F. H. Gardner, J. Amer. Med. Ass., <u>195</u>, 962 (1966).

421. M. J. Purves, Lancet, <u>2</u>, 1188 (1962).

422. C. Rich, J. Ensinck, and P. Ivanovitch, J. Clin. Invest., <u>43</u>, 545 (1964).

423. N. C. Leone, C. A. Stevenson, B. Beese, L. E. Hawes, and T. A. Dawber, Amer. Med. Ass. Arch. Ind. Health, <u>21</u>, 326 (1960).

424. D. S. Bernstein, N. Sadowsky, D. M. Hegsted, C. D. Guri, and F. J. Stare, J. Amer. Med. Ass., <u>198</u>, 499 (1966).

425. N. C. Leone, M. B. Shimkin, E. A. Arnold, C. A. Stevenson, E. R. Zimmerman, P. G. Geiser, and J. J. Lieberman, in Fluoridation as a Public Health Measure, Amer. Ass. Advan. Sci., Washington, D. C., 1964.

426. H. H. Messer, K. Wong, M. Wegner, L. Singer, and W. D. Armstrong, Nature (New Biology), 240, 218 (1972).

427. H. H. Messer, W. D. Armstrong, and L. Singer, Science, 177, 893 (1972).

428. J. S. McHarque, J. Agr. Res., 24, 781 (1923).

429. A. R. Kemmerer, C. A. Elvehjem, and E. B. Hart, J. Biol. Chem., 92, 623 (1931).

430. J. Waddell, H. Steenbock, and E. B. Hart, J. Nutr., 4, 53 (1931).

431. E. R. Orent and E. V. McCollum, J. Biol. Chem., 92, 651 (1931).

432. H. S. Wilgus, Jr., L. C. Norris, and G. F. Heuser, Science, 84, 252 (1936).

433. H. S. Wilgus, Jr., L. C. Norris, and G. F. Heuser, J. Nutr., 14, 155 (1937).

434. E. D. Weinberg, Appl. Microbiol., 12, 436 (1964).

435. D. E. Holtkamp and R. M. Hill, J. Nutr., 41, 307 (1950).

436. S. E. Smith and G. H. Ellis, J. Nutr., 34, 33 (1947).

437. T. B. Keith, R. C. Miller, W. T. S. Thorp, and M. A. McCarthy, J. Anim. Sci., 1, 120 (1942).

438. R. L. Atkinson, J. W. Bradley, J. R. Crouch, and J. H. Quisenberry, Poultry Sci., 46, 472 (1967).

439. National Research Council, Nutrient Requirements for Poultry, Nutrient Requirements for Domestic Animals, No. 1, Nat. Acad. Sci.-Nat. Res. Council, Washington, D. C., 1962.

440. W. H. Peterson and J. T. Skinner, J. Nutr., 4, 419 (1931).

441. H. A. Schroeder, J. J. Balassa, and I. H. Tipton, J. Chronic Dis., 19, 545 (1966).

442. R. Belz, Voeding, 21, 236 (1960).

443. B. B. North, J. M. Leichsenring, and L. M. Norris, J. Nutr., 72, 217 (1960).

444. I. H. Tipton, P. L. Stewart, and P. G. Martin, Health Phys., 12, 1683 (1966).

445. V. M. Lang, B. B. North, and L. M. Morse, J. Nutr., 85, 132 (1965).

446. G. W. Monier-Williams, in Trace Elements in Foods, Chapman and Hall, London, 1949.

447. D. M. Greenberg and W. A. Campbell, Proc. Nat. Acad. Sci. U.S., 26, 448 (1940).

448. D. M. Greenberg, H. D. Copp, and E. M. Cuthbertson, J. Biol. Chem., 147, 749 (1943).

449. W. T. Burnett, R. R. Bigelon, A. W. Kimbol, and C. W. Sheppard, Amer. J. Physiol., 168, 520 (1952).

450. A. J. Bertinchamps, S. T. Miller, and G. C. Cotzias, Amer. J. Physiol., 211, 217 (1966).

451. N. L. Kent and R. A. McCance, Biochem. J., 35, 877 (1941).

452. L. S. Maynard and S. Fink, J. Clin. Invest., 35, 83 (1956).

453. D. C. Borg and G. C. Cotzias, J. Clin. Invest., 37, 1269 (1958).

454. M. Kato, Quart. J. Exp. Physiol., 48, 355 (1963).

455. M. C. Scrutton, M. F. Utter, and A. S. Mildvan, J. Biol. Chem., 241, 3480 (1966).

456. S. J. Bach and D. B. Whitehouse, Biochem. J., 57, PXX1 (1954).

457. S. Edelbacher and H. Bauer, Naturwissenschaften, 26, 26 (1938).

458. D. C. Borg and G. C. Cotzias, Nature (London), 182, 1677 (1958).

459. A. J. Bertinchamps and G. C. Cotzias, Fed. Proc., 18, 469 (1959).

460. G. C. Cotzias and P. S. Papavasiliou, Nature (London), 195, 823 (1962).

461. A. C. Foradori, A. J. Bertinchamps, J. M. Gulebon, and G. C. Cotzias, J. Gen. Physiol., 50, 2255 (1967).

462. J. S. Wiberg and W. F. Newman, Arch. Biochem. Biophys., 72, 66 (1957).

463. H. Fore and R. A. Morton, Biochem. J., 51, 594, 598, 600, 603 (1952).

464. S. E. Smith, M. Medlicott, and G. H. Ellis, Arch. Biochem., 4, 281 (1944).

465. L. W. Wachtel, C. A. Elvehjem, and E. B. Hart, Amer. J. Physiol., 140, 72 (1943).

466. P. D. Boyer, J. H. Shaw, and P. H. Phillips, J. Biol. Chem., 143, 417 (1942).

467. L. L. Barnes, G. Sperling, and L. A. Maynard, Proc. Soc. Exp. Biol. Med., 46, 562 (1941).

468. M. E. Shils and E. V. McCollum, J. Nutr., 26, 1 (1943).

469. R. C. Miller, T. B. Keith, M. A. McCarthy, and W. T. S. Thorp, Proc. Soc. Exp. Biol. Med., 45, 50 (1950).

470. G. M. Neher, L. P. Doyle, D. M. Thrasher, and M. P. Plumlee, Amer. J. Vet. Res., 17, 121 (1956).

471. J. Grashuis, J. J. Lehr, L. L. E. Beuvery, and A. Beuvery-Asman, Meded. DeSchothorst, 540 (1953).

472. J. W. Lassiter and J. D. Morton, J. Anim. Sci., 27, 776 (1968).

473. M. Anke and B. Groppel, in Proc. First Int. Symp. Trace Element Metab. Anim., 1969 (C. F. Mills, ed.), Livingstone, Edinburgh, 1970.

474. M. Lyons and W. M. Insko, Jr., Ky. Agr. Exp. Sta. Bull., 371 (1937).

475. R. M. Loach, Jr. and A. M. Muenster, J. Nutr., 78, 51 (1962).

476. G. J. Everson, W. DeRafols, and L. S. Hurley, Fed. Proc. 23, 448 (1964).

477. R. E. Shrader and G. J. Everson, J. Nutr., 91, 453 1967).

478. H. Tsai and G. J. Everson, J. Nutr., 91, 447 (1967).

479. R. M. Leach, Jr., Fed. Proc., 26, 118 (1967).

480. R. M. Leach, Jr., A. M. Muenster, and E. M. Wien, Arch. Biochem. Biophys., 133, 22 (1969).

481. A. L. Daniels and G. J. Everson, J. Nutr., 9, 191 (1935).

482. P. J. Schaible, S. L. Bandemer, and J. A. Davidson, Mich. Agr. Exp. Sta., Tech. Bull., 159 (1938).

483. G. J. Everson, L. S. Hurley, and J. F. Geiger, J. Nutr., 68, 49 (1959).

484. O. G. Bentley and P. H. Phillips, J. Dairy Sci., 34, 396 (1951).

485. M. A. Rojas, I. A. Dyer, and W. A. Cassatt, J. Anim. Sci., 24, 664 (1965).

486. R. H. Grummer, O. G. Bentley, P. H. Phillips, and G. Bohstedt, J. Anim. Sci., 9, 170 (1950).

487. M. P. Plumlee, D. M. Thrasher, W. N. Beeson, F. N. Andrews, and H. E. Parker, J. Anim. Sci., 13, 996 (1954); 15, 352 (1956).

488. C. D. Caskey and L. C. Norris, Proc. Soc. Exp. Biol. Med., 44, 332 (1940).

489. L. S. Hurley and G. J. Everson, Proc. Soc. Exp. Biol. Med., 102, 360 (1959).

490. L. S. Hurley, G. J. Everson, and J. F. Geiger, J. Nutr., 66, 309 (1958); 67, 445 (1959).

491. C. D. Caskey, L. C. Norris, and G. F. Heuser, Poultry Sci., 23, 516 (1944).

492. R. M. Hill, D. E. Holtkamp, A. R. Buchanan, and E. K. Rutledge, J. Nutr., 41, 359 (1950).

493. L. S. Hurley, E. Wooten, and G. J. Everson, J. Nutr., 74, 282 (1961).

494. L. S. Hurley, D. E. Woolley, and P. S. Timiras, Proc. Soc. Exp. Biol. Med., 106, 343 (1961).

495. L. S. Hurley, E. Wooten, G. J. Everson, and C. W. Asling, J. Nutr., 71, 15 (1960).

496. R. E. Shrader and G. J. Everson, J. Nutr., 91, 453 (1967).

497. L. C. Erway and S. E. Mitchell, J. Hered., 64, 111 (1973).

498. G. J. Everson and R. D. Shrader, J. Nutr., 94, 89 (1968).

499. R. E. Shrader and G. J. Everson, J. Nutr., 94, 269 (1968).

500. P. M. Belyaev, J. Physiol. (U.S.S.R.), 25, 741 (1938).

501. A. H. Rubenstein, N. W. Levin, and G. A. Elliott, Nature (London), 194, 188 (1962).

502. G. O. Babenko and Z. V. Karplyuk, Ukr. Biokhim. Zh., 35, 732 (1963).

503. L. G. Kosenko, Klin. Med. (Moscow), 42, 113 (1964).

504. V. P. Zhuk, Bull. Exp. Biol. Med. (U.S.S.R.), 54, 1272 (1964).

505. S. Schiller and A. Dorfman, J. Biol. Chem., 227, 625 (1957).

506. R. J. Evans, M. Rhian, and C. I. Draper, Poultry Sci., 22, 88 (1943).

507. A. G. Hogan, L. R. Richardson, H. Patrick, and H. L. Kempter, J. Nutr., 21, 327 (1941).

508. T. H. Jukes, J. Biol. Chem., 134, 789 (1940); J. Nutr., 20, 445 (1940).

509. G. L. Curran, J. Biol. Chem., 210, 765 (1954).

510. B. H. Amdur, H. Rilling, and K. Bloch, J. Amer. Chem. Soc., 79, 2646 (1957).

511. T. T. Tchen, J. Amer. Chem. Soc., 79, 6344 (1957).

512. L. T. Bell and L. S. Hurley, Proc. Soc. Exp. Biol. Med., 145, 1321 (1974).

513. L. T. Bell and L. S. Hurley, Lab. Invest., 29, 723 (1973).

514. D. Keilin, Proc. Roy. Soc., 98B, 312 (1925).

515. H. R. Mahler and D. G. Elowe, J. Amer. Chem. Soc., 75, 5769 (1953).

516. D. A. Richert and W. W. Westerfield, J. Biol. Chem., 209, 179 (1954).

517. E. Beutler, Amer. J. Med. Sci., 234, 517 (1957).

518. E. Beutler, Acta Hematol., 21, 371 (1959).

519. E. Beutler, J. Clin. Invest., 38, 1605 (1959).

520. P. N. Davis, L. C. Norris, and F. J. Kratzer, J. Nutr., 94, 407 (1968).

521. W. J. Darby, in Handbook of Nutrition, 2nd Ed., McGraw-Hill (Blakiston), New York, 1951.

522. J. C. Hawksley, R. Lightwood, and U. M. Bailey, Arch. Dis. Child., 9, 359 (1934).

523. F. Lees and F. D. Rosenthal, Quart. J. Med., 27, 19 (1958).

524. G. Rybo, Acta Obstet. Gynecol. Scand., 45 (Suppl.), 7 (1966).

525. V. Laufberger, Bull. Soc. Chim. Biol., 19, 1575 (1937).

526. B. I. Allaire and A. Campagna, Obstet. Gynecol., 17, 605 (1961).

527. J. A. Pritchard and C. F. Hunt, Surg. Gynecol. Obstet., 106, 516 (1958).

528. T. H. Bothwell and C. A. Finch, in Iron Metabolism, Little, Brown, Boston, 1962.

529. C. Mukherjee and S. K. Mukherjee, J. Indian Med. Ass., 22, 345 (1953).

530. R. Hussain, R. B. Walker, M. Layrisse, P. Clark, and C. A. Finch, Amer. J. Clin. Nutr., 20, 842 (1967).

531. G. von Bunge, Hoppe-Seyler's Z. Physiol. Chem., 13, 399 (1899).

532. E. Ezekiel, J. Lab. Clin. Med., 70, 138 (1967).

533. V. A. Beal, A. J. Myers, and R. W. McCammon, Pediatrics, 30, 518 (1962).

534. P. Sturgeon, Pediatrics, 17, 341 (1956); 18, 267 (1956).

535. J. D. Farquhar, Amer. J. Dis. Child., 106, 201 (1963).

536. E. B. Hart, C. A. Elvehjem, H. Steenbock, G. Bohstedt, and J. M. Fargo, J. Nutr., 2, 227 (1930).

537. J. P. McGowan and A. Crichton, Biochem. J., 17, 204 (1923); 18, 265 (1924).

538. J. A. J. Venn, R. A. McCance, and E. M. Widdowson, J. Comp. Pathol. Ther., 57, 314 (1947).

539. J. W. Hibbs, H. R. Conrad, J. H. Vandersall, and G. Gale, J. Dairy Sci., 46, 1118 (1963).

540. J. A. Campbell and A. C. Gardiner, Vet. Rec., 72, 1006 (1960).

541. R. M. Richard, R. F. Shumard, A. L. Pope, P. H. Phillips, C. A. Herrick, and G. Bohstedt, J. Anim. Sci., 13, 274 and 674 (1954).

542. E. J. Underwood, in Trace Elements in Human and Animal Nutrition, 3rd Ed., Academic, New York, 1971, p. 47.

543. C. V. Moore, in Modern Nutrition in Health and Disease (R. S. Goodhart and M. E. Shils, eds.), Lea and Febiger, Philadelphia, 1973, p. 300.

544. R. A. MacDonald, Arch. Int. Med., 112, 184 (1963).

545. H. C. Sherman, in Chemistry of Food Nutrition, Macmillan, New York, 1935.

546. Nat. Health Med. Res. Council (Aust.), Spec. Rep. No. 1 (1945).

547. Health Bull. No. 23, India Press, New Delhi, 1951.

548. Committee on Iron Deficiency, J. Amer. Med. Ass., 203, 407 (1968).

549. A. E. Harper, Nutr. Rev., 31, 393 (1973).

550. E. B. Brown and B. W. Justus, Amer. J. Physiol., 194, 319 (1958).

551. B. W. Gabrio and K. Salomon, Proc. Soc. Exp. Biol. Med., 75, 124 (1950).

552. W. B. Stewart, C. L. Yuile, H. A. Clairborne, R. T. Snowman, and G. H. Whipple, J. Exp. Med., 92, 372 (1970).

553. C. W. Heath and A. J. Patek, Medicine, 16, 267 (1937).

554. W. L. Niccum, R. L. Jackson, and G. Stearns, Amer. J. Dis. Child., 86, 553 (1953).

555. D. J. Kroe, N. Kaufman, J. V. Klavins, and T. D. Kinney, Amer. J. Physiol., 211, 414 (1966).

556. D. Van Campen and E. Gross, J. Nutr., 99, 68 (1969).

557. S. Granick, J. Biol. Chem., 164, 737 (1946).

558. S. Granick, Physiol. Rev., 31, 489 (1951).

559. L. Hallberg and L. Sölvell, Acta Med. Scand., 181, 335 (1967).

560. C. V. Moore and R. Dubach, Trans. Ass. Amer. Physicians, 64, 245 (1951).

561. G. Pirzio-Biroli, T. H. Bothwell, and C. A. Finch, J. Lab. Clin. Med., 51, 37 (1958).

562. R. Hussain and V. N. Patwardhan, Indian J. Med. Res., 47, 676 (1959).

563. L. M. Sharpe, W. C. Peacock, R. Cook, and R. S. Harris, J. Nutr., 41, 433 (1950).

564. G. E. Cartwright and M. M. Wintrobe, in Modern Trends in Blood Diseases (J. F. Wilkinson, ed.), Butterworths, Washington, D. C., 1954, p. 183.

565. R. Dubach, S. T. Callender, and C. V. Moore, Blood, 3, 526 (1948).

566. R. E. Peterson and R. H. Ettinger, Amer. J. Med., 15, 518 (1953).

567. T. H. Bothwell, G. Pirzio-Biroli, and C. A. Finch, J. Lab. Clin. Med., 51, 24 (1958).

568. L. R. Weintraub, M. E. Conrad, and W. H. Crosby, Brit. J. Hematol., 11, 432 (1965).

569. G. A. Mendel, Blood, 18, 727 (1961).

570. G. A. Mendel, R. J. Wiler, and A. Mangalik, Blood, 22, 450 (1963).

571. L. R. Weintraub, M. E. Conrad, and W. H. Crosby, J. Clin. Invest., 43, 40 (1964).

572. R. Braude, A. G. Chamberlain, M. Kotarbinski, and K. R. Mitchell, Brit. J. Nutr., 16, 427 (1962).

573. M. E. Conrad, L. R. Weintraub, and W. H. Crosby, J. Clin. Invest., 43, 963 (1964).

574. R. P. Dallman, J. Nutr., 97, 475 (1969).

575. P. D. Dallman and H. C. Schwartz, Pediatrics, 35, 677 (1965).

576. P. D. Dallman and H. C. Schwartz, J. Clin. Invest., 44, 1631 (1965).

577. H. A. Salmon, J. Physiol. (London), 164, 17 (1962).

578. R. P. Cusack and W. B. Brown, J. Nutr., 86, 383 (1965).

579. S. K. Srivastava, G. G. Sanwal, and K. K. Tewari, Indian J. Biochem., 2, 257 (1965).

580. E. Beutler and R. K. Blaisdell, J. Lab. Clin. Med., 52, 694 (1958).

581. E. Beutler and R. K. Blaisdell, Blood, 15, 30 (1960).

582. H. Bortels, Arch. Mikrobiol., 1, 333 (1930).

583. R. A. Steinberg, J. Agr. Res., 52, 439 (1936).

584. D. I. Arnon and P. R. Stout, Plant Physiol., 14, 599 (1939).

585. E. C. de Renzo, E. Kaleita, P. Heytler, J. J. Oleson, B. L. Hutching, and J. H. Williams, J. Amer. Chem. Soc., 75, 753 (1953).

586. E. C. de Renzo, E. Kaleita, P. Heytler, J. J. Oleson, B. L. Hutching, and J. H. Williams, Arch. Biochem. Biophys., 45, 247 (1953).

587. D. A. Richert and W. W. Westerfield, J. Biol. Chem., 203, 915 (1953).

588. W. C. Ellis, W. H. Pfander, M. E. Muhner, and E. E. Pickett, J. Anim. Sci. 17, 180 (1958).

589. E. S. Higgins, D. A. Richert, and W. W. Westerfield, J. Nutr., 59, 539 (1956).

590. B. L. Reid, A. A. Kurnich, R. L. Svacha, and J. R. Crouch, Proc. Soc. Exp. Biol. Med., 93, 245 (1956).

591. I. H. Tipton, P. L. Stewart, and P. G. Martin, Health Phys., 12, 1683 (1966).

592. R. F. Miller, N. O. Price, and R. W. Engel, Fed. Proc., 18, 538 (1959).

593. D. Bertrand, C. R. Acad. Sci., 208, 2024 (1939).

594. H. TerMeulen, Nature (London), 130, 966 (1932).

595. W. W. Westerfeld and D. A. Richert, J. Nutr., 51, 85 (1953).

596. W. S. Ferguson, A. H. Lewis, and S. J. Watson, Nature (London), 141, 553 (1938).

597. L. T. Fairhall, R. D. Dunn, N. E. Sharpless, and E. A. Pritchard, U.S. Public Health Serv. Bull., 293 (1945).

598. M. C. Bell, B. G. Higgs, R. S. Lowry, and P. L. Wright, Fed. Proc., 23, 873 (1964).

599. R. K. Shirley, M. A. Jeter, J. P. Feaster, J. T. McCall, J. C. Cutler, and G. K. Davis, J. Nutr., 54, 59 (1954).

600. J. B. Nielands, F. M. Strong, and C. A. Elvehjem, J. Biol. Chem., 172, 431 (1948).

601. B. Rosoff and H. Spencer, Nature (London), 20, 410 (1964).

602. R. F. Miller, N. O. Price, and R. W. Engel, J. Nutr., 60, 539 (1956).

603. I. J. Cunningham, K. G. Hogan, and B. M. Lawson, N. Z. J. Agr. Res., 2, 145 (1959).

604. A. T. Dick, in Inorganic Nitrogen Metabolism (W. D. McElroy and B. Glass, eds.), Johns Hopkins Press, Baltimore, 1956, p. 445.

605. J. F. Scaife, N. Z. J. Sci. Technol., Sec. A, 38, 285 (1963).

606. J. F. Scaife, N. Z. J. Sci. Technol., Sec. A, 38, 293 (1963).

607. P. Andrews, R. C. Bray, and K. V. Shooter, Biochem. J., 93, 627 (1964).

608. P. G. Avis, F. Bergel, and R. C. Bray, J. Chem. Soc., 1219 (1956).

609. R. C. Bray, R. Peterson, and A. Ehrenberg, Biochem. J., 81, 178 (1956).

610. F. Bergel and R. C. Bray, Biochem. Soc. Symp., 15, 64 (1958).

611. S. P. Albrecht and E. C. Slater, Biochim. Biophys. Acta, 223, 457 (1970).

612. B. Mackler and B. Haynes, Arch. Biochem. Biophys., 146, 364 (1971).

613. H. J. Cohen, I. Fridovich, and K. V. Rajagopalan, J. Biol. Chem., 246, 374 (1971).

614. M. S. Seelig, Amer. J. Clin. Nutr., 26, 657 (1973).

615. P. Adler and J. Straub, Acta Med. Acad. Sci. Hung., 4, 221 (1953).

616. Z. Nagy and E. Polyik, Forgovosi Szemle, 48, 154 (1954).

617. T. L. Ludwig, W. B. Healy, and F. L. Losee, Nature (London), 186, 695 (1960).

618. W. B. Healy, T. G. Ludwig, and F. L. Losee, Soil Sci., 92, 359 (1961).

619. P. Adler, Ondontol. Rev., 8, 202 (1957).

620. B. J. Kruger, in The Effect of Trace Elements on Experimental Caries in the Rat, Univ. of Queensland Press, Brisbane, Australia, 1959.

621. W. Buttner, Arch. Oral Biol. Suppl., 6, 40 (1961).

622. W. Buttner, J. Dent. Res., 42, 453 (1963).

623. R. S. Malthus, T. G. Ludwig, and W. B. Healy, N. Z. Dent. J., 60, 291 (1964).

624. Y. Ericsson, Acta Odontol. Scand., 24, 405 (1966).

625. Y. M. Bala and V. M. Liftshits, Probl. Gematol. Perelv. Krovi, 10, 23 (1965).

626. T. H. Easterfield, T. Rigg, H. O. Askew, and J. A. Bruce, J. Agr. Sci., 19, 573 (1929).

627. F. H. Nielsen, in Newer Trace Metals in Nutrition, Marcel Dekker, New York, 1971, p. 215.

628. F. H. Nielsen and D. J. Higgs, Proc. Trace Substances, Environ. Health, 4, 241 (1971).

629. F. H. Nielsen and H. E. Sauberlich, Proc. Soc. Exp. Biol. Med., 134, 845 (1970).

630. F. H. Nielsen and D. A. Ollerich, Fed. Proc., 33, 1767 (1974).

631. F. H. Nielsen and H. H. Sandstead, Amer. J. Clin. Nutr., 27, 515 (1974).

632. F. W. Sunderman, Jr., S. Nomoto, R. Morang, M. W. Nechay, C. N. Burke, and S. W. Nielsen, J. Nutr., 102, 259 (1972).

633. N. L. Kent and R. A. McChance, Biochem. J., 35, 837 (1941).

634. N. L. Kent and R. A. McChance, Biochem. J., 35, 877 (1941).

635. H. A. Schroeder, J. J. Balassa, and I. H. Tipton, J. Chronic Dis., 15, 51 (1961).

636. K. R. Drinker, L. T. Fairhall, G. B. Ray, and C. K. Drinker, J. Ind. Hyg., 6, 307 (1924).

637. D. Gesell-Schlettwein and S. Mommsen-Straub, Int. 2, Vitaminforschung, 41, 429 (1971).

638. A. C. Titus, H. B. Elkins, H. G. Finn, and L. T. Fairhall, J. Ind. Hyg., 12, 306 (1930).

639. P. I. Nodiya, Gig. Sanit., 37, 108 (1972).

640. F. W. Sunderman, Jr., J. C. White, and F. W. Sunderman, Amer. J. Med., 34, 875 (1963).

641. G. Bertrand and M. Macheboeuf, C. R. Acad. Sci., 180, 1380 (1925).

642. G. Bertrand and M. Macheboeuf, C. R. Acad. Sci., 180, 1993 (1925).

643. G. Bertrand and M. Macheboeuf, C. R. Acad. Sci., 182, 1504 (1926).

644. G. Bertrand and M. Macheboeuf, C. R. Acad. Sci., 183, 5 (1926).

645. R. E. Tedeschi and F. W. Sunderman, Amer. Med. Ass. Arch. Ind. Health, 16, 486 (1957).

646. H. M. Perry, Jr. and E. F. Perry, J. Clin. Invest., 38, 1452 (1959).

647. H. M. Imbrus, J. Cholak, L. H. Miller, and T. Sterling, Arch. Environ. Health, 6, 286 (1963).

648. F. W. Sunderman, Jr., Amer. J. Clin. Pathol., 44, 182 (1965).

649. S. S. Phatak and V. N. Patwardhan, Indian J. Sci. Ind. Res. A, 9, 70 (1950).

650. S. S. Phatak and V. N. Patwardhan, Indian J. Sci. Ind. Res. A, 11, 172 (1952).

651. E. Horek and F. W. Sunderman, Jr., Clin. Chem., 19, 429 (1973).

652. J. C. Smith and B. Hackley, J. Nutr., 95, 541 (1968).

653. R. Monacelli, H. Tanaka, and J. H. Yoe, Clin. Chim. Acta, 1, 557 (1956).

654. H. J. Koch, E. R. Smith, N. F. Shimp, and J. Conner, Cancer, 9, 499 (1956).

655. L. M. Paixao and J. H. Yoe, Clin. Chim. Acta, 4, 507 (1959).

656. W. B. Herring, B. S. Leavell, L. M. Paixao, and J. H. Yoe, Amer. J. Clin. Nutr., 8, 846 (1960).

657. L. Hellerman and M. E. Perkins, J. Biol. Chem., 112, 175 (1935).

658. J. F. Speck, J. Biol. Chem., 178, 315 (1949).

659. L. T. Webster, Jr., J. Biol. Chem., 240, 4164 (1965).

660. K. Sugai, J. Biochem. (Tokyo), 36, 91 (1944).

661. W. J. Ray, Jr., J. Biol. Chem., 244, 3740 (1969).

662. F. Allison, Jr. and M. G. Lancaster, Ann. N. Y. Acad. Sci., 116, 936 (1964).

663. F. Allison, Jr., M. G. Lancaster, and J. L. Crosthwaite, Amer. J. Physiol., 43, 775 (1963).

664. J. E. Garvin, J. Cell. Physiol., 72, 194 (1968).

665. K. Fuwa, W. E. C. Wacker, R. Druyan, A. F. Bartholomay, and B. L. Vallee, Proc. Nat. Acad. Sci. U.S., 46, 1298 (1960).

666. G. L. Eichhorn, Nature, 194, 474 (1962).

667. P. C. Cheo, B. S. Friesen, and R. L. Sinsheimer, Proc. Nat. Acad. Sci. U.S., 45, 305 (1959).

668. W. E. C. Wacker, M. P. Gordon, and J. W. Huff, Biochemistry, 2, 716 (1963).

669. M. Tal, Biochim. Biophys. Acta, 169, 564 (1968).

670. M. Tal, Biochemistry, 8, 424 (1969).

671. M. Tal, Biochim. Biophys. Acta, 195, 76 (1969).

672. M. U. King, Nature (London), 201, 918 (1964).

673. G. L. Eichhorn, Nature (London), 194, 474 (1962).

674. W. E. C. Wacker and B. L. Vallee, J. Biol. Chem., 234, 3257 (1959).

675. S. R. Himmelhoch, H. A. Sober, B. L. Vallee, E. A. Peterson, and K. Fuwa, Biochemistry, 5, 2523 (1966).

676. S. Nomoto, M. D. McNeely, and F. W. Sunderman, Jr., Biochemistry, 10, 1647 (1971).

677. H. Kikkawa, J. Jap. Biochem. Soc., 27, 427 (1955).

678. H. Kikkawa, Z. Ogita, and S. Fujito, Science, 121, 43 (1955).

679. F. W. Sunderman, Jr., S. Nomoto, A. M. Pradhan, H. Levine, S. H. Bernstein, and R. Hirsch, N. Engl. J. Med., 283, 896 (1970).

680. M. D. McNeely, F. W. Sunderman, Jr., M. W. Nechay, and H. Levine, Clin. Chem., 17, 1123 (1971).

681. F. W. Sunderman, Jr., M. I. Decsy, and M. D. McNeely, Ann. N. Y. Acad. Sci., 199, 300 (1972).

682. M. D. McNeely, M. W. Nechay, and F. W. Sunderman, Jr., Clin. Chem., 18, 992 (1972).

683. M. W. Nechay and F. W. Sunderman, Jr., Clin. Chem., 19, 429 (1973).

684. K. Schwarz, Proc. Soc. Exp. Biol. Med., 77, 818 (1951); 78, 852 (1951).

685. K. Schwarz and C. M. Foltz, J. Amer. Chem. Soc., 79, 3293 (1957).

686. W. J. Hartley, C. Drake, and A. B. Grant, N. Z. J. Agr., 99, 259
      (1959).

687. J. W. McLean, G. G. Thompson, and J. H. Claxton, Nature (London),
      184, 251 (1959).

688. J. W. McLean, G. G. Thompson, and J. H. Claxton, N. Z. Vet. J., 7,
      47 (1959).

689. O. H. Muth, J. E. Oldfield, L. F. Remmert, and J. R. Schubert, Science,
      28, 1090 (1958).

690. J. F. Proctor, D. E. Hogue, and R. G. Warner, J. Anim. Sci., 17, 1183
      (1958).

691. R. G. Eggert, E. L. Patterson, W. T. Akers, and E. L. R. Stokstad, J.
      Anim. Sci., 16, 1037 (1957).

692. C. A. Grant and B. Thafvelin, Nord. Veterinuer Med., 10, 657 (1958).

693. W. J. Hartley and A. B. Grant, Fed. Proc., 20, 679 (1961).

694. P. L. Harris, M. I. Ludwig, and K. Schwarz, Proc. Soc. Exp. Biol. Med.,
      97, 686 (1958).

695. H. Dam, G. K. Nielsen, I. Prange, and E. Sondergaard, Nature (London),
      182, 802 (1958).

696. J. N. Thompson and M. L. Scott, J. Nutr., 97, 335 (1969); 100, 797
      (1970).

697. K. E. M. McCoy and P. H. Weswig, J. Nutr., 98, 383 (1967).

698. S. H. Wu, J. E. Oldfield, O. H. Muth, P. D. Whanger, and P. H. Weswig,
      Proc. West. Sec. Amer. Soc. Anim. Sci., 20, 85 (1969).

699. J. N. Thompson and M. L. Scott, in Proceedings of the 1967 Cornell
      Nutrition Conference for Feed Manufacturers, Cornell Univ. Press,
      Ithaca, New York, 1967, p. 130.

700. V. C. Morris and O. A. Levander, J. Nutr., 100, 1383 (1970).

701. D. Arthur, Can. Inst. Food Sci. Technol., 5, 165 (1972).

702. W. H. Allaway and J. F. Hodgson, J. Anim. Sci., 23, 271 (1964).

703. J. E. Oldfield, J. R. Schubert, and O. H. Muth, J. Agr. Food Chem.,
      11, 388 (1963).

704. R. M. Gardiner and P. C. Gorman, Aust. J. Exp. Agr. Anim. Husb., 3,
      284 (1966).

705. M. C. Nesheim and M. L. Scott, J. Nutr., 65, 601 (1958).

706. M. L. Scott, G. Olson, L. Krook, and W. R. Brown, J. Nutr., 91, 573
      (1967).

707. P. L. Wright and M. C. Bell, Amer. J. Physiol., 211, 6 (1966).

708. G. W. Butler and P. J. Peterson, N. Z. J. Agr. Res., 4, 484 (1961).

709. F. B. Cousins and I. M. Cairney, Aust. J. Agr. Res., 12, 927 (1961).

710. L. S. Jensen, E. D. Walter, and J. S. Dunlap, Proc. Soc. Exp. Biol.
      Med., 112, 899 (1963).

711. R. F. Burk, R. Whitney, H. Frank, and W. N. Pearson, J. Nutr., 95, 420 (1968).

712. L. L. Hopkins, Jr., A. L. Pope, and C. A. Baumann, J. Nutr., 88, 61 (1966).

713. P. L. Lopez, R. L. Preston, and W. H. Pfander, J. Nutr., 94, 219 (1968).

714. P. L. Wright and M. C. Bell, J. Nutr., 84, 49 (1964).

715. R. G. Buescher, M. C. Bell, and R. K. Berry, J. Anim. Sci., 19, 1251 (1960).

716. K. P. McConnell and R. S. Levy, Nature (London), 195, 774 (1962).

717. M. I. Smith, B. B. Westfall, and E. F. Stohlman, Pub. Health Rep., 52, 1171 (1937); 53, 1199 (1938).

718. A. L. Moxon and M. Rhian, Physiol. Rev., 23, 305 (1943).

719. K. P. McConnell and D. M. Roth, Biochem. Biophys. Acta, 62, 503 (1962).

720. K. P. McConnell and C. H. Wabnitz, J. Biol. Chem., 226, 765 (1957).

721. I. Rosenfeld, Proc. Soc. Exp. Biol. Med., 111, 670 (1962).

722. L. M. Cummings and J. M. Martin, Biochemistry, 6, 3162 (1967).

723. E. Hansson and S. O. Jacobson, Biochim. Biophys. Acta, 115, 285 (1966).

724. B. B. Westfall, E. F. Stohlman, and M. I. Smith, J. Pharmacol. Exp. Ther., 64, 55 (1938).

725. K. P. McConnell and D. M. Roth, J. Nutr., 84, 340 (1964).

726. V. Burton, R. F. Keeler, K. F. Swingle, and S. Young, Amer. J. Vet. Res., 23, 962 (1962).

727. W. G. Hoekstra, in Trace Element Metabolism in Animals, Vol. 2 (W. G. Hoekstra, J. W. Suttie, H. E. Ganther, and W. Mertz, eds.), University Park Press, Baltimore, 1974, p. 61.

728. P. D. Whanger, N. D. Pederson, and P. H. Weswig, in Trace Element Metabolism in Animals, Vol. 2 (W. G. Hoekstra, J. W. Suttie, H. E. Ganther, and W. Mertz, eds.), University Park Press, Baltimore, 1974, p. 571.

729. K. R. Millar, N. Z. J. Agr. Res., 15, 547 (1972).

730. A. T. Diplock, in Trace Element Metabolism in Animals, Vol. 2 (W. G. Hoekstra, J. W. Suttie, H. E. Ganther, and W. Mertz, eds.), University Park Press, Baltimore, 1974, p. 147.

731. O. A. Levander, V. C. Morris, and D. J. Higgs, in Trace Element Metabolism in Animals, Vol. 2 (W. G. Hoekstra, J. W. Suttie, H. E. Ganther, and W. Mertz, eds.), University Park Press, 1974, p. 584.

732. E. E. Edwin, A. T. Diplock, J. Bunyan, and J. Green, Biochem. J., 79, 108 (1961).

733. J. Green, A. T. Diplock, J. Bunyan, E. E. Edwin, and D. McHale, Nature, 190, 318 (1961).

734. J. Green, A. T. Diplock, J. Bunyan, and E. E. Edwin, Biochem. J., 79, 108 (1961).

735. G. D. Paulson, A. L. Pope, and C. A. Baumann, Proc. Soc. Exp. Biol. Med., 122, 321 (1966).

736. P. D. Whanger, O. H. Muth, J. E. Oldfield, and P. H. Weswig, J. Nutr., 97, 553 (1969).

737. P. D. Whanger, P. H. Weswig, O. H. Muth, and J. E. Oldfield, J. Nutr., 99, 331 (1969).

738. O. H. Muth, J. E. Oldfield, L. F. Remmert, and J. R. Schubert, Science, 28, 1090 (1958).

739. H. E. Oksanen, in Selenium in Biomedicine (O. H. Muth, ed.), Avi Publishing Co., Westport, Connecticut, 1967, p. 215.

740. H. Dam, J. Nutr., 27, 193 (1944).

741. M. C. Nesheim and M. L. Scott, Fed. Proc., 20, 674 (1961).

742. E. L. Patterson, R. Milstrey, and E. R. L. Stokstad, Proc. Soc. Exp. Biol. Med., 95, 621 (1957).

743. R. M. Salisbury, J. Edmondson, W. S. H. Poole, F. C. Bobby, and H. Bernie, Worlds Poultry Cong., Proc. 12th, 1962, p. 379.

744. K. Schwarz, J. G. Bieri, G. M. Briggs, and M. L. Scott, Proc. Soc. Exp. Biol. Med., 95, 621 (1957).

745. E. D. Andrews, W. J. Hartley, and A. B. Grant, N. Z. Vet. J., 16, 3 (1968).

746. C. Drake, A. B. Grant, and W. J. Hartley, N. Z. Vet. J., 8, 4 and 7 (1960).

747. G. B. Jones and K. O. Godwin, Aust. J. Agr. Res., 14, 716 (1963).

748. G. F. Wilson, N. Z. J. Agr. Res., 7, 432 (1964).

749. W. J. Hartley, in Selenium in Biomedicine (O. H. Muth, ed.), Avi Publishing Co., Westport, Connecticut, 1967, p. 79.

750. K. E. Hart and M. M. Mackinnon, N. Z. Vet. J., 6, 118 (1958).

751. K. E. Hart and M. M. Mackinnon, N. Z. Vet. J., 7, 18 (1959).

752. D. L. Mace, J. A. Tucker, C. B. Bills, and C. J. Ferreira, Calif. Dep. Agr., Bull., 1, 63 (1963).

753. W. J. Hartley, Proc. N. Z. Soc. Anim. Prod., 23, 20 (1963).

754. L. S. Jensen, Proc. Soc. Exp. Biol. Med., 128, 970 (1968).

755. R. J. Shamberger, Experientia, 22, 116 (1966).

756. R. J. Shamberger, J. Nat. Cancer Inst., 44, 931 (1970).

757. R. J. Shamberger and C. E. Willis, C. R. C. Crit. Rev. Clin. Lab. Sci., 2, 211 (1971).

758. R. J. Shamberger, S. Tytko, and C. E. Willis, Proc. Seventh Ann. Conf. Trace Sub. Environ. Health, VII, 35 (1974).

759. R. J. Shamberger, T. L. Andreone, and C. E. Willis, Proc. Amer. Ass. Cancer Res., 15, 26 (1974).

760. R. J. Shamberger, T. L. Andreone, and C. E. Willis, J. Nat. Cancer Inst., (1974) (in press).

761. R. J. Shamberger, F. F. Baughman, S. L. Kalchert, C. E. Willis, and G. C. Hoffman, Proc. Nat. Acad. Sci. U.S., 70, 1461 (1973).

762. R. J. Shamberger, in Trace Element Metabolism in Animals, Vol. 2 (W. G. Hoekstra, J. W. Suttie, H. E. Ganther, and W. Mertz, eds.), University Park Press, Baltimore, 1974, p. 511.

763. R. J. Shamberger, E. Rukovena, A. K. Longfield, S. A. Tytko, S. Deodhar, and C. E. Willis, J. Nat. Cancer Inst., 50, 863 (1973).

764. C. C. Clayton and C. A. Baumann, Cancer Res., 9, 575 (1949).

765. J. R. Harr, J. H. Exon, P. D. Whanger, and P. H. Weswig, Clin. Toxicol., 5, 187 (1972).

766. J. R. Shapiro, Ann. N. Y. Acad. Sci., 192, 215 (1972).

767. J. E. Spallholz, J. L. Martin, M. L. Gerlach, and R. H. Heinzerling, Proc. Soc. Exp. Biol. Med., 143, 685 (1973).

768. D. V. Frost, Ann. Rev. Pharmacol., 15, 259 (1974).

769. D. Ingvoldstad, The Bulletin of the Selenium-Tellurium Development Ass., Inc., No. 12, pp. 1-4 (1972).

770. K. O. Godwin, Quart. J. Exp. Physiol., 50, 282 (1965).

771. K. O. Godwin and F. J. Fraser, Quart. J. Physiol., 51, 94 (1966).

772. H. M. J. Perry, J. Amer. Diet. Ass., 62, 631 (1973).

773. H. A. Schroeder, Med. Clin. North Amer., 58, 381 (1974).

774. H. M. Perry, M. W. Erlanger, and E. P. Perry, in Trace Substances in Environmental Health, Vol. VIII (D. D. Hemphill, ed.), Univ. Missouri Press, Columbia, 1974 (in press).

775. R. J. Shamberger, S. A. Tytko, and C. E. Willis, in Trace Substances in Environmental Health, Vol. VIII (D. D. Hemphill, ed.), Univ. Missouri Press, Columbia, 1975 (in press).

776. E. L. Wynder and B. S. Reddy, Amer. J. Dis., 19, 937 (1974).

777. E. M. Carlisle, Science, 167, 279 (1970).

778. E. M. Carlisle, Fed. Proc., 30, 462 (1971).

779. E. M. Carlisle, Fed. Proc., 31, 700 (1972).

780. E. M. Carlisle, Science, 178, 619 (1972).

781. K. Schwarz and D. B. Milne, Nature, 239, 333 (1972).

782. E. M. Carlisle, Fed. Proc., 32, 930 (1973).

783. F. H. Nielsen and H. H. Sandstead, Amer. J. Clin. Nutr., 27, 515 (1974).

784. K. Schwarz, in Trace Element Metabolism in Animals, Vol. 2 (W. G. Hoekstra, J. W. Suttie, H. E. Ganther, and W. Mertz, eds.), University Park Press, Baltimore, 1974, p. 355.

785. J. G. Leslie, T. K. Kung-Ying, and T. H. McGavack, Proc. Soc. Exp. Biol. Med., 110, 218 (1962).

786. H. Brown, J. Biol. Chem., 75, 789 (1927).

787. R. C. MacCardle, M. F. Engman, Jr., and M. F. Engman, Sr. Arch. Dermatol. Syphilol., 47, 335 (1943).

788. L. P. H. Jones and K. A. Handreck, Advan. Agron., 19, 107 (1967).

789. J. Loeper, J. Loeper, and A. Lemaire, Presse Med., 74, 865 (1966).

790. Y. Charnot and G. Peres, Ann. Endocrinol., Paris, $\underline{32}$, 397 (1971).

791. M. C. Nottle and J. M. Armstrong, Aust. J. Agr. Res., $\underline{17}$, 165 (1966).

792. R. Connell, F. Whiting, and S. A. Forman, Can. J. Comp. Med. Vet. Sci., $\underline{23}$, 41 (1959).

793. F. Whiting, R. Connell, and S. A. Forman, Can. J. Comp. Med. Vet. Sci., $\underline{22}$, 232 (1958).

794. K. G. Parker, J. Range Manage., $\underline{10}$, 105 (1957).

795. K. F. Swingle, Amer. J. Vet. Res., $\underline{14}$, 493 (1953).

796. K. F. Swingle and H. Marsh, Amer. J. Vet. Res., $\underline{14}$, 16 (1953).

797. R. F. Keeler and S. A. Lovelace, Amer. J. Vet. Res., $\underline{22}$, 617 (1961).

798. H. Micheels, Rev. Sci. (Paris), $\underline{5}$, 427 (1906).

799. B. B. Cohen, Plant Physiol., $\underline{15}$, 755 (1940).

800. K. Schwarz, D. B. Milne, and E. Vinyand, Biochem. Biophys. Res. Commun., $\underline{40}$, 22 (1970).

801. R. A. Kehoe, J. Cholak, and R. V. Storey, J. Nutr., $\underline{19}$, 579 (1940).

802. H. A. Schroeder, J. J. Balassa, and I. H. Tipton, J. Chronic Dis., $\underline{17}$, 483 (1964).

803. I. H. Tipton, P. L. Stewart, and P. G. Martin, Health Phys., $\underline{12}$, 1683 (1969).

804. G. W. Monier-Williams, in Trace Elements in Food, Chapman and Hall, London, 1949.

805. H. M. Perry, Jr. and E. F. Perry, J. Clin. Invest., $\underline{38}$, 1452 (1959).

806. M. Budikova, O. Charamza, and O. Kuchar, Bratisl. Lek. Listy, $\underline{56}$, 708 (1971).

807. J. Kuba, O. Charamza, E. Klaus, and M. Sevcik, Radiobiol. Radiother., $\underline{12}$, 501 (1971).

808. M. Hegesippe, J. Beydon, A. Bardy, and C. Panneciere, J. Nucl. Biol. Med., $\underline{17}$, 93 (1973).

809. D. Bertrand, Ann. Inst. Pasteur, $\underline{68}$, 226 (1942).

810. D. I. Arnon and G. Wessel, Nature, $\underline{172}$, 1039 (1953).

811. I. Roitman, L. R. Travassos, H. P. Azevedo, and A. Cury, Sabouraudia, $\underline{7}$, 15 (1969).

812. A. Nason, in Trace Elements (C. A. Lamb, O. G. Gentley, and J. M. Beattie, eds.), Academic, New York, 1958, pp. 269-296.

813. C. K. Horner, D. Burck, F. Allison, and M. S. Sherman, J. Agr. Res., $\underline{65}$, 173 (1942).

814. H. Takahashi and A. Nason, Biochim, Biophys. Acta, $\underline{23}$, 433 (1957).

815. L. L. Hopkins, Jr. and H. E. Mohr, Fed. Proc., $\underline{30}$, 462 (1971).

816. K. Schwarz and D. B. Milne, Science, $\underline{174}$, 426 (1971).

817. H. A. Schroeder, J. J. Balassa, and I. H. Tipton, J. Chronic Dis., $\underline{16}$, 1047 (1963).

818. F. H. Nielsen and H. H. Sanstead, Amer. J. Clin. Nutr., $\underline{27}$, 515 (1974).

819. C. A. Strasia, Ph.D. Thesis, Univ. of Michigan, Ann Arbor, 1971.

820. R. Söremark, J. Nutr., 92, 183 (1967).

821. D. Schlettwein-Gsell, Int. J. Vit. Nutr. Res., 43, 242 (1973).

822. W. H. Allaway, J. Kubota, F. L. Losee, and M. Roth, Arch. Environ. Health, 16, 342 (1968).

823. E. M. Butt, R. E. Nusbaum, T. C. Gelmour, S. L. Didio, and Sister Mariano, Arch. Environ. Health, 8, 52 (1964).

824. G. L. Curran, D. L. Azarnoff, and R. E. Bolinger, J. Clin. Invest., 38, 1251 (1959).

825. N. A. Talvitie and W. G. Wagner, Amer. Med. Ass. Arch. Ind. Hyg. Occup. Med., 9, 414 (1954).

826. H. M. Perry, Jr. and E. F. Perry, J. Clin. Invest., 38, 1452 (1959).

827. R. Söremark and S. Ullberg, in Use of Radioisotopes in Animal Biology and the Medical Sciences (N. Fried, ed.), Academic, New York, 1962, p. 103.

828. J. N. Hathcock, C. H. Hill, and G. Matrone, J. Nutr., 82, 106 (1964).

829. L. L. Hopkins and B. E. Tilton, Amer. J. Physiol., 211, 169 (1966).

830. F. Bernheim and M. L. C. Bernheim, J. Biol. Chem., 128, 79 (1939).

831. G. M. Martin, E. P. Benditt, and N. Eriksen, Nature, 186, 884 (1960).

832. H. Pezzano and L. Coscia, Acta Physiol. Lat. Amer., 20, 403 (1971).

833. J. T. Mountain, F. R. Stockwell, and H. E. Stokinger, Proc. Soc. Exp. Biol., 92, 582 (1956).

834. C. E. Lewis, Amer. Med. Ass. Arch. Ind. Health, 19, 419 (1959).

835. G. L. Curran and R. L. Costello, J. Exp. Med., 103, 49 (1956).

836. V. V. Korkov, Farmakol. Toksikol., 28, 83 (1965).

837. G. L. Curran and R. E. Burch, in Proc. First Ann. Conf. Trace Substances Environ. Health (D. D. Hemphill, ed.), Univ. of Missouri, 1967, p. 96.

838. E. G. Dimond, J. Caravaca, and A. Benchimol., Amer. J. Clin. Nutr., 12, 49 (1963).

839. J. Somerville and B. Davies, Amer. Heart J., 64, 54 (1962).

840. D. L. Azarnoff and G. L. Curran, J. Amer. Chem. Soc., 79, 2968 (1967).

841. D. L. Azarnoff, F. E. Brock, and G. L. Curran, Biochim. Biophys. Acta, 51, 397 (1961).

842. F. Bernheim and M. L. C. Bernheim, J. Biol. Chem., 127, 353 (1939).

843. G. L. Curran, J. Biol. Chem., 210, 765 (1954).

844. L. L. Hopkins, Jr. and H. E. Mohr, Fed. Proc. 33 (1974).

845. L. L. Hopkins, Jr., in Trace Element Metabolism in Animals, Vol. 2 (W. G. Hoekstra, J. W. Suttie, H. E. Ganther, and W. Mertz, eds.), University Park Press, Baltimore, 1974, p. 397.

846. M. J. Meeks, R. R. Landolt, and W. V. Kessler, J. Pharm. Sci., 60, 482 (1971).

847. R. Masironi, Bull. WHO, 43, 687 (1970).

848. H. A. Schroeder, J. Chronic Dis., 12, 586 (1960).

849. J. Kobayashi, Ber. Ohara Inst. Iandiv. Biol., 2, 12 (1957).

850. H. A. Schroeder, J. Chronic Dis., 12, 586 (1960).

851. J. N. Morris, M. D. Crawford, and J. A. Heady, Lancet, 1, 860 (1961).

852. J. H. Dingle, Illinois Med. J., 125, 25 (1964).

853. G. Biörck, H. Bostrom, and A. Widström, Acta Med. Scand., 178, 239 (1965).

854. R. Mulchay, Brit. Med. J., 1, 861 (1966).

855. H. Boström and P. O. Wester, Acta Med. Scand., 181, 465 (1967).

856. T. Crawford and M. D. Crawford, Lancet, 1, 229 (1967).

857. M. D. Crawford, M. J. Gardner, and J. N. Morris, Lancet, 1, 827 (1968).

858. K. Biersteker, T. Soc. Geneeska, 45, 658 (1967).

859. T. Anderson, W. LeRiche, and J. Mackay, N. Engl. J. Med., 280, 805 (1969).

860. R. D. Lindeman and Assenzo, Amer. J. Pub. Health, 54, 1071 (1964).

861. H. A. Schroeder and L. A. Kraemer, Arch. Environ. Health, 28, 303 (1974).

862. F. Lowater and M. M. Murray, Biochem. J., 31, 837 (1937).

863. R. Söremark and N. Anderson, Acta Ondontol. Scand., 20, 81 (1962).

864. P. R. Thomassen and H. M. Leicester, J. Dent. Res., 43, 346 (1964).

865. O. Rygh, Bull. Soc. Chim. Biol., 31, 1052, 1403, 1408 (1949).

866. O. Rygh, Bull. Soc. Chim. Biol., 33, 133 (1953).

867. O. Rygh, Research (London), 2, 340 (1949).

868. C. F. Geyer, J. Dent. Res., 32, 590 (1953).

869. B. J. Kruger, J. Aust. Dent. Ass., 3, 236 (1958).

870. J. W. Hein and J. Wisotzky, J. Dent. Res., 34, 756 (1955).

871. W. Buttner, J. Dent. Res., 42, 453 (1963).

872. H. R. Mühlemann and K. G. König, Helv. Odontol. Acta, 8, 79 (1964).

873. J. C. Muhler, J. Dent. Res., 36, 787 (1957).

874. G. Tank and C. A. Storvick, J. Dent. Res., 39, 473 (1960).

875. D. M. Hadjimarkos, Nature (London), 209, 1137 (1966).

876. D. M. Hadjimarkos, Advan. Oral Biol., 3, 253 (1968).

877. F. H. Nielsen and D. A. Ollerich, Fed. Proc., 32, 929 (1973).

878. J. D. Summers and E. T. Moran, Jr., Poultry Sci., 51, 1760 (1972).

879. M. Crandall and J. H. Caulton, Exp. Cell Res., 82, 159 (1973).

880. R. L. Costello and L. W. Hedgecock, J. Bacteriol., 77, 794 (1959).

881. R. L. Costello and L. W. Hedgecock, quoted by G. L. Curran in Metal Binding in Medicine (M. J. Seven and L. A. Johnson, eds.), Lippincott, Philadelphia, 1960, p. 216.

882. Y. M. Bala and L. M. Kopylova, Probl. Tuberkuleza (Moskva), 49, 63 (1971).

883. J. Raulin, Ann. Sci. Nat. Bot. Biol. Vegetale, 11, 93 (1869).

884. A. L. Sommer and C. B. Lipman, Plant Physiol., I, 231 (1926).

885. A. L. Sommer, Plant Physiol., 3, 231 (1928).

886. V. Birckner, J. Biol. Chem., 38, 191 (1919).

887. W. R. Todd, C. A. Elvehjem, and E. B. Hart, Amer. J. Physiol., 107, 146 (1934).

888. H. F. Tucker and W. D. Salmon, Proc. Soc. Exp. Biol. Med., 88, 613 (1955).

889. B. L. O'Dell and J. E. Savage, Poultry Sci., 36, 489 (1957).

890. B. L. O'Dell, P. M. Newberne, and J. E. Savage, J. Nutr., 65, 503 (1958).

891. A. S. Prasad, in Zinc Metabolism (A. S. Prasad, ed.), Thomas, Springfield, Illinois, 1966, p. 250.

892. A. S. Prasad, J. A. Halsted, and M. Nadimi, Amer. J. Med., 31, 532 (1961).

893. A. S. Prasad, A. Miale, Z. Farid, H. H. Sandstead, A. Schulert, and W. J. Darby, Arch. Intern. Med., 111, 407 (1963).

894. P. Dynna and G. N. Havre, Acta Vet. Scand., 4, 197 (1963).

895. S. Haaranen, Nord. Veterinaer Med., 14, 265 (1962); 15, 536 (1963).

896. S. P. Legg and L. Sears, Nature (London), 186, 1061 (1960).

897. R. M. Forbes and M. Yohe, J. Nutr., 70, 53 (1960).

898. R. W. Luecke, B. E. Rukson, and B. V. Baltzer, in Proc. First Int. Symp. Trace Element Metab. Anim., 1969 (C. F. Mills, ed.), Livingstone, Edinburgh, 1970, p. 471.

899. H. Swenerton and L. S. Hurley, J. Nutr., 95, 8 (1968).

900. E. R. Miller, D. O. Liptrap, and D. E. Ullrey, in Proc. First Int. Symp. Trace Element Metab. Anim., 1969 (C. F. Mills, ed.), Livingstone, Edinburgh, 1970, p. 377.

901. W. H. Smith, M. P. Plumlee, and W. M. Beeson, Science, 128, 1280 (1960).

902. M. W. Moeller and H. M. Scott, Poultry Sci., 37, 1227 (1958).

903. R. H. Robertson and P. J. Schaible, Poultry Sci., 37, 1321 (1958); 39, 837 (1960).

904. R. J. Young, H. M. Edwards, and M. B. Gillis, Poultry Sci., 37, 1100 (1958).

905. J. M. Pensack, J. N. Henson, and P. D. Bogdonoff, Poultry Sci., 37, 1232 (1958).

906. C. F. Mills, A. C. Dalgarno, R. B. Williams, and J. Quarterman, Brit. J. Nutr., 21, 751 (1967).

907. E. J. Underwood and M. Somers, Aust. J. Agr. Res., 20, 889 (1969).

908. W. J. Miller, C. M. Clifton, and N. W. Cameron, J. Dairy Sci., 46, 715 (1963).

909. R. A. McCance and E. M. Widdowson, Biochem. J., <u>36</u>, 692 (1942).

910. H. H. Sandstead, A. S. Prasad, A. S. Schulert, Z. Farid, A. Miale, S. Bassily, and W. J. Darby, Amer. J. Clin. Nutr., <u>20</u>, 422 (1967).

911. H. A. Schroeder, A. P. Nason, I. H. Tipton, and J. J. Balassa, J. Chronic Dis., <u>20</u>, 179 (1967).

912. H. M. Trimble and F. I. Scoular, J. Nutr., <u>52</u>, 209 (1954).

913. R. W. Engel, R. F. Miller, and N. O. Price, in Zinc Metabolism (A. S. Prasad, ed.), Thomas, Springfield, Illinois, 1966, p. 326.

914. A. E. Harper, Nutr. Rev., <u>31</u>, 393 (1973).

915. J. Kubota, V. A. Lazar, and F. L. Losee, Arch. Environ. Health, <u>16</u>, 788 (1966).

916. J. G. Reinhold, Amer. J. Clin. Nutr., <u>24</u>, 1024 (1971).

917. E. J. Dahmer, B. W. Coleman, and R. H. Grummer, J. Anim. Sci., <u>35</u>, 1181 (1972).

918. M. E. Bartholomew, R. Tupper, and A. Wormall, Biochem. J., <u>73</u>, 256 (1959).

919. R. E. Thiers and B. L. Vallee, J. Biol. Chem., <u>226</u>, 911 (1957).

920. G. Weitzel, Angew. Chem., <u>68</u>, 566 (1966).

921. D. Keilin and T. Mann, Nature (London), <u>144</u>, 442 (1939).

922. J. M. Orten, in Zinc Metabolism (A. S. Prasad, ed.), Thomas, Springfield, Illinois, 1966, p. 38.

923. B. L. Vallee, Physiol. Rev., <u>39</u>, 443 (1959).

924. E. Schneider and C. A. Price, Biochim. Biophys. Acta, <u>55</u>, 406 (1962).

925. A. Nason, N. D. Kaplan, and H. A. Oldewurtel, J. Biol. Chem., <u>201</u>, 435 (1953).

926. M. Fujioka and I. Lieberman, J. Biol. Chem., <u>239</u>, 1164 (1964).

927. H. H. Sandstead and R. A. Rinaldi, J. Cell. Physiol., <u>73</u>, 81 (1969).

928. M. Somers and E. J. Underwood, Aust. J. Biol. Sci., <u>22</u>, 1229 (1969).

929. P. J. Buchanan and J. M. Hsu, Fed. Proc., <u>27</u>, 483 (1968).

930. R. B. Williams, C. F. Mills, J. Quarterman, and A. C. Dalgarno, Biochem. J., <u>95</u>, 29P (1965).

931. R. B. Williams and J. K. Chesters, in Proc. First Int. Symp. Trace Element Metab. Anim., 1969 (C. F. Mills, ed.), Livingstone, Edinburgh, 1970, p. 64.

932. A. S. Prasad and D. Oberleas, J. Lab. Clin. Med., <u>83</u>, 634 (1974).

933. R. C. Theur and W. G. Hoekstra, J. Nutr., <u>89</u>, 448 (1966).

934. P. K. Ku, D. E. Ullrey, and E. R. Miller, in Proc. First Int. Symp. Trace Element Metab. Anim., 1969 (C. F. Mills, ed.), Livingstone, Edinburgh, 1970, p. 158.

935. A. S. Prasad and D. Oberleas, J. Lab. Clin. Med., <u>82</u>, 461 (1973).

936. M. W. Terhune and H. H. Sandstead, Science, <u>177</u>, 68 (1972).

937. B. J. Poiesz, Biochem. Biophys. Res. Commun., <u>56</u>, 959 (1974).

938. E. Hove, C. A. Elvehjem, and E. B. Hart, Amer. J. Physiol., 119, 768
      (1937); 124, 750 (1938).

939. E. Hove, C. A. Elvehjem, and E. B. Hart, J. Biol. Chem., 136, 425
      (1940).

940. B. L. Vallee and H. Neurath, J. Biol. Chem., 217, 253 (1955).

941. D. G. Hendricks and A. W. Mahoney, J. Nutr., 102, 1079 (1972).

942. J. Quarterman, C. F. Mills, and W. R. Humphries, Biochem. Biophys.
      Res. Commun., 25, 354 (1966).

943. A. M. Huber and S. N. Gershoff, J. Nutr., 103, 1739 (1973).

944. J. Quarterman, Biochem. J., 102, 41P (1967).

945. R. H. Follis, Jr., H. G. Day, and E. V. McCollum, J. Nutr., 22, 223
      (1941).

946. W. J. Miller, J. D. Morton, W. J. Pitts, and C. M. Clifton, Proc. Soc.
      Exp. Biol. Med., 118, 427 (1965).

947. D. M. Blackmon, W. J. Miller, and J. D. Morton, Vet. Med., 62, 265
      (1967).

948. F. H. Kratzer, P. Vohra, J. B. Allred, and P. N. Davis, Proc. Soc.,
      Exp. Biol. Med., 98, 205 (1958).

949. M. L. Scott, E. R. Holm, and R. E. Reynolds, Poultry Sci., 38, 1344
      (1959).

950. M. R. Spivey-Fox and B. N. Harrison, Proc. Soc. Exp. Biol. Med., 116,
      256 (1964).

951. M. R. Spivey-Fox and B. N. Harrison, J. Nutr., 86, 89 (1965).

952. J. C. Smith, Jr., E. G. McDaniel, and F. F. Fan, Science, 181, 954
      (1973).

953. J. K. Miller and W. J. Miller, J. Dairy Sci., 43, 1854 (1960).

954. J. K. Miller and W. J. Miller, J. Nutr., 76, 467 (1962).

955. L. S. Hurley and H. Swenerton, Proc. Soc. Exp. Biol. Med., 123, 692
      (1966).

956. E. R. Miller, R. W. Luecke, D. E. Ullrey, B. V. Baltzer, B. L. Brad-
      ley, and J. A. Hoefer, J. Nutr., 95, 278 (1968).

957. T. R. Zeigler, M. L. Scott, R. McEvoy, R. H. Greenlaw, F. Huegin,
      and W. H. Strain, Proc. Soc. Exp. Biol. Med., 109, 239 (1962).

958. W. J. Pories, J. H. Henzel, and J. A. Hennessen, in Proc. First Ann.
      Conf. Trace Substances Environ. Health, 1967, p. 114 (1968).

959. W. J. Pories and W. H. Strain, in Zinc Metabolism (A. S. Prasad, ed.),
      Thomas, Springfield, Illinois, 1966, p. 378.

960. H. H. Sandstead and G. H. Shepard, Proc. Soc. Exp. Biol. Med., 128,
      687 (1968).

961. E. D. Savlov, W. H. Strain, and F. Huegin, J. Surg. Res., 2, 209
      (1962).

962. N. R. Calhoun and J. C. Smith, Lancet, 2, 682 (1968).

963. A. Rahmat, J. N. Norman, and G. Smith, Brit. J. Surg., 61, 271 (1974).

964. J. Murray and S. Rosenthal, Surg. Gynecol. Obstet., 126, 1298 (1968).

965. E. P. Quarantillo, Jr., Amer. J. Surg., 121, 661 (1971).

966. F. Fernandez-Madrid, A. S. Prasad, and D. Oberleas, J. Lab. Clin. Med., 78, 853 (1971).

967. R. I. Henkin, in Trace Element Metabolism in Animals, Vol. 2 (W. G. Hoekstra, J. W. Suttie, H. E. Ganther, and W. Mertz, eds.), University Park Press, Baltimore, 1974, p. 647.

968. M. J. Millar, M. I. Fischer, P. V. Elcoate, and C. A. Mawson, Can. J. Biochem. Physiol., 36, 557 (1958); 38, 1457 (1960).

969. B. Wetterdal, Acta Radiol., Suppl., 156 (1958).

970. W. J. Miller, D. M. Blackmon, R. P. Gentry, G. W. Powell, and H. E. Perkins, J. Dairy Sci., 49, 1446 (1966).

971. W. J. Pitts, W. J. Miller, O. T. Fosgate, J. D. Morton, and C. M. Clifton, J. Dairy Sci., 49, 455 (1966).

972. W. J. Miller, W. J. Pitts, C. M. Clifton, and S. C. Schmittle, J. Dairy Sci., 47, 556 (1964).

973. J. Friberg and O. Nilsson, Upsala J. Med. Sci., 79, 63 (1974).

974. J. Apgar, Amer. J. Physiol., 125, 160, 1478 (1968).

975. D. L. Blamberg, U. B. Blackwood, W. C. Supplee, and G. F. Combs, Proc. Soc. Exp. Biol. Med., 104, 217 (1960).

976. E. W. Kienholz, D. E. Turk, M. L. Sunde, and W. G. Hoekstra, J. Nutr., 75, 211 (1961).

977. W. G. Hoekstra, E. C. Faltin, C. W. Lin, H. F. Roberts, and R. H. Grummer, J. Anim. Sci., 26, 1348 (1967).

978. H. H. Sandstead, S. R. Glasser, and D. D. Gillespie, Fed. Proc., 29, 297 (1970).

979. L. S. Hurley, Amer. J. Clin. Nutr., 22, 1332 (1969).

980. H. Swenerton and L. S. Hurley, Science, 173, 62 (1971).

981. P. B. Mutch and L. S. Hurley, J. Nutr., 104, 828 (1974).

982. W. J. Pories, J. H. Henzel, C. G. Rob, and W. H. Strain, Lancet, 2, 121 (1967).

983. J. H. Henzel, B. Holtman, F. W. Keitzer, M. S. DeWeese, and E. Lichti, Proc. Second Conf. Trace Substances Environ. Health, 1968, p. 83 (1968).

984. N. F. Volkov, Fed. Proc., 22 (Trans. Suppl.), 897 (1963).

985. W. E. Wacker, D. D. Ulmer, and B. L. Vallee, New Engl. J. Med., 255, 449 (1956).

986. W. H. Strain, F. Huegin, C. A. Lankau, W. P. Beiliner, R. K. McEvoy, and W. J. Pories, Int. J. Radiat. Isotopes, 15, 231 (1964).

987. A. M. Handjani, J. C. Smith, Jr., J. B. Herrmann, and J. A. Halsted, Chest, 65, 185 (1974).

988. L. M. Klevay, Nutr. Rep. Int., 9, 393 (1974).

989. N. W. H. Addink, Nature (London), 186, 253 (1960).

990. N. W. H. Addink and L. J. P. Frank, Cancer, 12, 544 (1959).

991. I. Vikbladh, Scand. J. Clin. Lab. Invest., 2, 143 (1950).

992. J. G. Gibson, B. L. Vallee, R. G. Fluharty, and J. E. Nelson, Proc. Sixth Int. Congr. Cancer Res., 1954, p. 1102.

993. S. Szmigielski and J. Litwin, Cancer, 17, 1381 (1964).

994. J. K. Chesters, Biochem. J., 130, 133 (1972).

995. N. A. Berger and A. M. Skinner, J. Cell Biol., 61, 45 (1974).

996. D. E. Poswillo and B. Cohen, Nature (London), 231, 447 (1971).

997. W. DeWys, W. J. Pories, M. C. Richter, and W. H. Strain, Proc. Soc. Exp. Biol. Med., 135, 17 (1970).

998. J. T. McQuitty, Jr., W. D. DeWys, L. Monaco, W. H. Strain, C. G. Rob, J. Apgar, and W. J. Pories, Cancer Res., 30, 1387 (1970).

999. D. H. Barr and J. W. Harris, Proc. Soc. Exp. Biol. Med., 144, 284 (1973).

1000. J. R. Duncan, I. E. Dreosti, and C. F. Albrecht, J. Nat. Cancer Inst., 53, 277 (1974).

1001. I. L. Mulay, R. Roy, B. E. Knox, N. H. Suhr, and W. E. Delaney, J. Nat. Cancer Inst., 47, 1 (1971).

1002. H. Rubin, Proc. Nat. Acad. Sci., U.S., 69, 712 (1972).

1003. I. Lieberman and P. Ove, J. Biol. Chem., 237, 1634 (1962).

1004. U. Weser, S. Seeber, and P. Warnecke, Experientia, 25, 489 (1969).

1005. W. B. Herring, B. S. Leavell, M. Paixao, and J. H. Yoe, Amer. J. Clin. Nutr., 8, 846 (1960).

1006. T. R. Talbot and J. F. Ross, Lab. Invest., 9, 174 (1964).

1007. B. L. Vallee and J. G. Gibson, J. Biol. Chem., 176, 445 (1948).

1008. B. L. Vallee and J. G. Gibson, Blood, 4, 455 (1949).

1009. J. A. Halsted, B. Hackley, C. Rudzki, and J. C. Smith, Gastroenterology, 54, 1098 (1968).

1010. A. M. Kahn, H. W. Helwig, A. G. Redeker, and T. B. Reynolds, Amer. J. Clin. Pathol., 44, 426 (1965).

1011. A. S. Prasad, D. Oberleas, and J. A. Halsted, J. Lab. Clin. Med., 66, 508 (1965).

1012. B. L. Vallee, W. E. C. Wacker, A. F. Bartholomay, and F. L. Hoch, Ann. Intern. Med., 50, 1077 (1959).

1013. F. W. Sunderman, Jr., Human Pathol., 4, 549 (1973).

1014. P. J. Schechter, W. T. Friedewald, D. A. Bronzert, M. S. Raff, and R. I. Henkin, Intern. Rev. Neurobiol. (Suppl. 1), 125 (1972).

1015. I. K. Cohen, P. J. Schechter, and R. I. Henkin, J. Amer. Med. Ass., 223, 914 (1973).

1016. S. L. Husain, Lancet, 1, 1069 (1969).

1017. M. W. Greaves and A. W. Skillern, Lancet, 2, 889 (1970).

1018. G. R. Serjeant, R. E. Galloway, and M. C. Gueri, Lancet, 2, 891
       (1970).

1019. T. Hallbrook and E. Lanner, Lancet, 2, 780 (1972).

1020. C. Cohen, Brit. Med. J., 2, 561 (1968).

1021. D. F. Abbott, A. N. Exton-Smith, P. H. Millard, and J. M. Temperly,
       Brit. Med. J., 2, 763 (1968).

1022. A. Barbeau, Trans. Amer. Neurol. Ass., 98, 1 (1973).

1023. H. H. Sandstead, Y. Y. Al-Ubaidi, E. Halas, and G. Fosmire, in Trace
       Element Metabolism in Animals, Vol. 2 (W. G. Hoekstra, J. W. Suttie,
       H. E. Ganther, and W. Mertz, eds.), University Park Press, Baltimore,
       1974, p. 745.

1024. R. I. Henkin, in Trace Element Metabolism in Animals, Vol. 2 (W. G.
       Hoekstra, J. W. Suttie, H. E. Ganther, and W. Mertz, eds.), University
       sity Park Press, Baltimore, 1974, p. 652.

1025. D. J. Mahler, J. R. Walsh, and G. D. Haynie, Amer. J. Clin. Pathol.,
       56, 17 (1971).

1026. R. D. Korant, J. C. Kauer, and B. E. Butterworth, Nature, 248, 588
       (1974).

QUANTITATIVE ANALYSIS FOR ENVIRONMENTAL AND BIOLOGICAL CONCENTRATIONS OF HEAVY METALS

Clifton E. Meloan
Kansas State University
Manhattan, Kansas

There are many methods possible for determining trace elements in the environment. However, because of cost, sensitivity, and the nature of the sample, the choice narrows rapidly. Colorimetric methods have long been a standby but are falling by the wayside because they are not sensitive enough to meet current requirements and they generally require a considerable number of separation steps if mixtures are present, which is usually the case. Of the electroanalytical methods, only stripping has found much application, but few metals can be determined at once and then after considerable work-up. Gas chromatography and liquid chromatography of metals are still in the development stages. The result is that during the past few years the most attention has been focused on atomic absorption, atomic fluorescence, flame emission, x-ray fluorescence, electron probe, ion probe, spark source mass spectroscopy, and neutron activation analysis (Fig. 1).

As our knowledge of the effects of trace elements in the environment has increased, tremendous pressure has been placed on the research scientist and quality control groups to determine these elements at ever decreasing levels. This has been done in many cases with the result that our ability to determine the presence of elements at low concentration has outstripped our ability to comprehend what the results mean. Consequently, much apprehension and suspicion of chemicals have been generated in the minds of the general public every time a new paper is published.

It is becoming more obvious that it is no longer adequate to determine the concentration of one element, but we are finding that it is the relative ratios of combinations of elements that is important. For example, copper

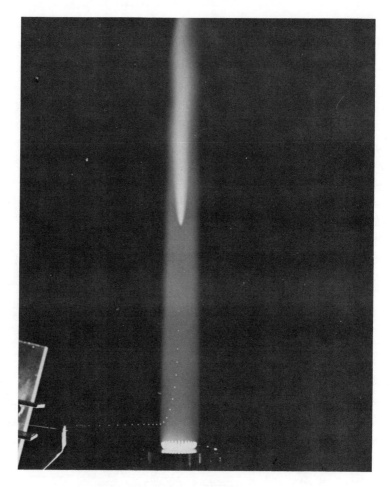

FIG. 1. The isolated drop nebulizer in operation [3].

poisoning in animals can be cured by adding one-sixth the amount of molybdenum and it has been shown that mercury poisoning in rats can be stopped
by adding 1/20 of its amount of selenium. Figure 2 shows the interrelation
of several elements in animals.

What elements are we interested in? Not many years ago, interest centered around lead and arsenic, unless you were a toxicologist. Now, however,
this list is being rapidly expanded. As an example, let us look at the
coatings industry and see how what started out to be a "heavy metals" survey
has expanded almost unbelievably.

Some of the more common elements that have been or are currently being
used in coatings or allied products in concentrations greater than 100 ppm

(0.01%) are Sb, As, Ba, Cd, Cr, Co, Cu, Fe, Pb, Mn, Hg, Mo, Ni, Sr, Sn, Ti, Zn, Zr, Ce, La, and V. This is only a part of the problem, however. Notice that Al is not on the list. While Al is not used in coatings, it is a very popular can material, and therefore its presence must be monitored in the coating and in the product the coating is designed to protect. In addition, if anything goes wrong with the product in a container, the coating is one of the first items to be suspected. This means that any element present that controls the quality of the product must be monitored at some time or another. Beer, for example, requires that Al, Na, Ca, Mg, K, Cu, Zn, and Fe be monitored at the ppm (0.0001%) level for quality control. We now have added Na, Ca, Mg, and K to the original list and pushed the required levels down 100-fold.

The net effect is that in the current climate of fear and suspicion of chemicals, added to the sincere interest of basic research scientists concerning the pathways of trace elements, we must be prepared to examine almost the entire periodic table at ppb (0.0000001%) levels.

In the space allotted we will attempt not only to describe the principle of operation of those instruments that are currently being used extensively but also to present a brief discussion of one or two instruments that promise

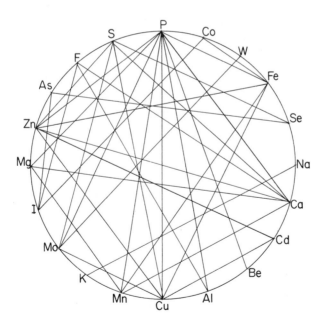

FIG. 2. Mineral interrelationships in animals [4].

to have utility in the near future. Two books are highly recommended for
the first few techniques discussed [1,2].

FLAME EMISSION

The first three techniques to be described will be flame emission,
atomic absorption, and atomic fluorescence. These will be developed along
historical lines in order to show how and why they are developed.

Flame emission spectroscopy is a process whereby a sample in solution
is aspirated into a flame, the atoms and molecules are excited by the thermal energy of the flame, and the radiation from the resulting reversion is
separated by a monochromator and detected.

Those who have had some experience in this field might ask, "Why flame
emission? Flame photometry went out long ago." Flame photometry, yes, but
recent developments such as using fuel-rich flames, being able to use only
selected portions of the flame, and using photomultiplier detectors have put
flame emission right back in the picture. It is now possible to determine
15 to 20 elements previously not detectable and to increase the sensitivity
of many of the previously determined elements. Flame emission spectroscopy
is more sensitive than atomic absorption (described later) for about half
of the elements (see Table 3), and you need only one source. Figure 3 is
a diagram of the basic components required for flame emission spectroscopy.

Almost everyone who has taken a course in chemistry has taken a spatula
full of various salts, held them in the flame of a Bunsen burner, and watched
the various colors being emitted. If one does this systematically, one finds
that only the alkalies, alkaline earths, and a few other elements give off
colored radiation. Figure 4 is an energy diagram to help explain the process in this phenomenon.

The heat energy from the flame raises an electron from the ground state
to an excited state (element X in Fig. 4). If the excited-state electron
drops back to the ground state in one step, the radiation given off is called
a resonance line. (Note: We get "lines" because the radiation is passed
through slits.) There will be a line for each energy level in the system.
Lines are used rather than squares or circles because lines require less
separation to be clearly seen. If the electron loses its energy in steps,
some of the energy may be given off in the ultraviolet, visible, and infrared regions. The atom may lose its energy by simply colliding with other
atoms, and the electron can drop back into the ground energy level without

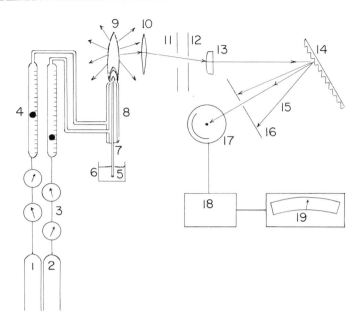

FIG. 3. Schematic diagram of the major components of a flame emission spectrophotometer:

1. H_2, C_2H_2
2. O_2, air, or N_2O
3. Pressure gauges
4. Flow meters
5. Sample solution
6. Sample holder
7. Capillary

8. Nebulizer
9. Flame
10. Condensing lens
11. Mask
12. Entrance slits
13. Collimating lens

14. Diffraction grating
15. Diffracted beam
16. Exit slits
17. Phototube detector
18. Amplifier
19. Readout meter or recorder

giving off any radiation at all. With the alkali and alkaline earth metals,
the energy required to excite the atoms is relatively low, and there is
enough energy in a gas/air flame ($900°$ to $1200°C$) to do this.

Each metal has a different set of energy levels since each metal has
a different nuclear charge and a different number of electrons. Compare
elements X, Y, and Z in Fig. 4. The wavelengths of emitted radiation will
therefore be different for each element because of these basic differences
of charge and number of electrons. The colors resulting (i.e., yellow for
sodium, violet for potassium, green for barium, and red for strontium) can
be used for qualitative analysis. If the intensity of this radiation is
measured, then quantitative analysis is possible. One may ask why iron or
zinc does not give off colored radiation when heated in a burner. The
question is answered by the fact that both iron and zinc require more energy to reach the first energy state than is possible to obtain with a

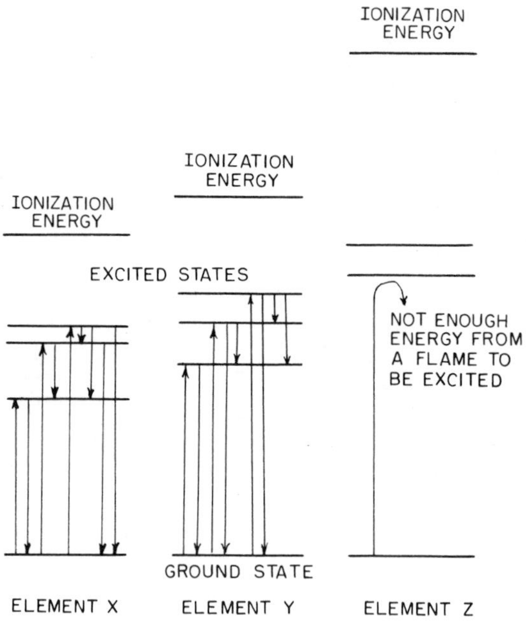

FIG. 4. Comparison of levels of excitation energy produced in a flame.

low-temperature burner. This is illustrated by element Z in the comparison of excitation energy levels.

The purpose of a flame emission spectrophotometer is to provide a flame, the temperature of which is hot enough to excite as many elements as possible (currently about 60), to determine which wavelengths are given off and what their intensities are. By so doing, it is possible to determine which elements are present as well as their concentration, usually in the ppm region and in some cases in the ppb range.

The Overall Process

Figure 5 is a diagram of the overall process that takes place during a flame emission, atomic absorption, or atomic fluorescence determination. The type of technique is determined by where and how the measurement is made.

The processes are described as follows:

1. The sample is broken into droplets (nebulized and mixed with the fuel).
2. The solvent is evaporated, leaving dry salt particles.
3. The dry salt is vaporized and then dissociated.
4. The dissociated ions form either compounds, neutral atoms, or remain as ions (atomization).

5. These species are excited primarily by bombardment by the gas molecules in the flame (thermal energy).

6. When the excited atom or molecule reverts to the ground state (in about 10^{-8} sec) without colliding with other particles, radiation is given off, producing a series of lines for an atom and one or more bands for a molecule. Bands are several lines very close together (see Fig. 66).

Neutral atoms are generally preferred because the energy required to reach the first excited state is less than that required for exciting ions to the first excited state. This means that all other things being equal, a more intense emission should be obtained from neutral atoms. Molecular spectra are also easy to obtain, but the bands obtained are harder to handle and cause more interference than do the line spectra of atoms.

The Individual Components

We will now discuss the individual components that make up a flame emission apparatus. These will be discussed in the order shown in Fig. 3.

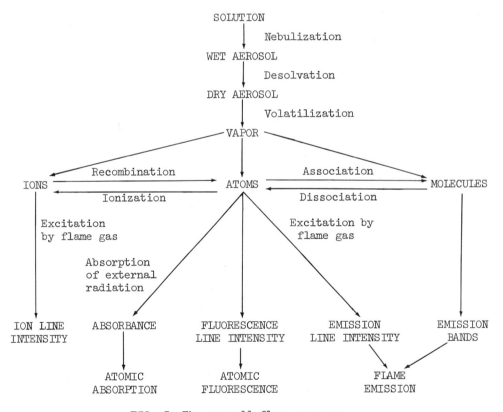

FIG. 5. The overall flame process.

Fuels. What is needed is a hot flame, generally fuel rich, with a slow burning rate. A hot flame is desired to reduce compound formation and increase the concentration of excited neutral atoms. A fuel-rich flame is useful in reducing metal oxides to the metal, thereby increasing the number of elements that can be determined as well as increasing the concentration of neutral atoms. A slow burning rate is desired because it reduces the possibility of flashback and allows more time for the element to be in the flame. Flashback occurs when the rate at which the flame burns is faster than the rate at which the fuel is fed to the burner tip. The flame then enters the mixing chamber (Fig. 26) and causes an explosion. Not much damage is ever done, but it ruins the analysis and is frightening. Table 1 lists several flames for comparison.

Notice the slow burning velocity of natural gas and methane. This is why you can have a small pilot light on your furnace and water heater without its causing much concern.

The hydrogen flame is now used only for As, Sb, and Sn. These elements have high excitation potentials and the hydrogen flame produces intermediate which cause overexcitation and can excite these elements. It is a cool flame, and even under fuel-rich conditions it does not have the reducing power of acetylene flames. These flames are less efficient in atomization, exhibit more chemical interferences, and are less efficient in excitation for most elements. The major advantage is the low background, but this is not enough to make it a flame of choice.

TABLE 1. Characteristics of Several Flames[a]

Fuel	Oxidant	Temperature (Stoichiometric Mixture)	Burning Velocity (cm/sec)
Acetylene	Air	2155-2400	160-266
Acetylene	O_2	3060-3155	800-2480
Acetylene	N_2O	2600-2800	160
H_2	Air	2000-2050	320-440
H_2	O_2	2550-2700	900-3680
CH_4	Air	1875	70
Natural gas	Air	1700-1900	55

[a]From Ref. 1.

It is recommended that an air-natural gas flame be used for alkalies because its cool flame reduces ion formation. Use an ion suppressor (Li salt) to further reduce ionization.

The two most common fuel-oxidizer combinations are acetylene-O_2 and acetylene-air-nitrous oxide. The former has a high burning rate which means the burner ports must be small to avoid flashback. It has a high temperature which increases atomization and provides a high population of excited states. The higher temperature eliminates many of the chemical interferences, but it has a rather high background.

The discovery of the nitrous oxide-acetylene flame has permitted the analyses of about 25 more elements because fewer oxides are formed in the flame. These elements include the rare earths and Al, Be, Ti, V, Si, and Hf. The new reaction provides an atmosphere 33% in O_2. This is a very hot flame yet has a low burning velocity. The low velocity permits the elements to be in the flame longer thereby increasing the emitted radiation.

$$10N_2O \rightleftarrows 10N_2 + 5O_2 \qquad (\Delta H = -101.5 \text{ kcal}) \tag{1}$$

$$2C_2H_2 + 5O_2 \rightleftarrows 4CO_2 + 2H_2O \qquad (\Delta H = -300.1 \text{ kcal}) \tag{2}$$

Pressure Gauges. These are the coarse pressure gauges on the gas cylinders. The acetylene gauge is the most important to watch. If the tank gets below about 70 psi on the coarse gauge, then the acetone that has been placed in the tank to prevent the acetylene from polymerizing will start to enter the flame. This is indicated by a yellow flame. Do not set the second gauge (low pressure) greater than 15 psi when using acetylene. Acetylene escaping from a broken hose at greater than 15 psi has been known to spontaneously explode in air.

Flow Meters. Flow meters are used to accurately measure the volume of each gas going to the flame. For example, N_2O flow rates are 6 to 7 liters per min. A fuel-rich O_2-C_2H_2 flame would be 2.7 liters of O_2 to 3.4 liters of C_2H_2. Flow meters are required if you intend to do reproducible work. Floating-ball flow meters called rotameters are usually used.

Sample Solutions. Solutions should be adjusted to be about a maximum of 100 ppm. If the solutions are more concentrated than that, then the burner plugs up quite easily and self-absorption within the flame causes a loss in sensitivity. Self-absorption is caused when the radiation from one atom is absorbed by another atom of the same kind. This is quite prevalent at high concentrations of atoms. At very high concentrations, self-absorption may be so prevalent that the center of an intense line is reduced in intensity and may even be reduced so far that two lines appear, a process called reversal. It is good technique to make standards up as 1000 ppm solutions and dilute them just before using or surface adsorption problems with the container may result. The author once had a 20-ppm La solution just "disappear" overnight because it had been stored in a glass bottle.

Nebulizer burners. The purpose of the nebulizer is to break up the sample solution into very small drops and mix them with the flame gases. There are several terms that are commonly used to describe burners. These are defined below.

Diffusion burner: The mixing of the gases occurs at the top of the burner by a diffusion process. The Beckman burner (Fig. 6) is an example.

Premix burner: The fuel and oxidizer are mixed in the burner tube before it gets to the flame (Fig. 7). A Bunsen burner is an example.

Turbulent flow burner: The flow of gases into the flame and in the flame is turbulent because of the way the gases are mixed and because of large solvent droplets. The Beckman burner is an example.

Laminar flow burner: The flow of gases into the flame is perpendicular to the flame front, the flames are smooth, and the zones of the flame are better defined because of this. The Lundegardh burner (Fig. 26) is an example.

Total consumption burner: None of the sample aspirated is recovered. The Beckman burner is an example.

Most burners are the direct introduction type and work like a hand fly-spray. A stream of gas passes over a capillary causing a reduced pressure

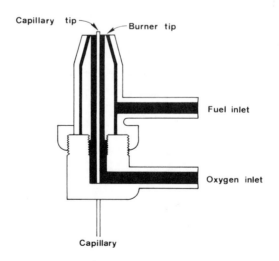

FIG. 6. A Beckman burner.

806

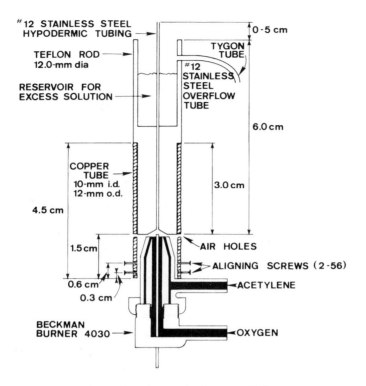

FIG. 7. A premix burner [5].

which draws up the sample into the flame. The Beckman burner is the classic in the field. It is a diffusion, turbulent-flow, total-consumption burner. It is good for O_2-H_2 flames because the small capillary makes flashback difficult.

Capillary feed-type burners can handle much more sample than will ordinarily feed into them. This difficulty is overcome by pumping the sample into the burner. These are called mechanical feed burners, and their advantages are higher emission intensity and the production of a constant feed rate regardless of the sample's viscosity.

The Beckman burner was designed for O_2-rich or stoichiometric flames. With fuel-rich flames a deposit tends to form at the capillary-oxygen opening which when heated produces an enhanced background as well as reducing the nebulization efficiency. In addition, the turbulent mixing also produces high background noise. These difficulties can be overcome by the burner shown in Fig. 7. The added tube provides a premixing chamber after the sample is nebulized which drastically reduces the deposit formation and increases the sensitivity of detection an order of magnitude or more.

Several other types of burners are discussed in the atomic absorption section.

Handling Techniques. The nebulizer is probably the most critical part of a flame emission spectrophotometer and the part given the roughest treatment by inexperienced operators. It is essential that the inner capillary be centered in the gas stream in order to produce a concentric flame. Three set screws hold the capillary in place, and their heads are covered with lacquer to keep them from loosening. Cleaning the burner with an organic solvent will dissolve the lacquer, and the screws will vibrate loose. A good detergent is the cleanser of choice.

The burner often plugs up, particularly if heavy salt concentrations are being used. The first assumption by the inexperienced operator is that the capillary is plugged and the remedy is to run a cleaning wire through it. Only the wire supplied with the instrument should be used since its tip is polished round. A homemade cleaning wire, prepared by cutting a piece of wire, has a sharp chisel tip that scratches the inside wall of the capillary. This will then cause an uneven flame to form. The capillary is usually not what is plugged, but it is the O_2 opening. A sonic cleaner will usually clean this without damage. If fuel-rich flames have been used, then the greasy carbon deposit can sometimes be removed with $CHCl_3$-acetone.

The Flame. Figure 8 presents some of the general facts about flames. Figure 9, the isolated drop nebulizer, shows how much of the information about the sequence of events was determined. A photograph of it in operation is shown in Fig. 1.

A vibrator breaks a stream of solution into drops. A pulsating electrode puts a charge on every fifth, or tenth, or any fraction of the drops. These charged drops are then separated by a deflection plate that is oppositely charged. The droplet generator is capable of producing droplets from less than 10 μm in diameter to greater than 200 μm in diameter. The droplets can be introduced into the flame at any frequency from 1/sec to 200,000/sec and are reproducible to 0.1%.

Hydrocarbon flames are very suitable (especially C_2H_2) because the C_2, CH, and CN radicals participate in reactions which make possible the liberation of metal atoms from relatively stable oxides and because of their lower flame velocity, they can be used with premix burners. Generally, their background emission is much higher than hydrogen flames.

The following species have been identified in air-hydrocarbon flames: O_2, N_2, CO_2, CO, H_2O, C_2H_2, CH_3-CH, CHO, CH, CH_2, CH_3, C_2H, C_2, C_3, C_5, H_2,

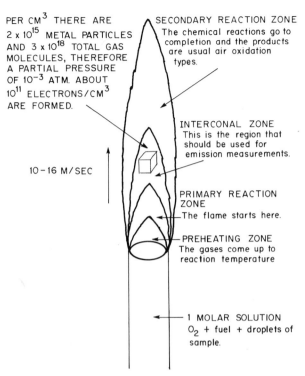

FIG. 8. Some facts about the flame.

H, O, OH, HO_2, CHO^+, $C_2O_2H^+$, $C_3H_3^+$, NO^+, CO^+, OH^+, H_2O^+. H_3O^+, $H_5O_2^+$, and $H_7O_3^+$.

The oxidation of acetylene produces the following reactions:

$$H + O_2 \rightarrow OH + O \tag{3}$$

$$OH + C_2H_2 \rightarrow H_2O + C_2H \tag{4}$$

$$O + C_2H_2 \rightarrow OH + C_2H \tag{5}$$

$$C_2H + C_2H_2 \rightarrow C_4H_2 + H \tag{6}$$

$$C_2H + O_2 \rightarrow CO_2 + CH^* \tag{7}$$

$$CH^* + O \rightarrow CO^* + H \tag{8}$$

$$C_2H + O \rightarrow CO + CH^* \tag{9}$$

If water is present,

$$H_2O + O_2 \rightarrow HO_2 + OH \tag{10}$$

$$HO_2 + H_2O \rightarrow H_2O_2 + OH \tag{11}$$

$$HO_2 + HO_2 \rightarrow H_2O_2 + O_2 \tag{12}$$

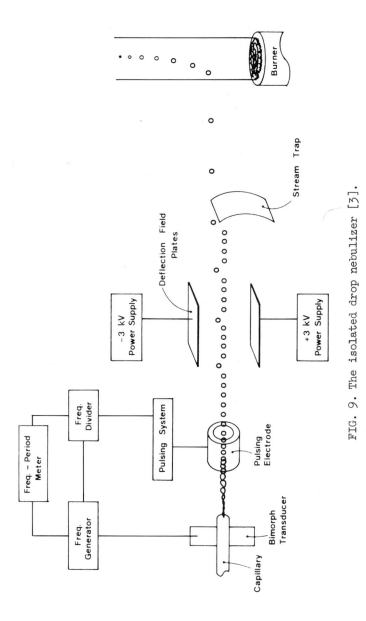

FIG. 9. The isolated drop nebulizer [3].

$$OH + H_2 \rightarrow H_2O + H \tag{13}$$

$$H + HO_2 \rightarrow 2OH \tag{14}$$

OH and H are the most important radicals, and the reaction $H + H_2O \rightleftarrows OH + H_2$ controls the H and OH equilibrium. The reaction $CO + O + M \rightarrow CO_2 + M + h\nu$ gives rise to the blue color of these flames.

It is the recombination of the free radicals that produces the heat energy for the flame. The reaction zone is about 0.1 mm, and the temperature increases about 2000 K in H_2 flames. A temperature gradient of about 100,000 K/cm therefore exists in the primary combustion zone. This heat energy causes the free radicals to be thrown in all directions, and their rate of recombination or reaction determines the burning velocity. A gas with a burning velocity of 250 cm/sec will produce gases leaving the flame at 1600 cm/sec; the average time to pass through the reaction zone is 10^{-5} sec. A flame burns smoothly when the burning rate downward equals the gas flow rate upward. If the burning rate downward is too fast, then flashback occurs. If the burning rate downward is too slow or the gas flow too fast, then the flame is blown out. Actually, the flow rate of the gas should be about five times the combustion rate to keep the burner head from overheating due to the flame front setting on it.

Desolvation. For a 10-μm diameter particle in an air-acetylene flame, it takes about 3 msec to evaporate the solvent. This is a flame distance of nearly 3 mm. The desolvation rate is faster in turbulent flow burners because the transfer of heat to the droplet is speeded up by convection. The addition of organic solvents will also increase the rate of desolvation because of the additional heat of combustion.

About 6% of the total flame heat is required to heat the H_2O and another 15% of the total heat is used to dissociate water. With a total consumption burner this can amount to a 600°C reduction in flame temperature. For a premix chamber type where the large water droplets are removed prior to combustion, the flame temperature is reduced only about 10°C, which is negligible.

Turbulent flow burners lose a lot of droplets (about 95%) because of their large size, yet turbulent flow burners may have a higher metal concentration over premix types by an order of magnitude.

Volatilization. Once the solvent has been evaporated from the salt, the salt must then be heated to a temperature sufficient to vaporize and finally dissociate it. A time delay of 1 msec has been found between complete desolvation of a 50 μm droplet of 10 ppm NaCl and the appearance of

Na emission. NaCl melts at 1100 K and boils at 1750 K. According to Dean, "It should be stressed that an m.p. or b.p. below the flame temperature is not necessary for complete volatilization. The final partial pressure is so very low it generally volatilizes."

Higher solution concentrations result in a larger average particle diameter and may thus retard complete volatilization. Therefore you want small drops and low concentration. Remember, the nonvolatilized particles are incandescent and raise the intensity of the background.

In many cases it makes quite a difference what form the metal salt is in. Magnesium will be used as an example.

$$MgSO_4 \xrightarrow{\text{1160 K}} MgO + SO_2 + SO_3$$
$$\text{(m.p. 3075 K)}$$
$$\text{(b.p. 3850 K)}$$

(Therefore a very hot flame is needed.)

$$MgCl_2 \cdot 6H_2O \xrightarrow{\text{430 K}} MgCl_2 \cdot H_2O \begin{cases} MgCl_2 + H_2O \\ MgO + 2HCl \end{cases}$$
$$\text{(m.p. 1685 K)}$$

(Can use a cool flame.)

$$Mg(NO_3)_2 \cdot 2H_2O \xrightarrow[\text{slow heat}]{594° C} MgO$$
$$\text{(m.p. 129° C)}$$

fast heat melts and vaporizes before MgO forms

About 0.03% of the total flame energy is required for volatilization and/or sublimation.

Dissociation. About 0.3% of the total flame energy is required to dissociate the metal salts. Metal compounds in flames are usually di- (CaO) or triatomic ($LiOH$). More complex compounds such as K_2SO_4 or organometallics are not stable at flame temperatures. Dimers such as Na_2 are not important since their concentration is proportional to the atomic concentration which is low.

Hydrides are not important because none are appreciably stable at flame temperatures.

Most metals exist as either oxides or hydroxides in the flame. Most elements except the alkalies exist as the oxides. LaO, UO_2, and TiO are refractory oxides and require a fuel-rich flame to reduce them. OH compounds are formed by the alkalies and alkaline earths.

TABLE 2. Typical Dissociation Constants[a]

Compound	Fuel Rich	Stoichiometric
FeO	0.95	0.7
CaO	0.60	0.2
AlO	0.08	0.008
BaO	0.03	0.003

[a]From Ref. 6.

The degree of dissociation α is independent of the absolute metal concentration because even if a 1 M solution is present in the sample, when this is sprayed in the flame, the metal concentration will be less than 0.1% of the total concentration of the flame molecules. Table 2 shows some typical dissociation constants and how the fuel/oxidizer ratio affects them. A large number is desired. The dissociation constant K_p^d can be changed 10-fold by changing the dissociation energy 0.5 eV or the temperature $250°$ C.

Atomization. Once the metal salt has been dissociated, it is necessary to obtain as many neutral atoms as possible. This generally involves the reaction of a positive ion with an electron; therefore conditions which provide large numbers of electrons are desired. A flame such as an air-acetylene flame will have a concentration of about 10^{10} to 10^{11} ions/cm^3 immediately above the reaction zone and a similar number of electrons.

There are many electrons present naturally in the flame due to the combustion reactions. The addition of an organic compound sharply increases the electron concentration.

$$2CH \rightarrow C_2 + H_2 \tag{15}$$

$$C_2 + OH \rightarrow CO + CH \tag{16}$$

$$CH + O \rightarrow CHO^+ + e^- \tag{17}$$

$$CHO^+ + H_2O \rightarrow CO + H_3O^+ \tag{18}$$

$$C_2 + OH \rightarrow CO + CH \tag{19}$$

This series of reactions producing the high electron concentration is restricted to a few millimeters above the reaction zone even though C_2 and CH are found throughout the flame. This production of electrons is another reason for using acetylene flames and also why the use of organic solvents is considered.

At high flame temperatures a free metal atom may be split into a + ion and an electron. Double ions have not been reported in flames, but a few compound ions are known, $SrOH^+$ and H_3O^+ being examples. Negative halogen ions may be formed such as Cl^-. OH^- is not important outside of the reaction zone. Carbon particles produce free electrons.

The sum of the + ions must equal the sum of the - ions plus the electrons in order to maintain a charge balance. Advantage is taken of this in order to reduce the ion concentration of the desired metal, thus producing more neutral atoms. This is done by adding another easily ionizable metal, usually an alkali such as Li,

$$[M_1^+] \quad + \quad [M_2^+] \quad = [e^-] \tag{20}$$
$$\text{(desired)} \quad \text{(added)}$$

This not only produces more electrons, but the sum of the positive ions must equal the negative charge so that the desired metal ion concentration is reduced.

The addition of a halogen increases ionization because the halogen uses up the electrons, so more must be produced, thus creating more + ions.

$$[M_1^+] = [e^-] + [X^-] \tag{21}$$

Excitation. Once neutral metal atoms have been produced, it is necessary to raise them to the excited state. There are three basic excitation processes: radiation, chemiluminescence, and collisional. Only collisional is of major significance.

Radiative. In this process a ray of radiation from one of the flame processes is absorbed by the metal atom raising the atom to an excited state.

$$M + h\nu \rightleftarrows M^* \tag{22}$$

This is not an efficient process.

Chemiluminescence. In this situation the energy from a chemical reaction is responsible for the excitation.

$$M + X + Y \rightleftarrows M^* + XY \tag{23}$$

Collision. This is the most important process for exciting neutral metal atoms. In this process a collision between the metal (M) and one or more of the molecules in the flame gas (G) provides the energy for the excitation.

$$M + G \rightarrow M^* + G \tag{24}$$

The reason for its importance is that gas molecules possess many densely spaced rotational and vibrational energy levels, so there is a greater probability that a gas molecule will have the correct energy for the excitation. The conversion of vibrational energy to electronic energy is fast. Any discrepancies go into translational and rotational energy. Even then, this is not very efficient. In the 10^{-5} sec a metal atom is in the reaction zone it will undergo 10^4 to 10^5 collisions, yet only a few atoms out of several thousand are ever excited. Therefore, only a few collisions are "just right."

Noble gases are bad for excitation because they possess only translational energy. The transition from translational energy to electronic energy is efficient only if the concentration of noble gas is large.

Background Emission. Because flame emission methods are single-beam operations, the effect of background is very important. In the H_2-O_2 flame the background from the OH band and from H_2O may cause some problems in certain areas of the spectrum (Fig. 10). Figures 11 and 12 show the background for both the premixed and turbulent-flow O_2-C_2H_2 flames.

Effect of Flame Composition. Figures 13 and 14 show some of the differences between regular and fuel-rich flames. A fuel-rich flame is about $150°$ C cooler than the normal stoichiometric flame.

Condensing Lens. This is a spherical quartz lens used to focus the emitted radiation onto the entrance slits.

Mask. This is a metal or cardboard plate usually placed just ahead of the entrance slit that blots out all of the flame except the region of interest. This eliminates much of the background emission.

Entrance Slits. The purpose of these slits is to produce line spectra. This permits higher resolution. To see that this is so, place two quarters one on top of the other and then place two toothpicks one on top of the other. Move the top one of each until you can clearly say that there are two there. Do you see that the toothpicks (lines) are much easier to resolve than the quarters (circles)? The ability to separate two lines is called resolution ($R = \lambda/\Delta\lambda$).

"The response to the flame background and to band spectra varies as the square of the slit width, whereas the response to a spectral line is linear with slit width. The net effect of decreasing the slit width is to produce a larger signal-to-background ratio when working with spectral lines," Dean [2].

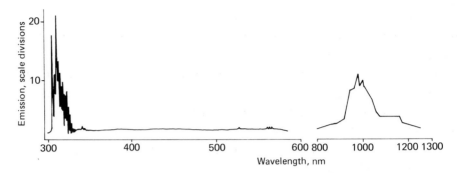

FIG. 10. OH and H₂O emissions [1].

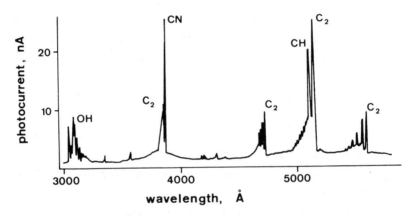

FIG. 11. A premixed O₂-C₂H₂ flame background [1].

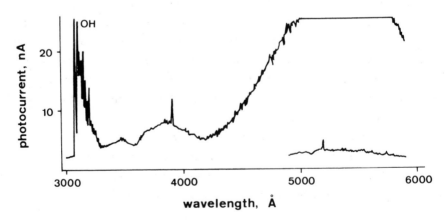

FIG. 12. A turbulent flow O₂-C₂H₂ flame background [1].

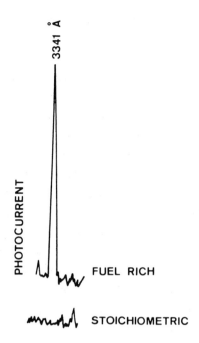

FIG. 13. A partial titanium spectrum [1].

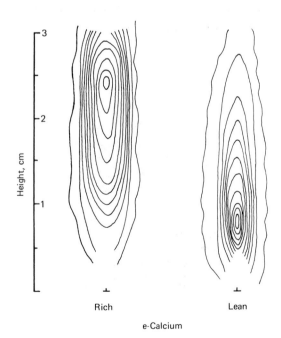

FIG. 14. Comparison of rich and lean flames [7].

Collimating Lens. The collimating lens is used to provide a flat focal plane when the radiation reaches the monochromator. It essentially straightens out the curvature produced by the condensing lens.

Monochromators. The vast majority of instruments now employ reflection diffraction gratings as the monochromator. Figure 15 is a diagram of how this device separates a beam of many wavelengths into different regions of space. It is based on Huygen's principle which states that if a plane wave is interrupted, the point of interruption will act as a secondary source for radiation. Notice in the figure that the new radiation from point 1 can be reinforced by the new radiation from point 2. Notice that if these places of reinforcement are connected, the original beam is bent in another direction or is diffracted. A different wavelength would reinforce at a different angle and therefore be separated from the first wavelength.

Notice also that if the first wavelength was 9000 Å, a wavelength of 4500, 3000, 2250, or any multiple of 9000 Å would also be reinforced at the same angle. This produces what we call the order of the spectrum. The longest wavelength is called the first order (9000 Å), one-half of it or 4500 Å is the second order, and so on. Filters must sometimes be used to to remove these extra orders if they are of high intensity.

A term usually associated with monochromators is dispersion. This is a measure of the angular separation of two light rays which differ in λ by

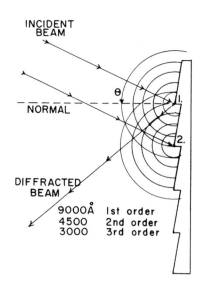

FIG. 15. A reflection diffraction grating.

a given amount, $d\theta/d\lambda$. Values are usually given in Å/mm (reciprocal linear dispersion). A value of 4 Å/mm will be a high-dispersion instrument, while a value of 37 Å/mm would be considered a low dispersion.

The slit system and the monochromator combine to reduce stray light, extraneous light, and spectral interferences:

Stray light is the internal scattering of radiation within the instrument.

Extraneous light is caused by room lights. Fluorescent lights produce an Hg 4358 and 4047 Å line that interferes with Pb 4057.8 Å. Zn, S, Ca, and W lines also are emitted by fluorescent lights.

Spectral interference is any radiation that coincides or overlaps that of the desired element.

Exit Slits. Once the monochromator has separated the beam into its component parts the exit slit is used to permit only the desired wavelength to pass to the detector. The exit slit is usually the same size opening as the entrance slit (a few micrometers), and because of the curved lens used in the optics, the slits are curved to maintain uniform intensity. The radius of curvature is one-half the distance between the entrance and exit slits.

Detectors. The detector and at least the preamplifier (voltage) are usually combined by using a photomultiplier tube such as the 1P28 shown in Fig. 16.

In the multiplying phototubes, the incident radiation strikes the cathode, which is coated with a mixture of cesium and silver or bismuth-oxygen and silver for the far ultraviolet (UV). The photon of radiation causes electrons to be released from the cathode surface. These electrons are attracted to the first dynode by applying 75-100 V (+) to the dynode. Each electron is accelerated and its energy increased to the point that when it strikes the first dynode, it has enough energy to cause three or four more electrons to be released. This process is repeated until dynode 10 (the anode) is reached. By now, several million electrons have been released, and there is a corresponding amplification of the original signal.

General Technique

Flame emission spectroscopy is a very sensitive technique, so sensitive in fact that good operators find that what would seem to be insignifi-

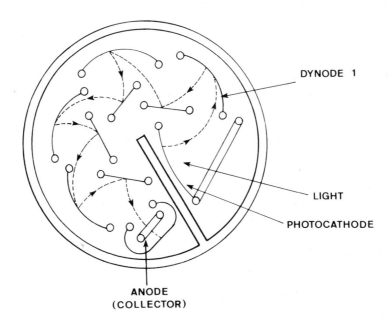

FIG. 16. Schematic diagram of a 1P28 photomultiplier tube.

cant activities are really a problem. The following is an excerpt from
John Dean, Flame Photometry [8]:

> The handling of soap powder in a distant part of the laboratory may
> pollute the air for hours. Tobacco smoke contributes potassium in
> considerable quantities. Operation near the seacoast is difficult
> during ocean winds. Normal walking along the floor covering and
> movement of the body clothing create contaminants.
>
> Fingerprints on glassware and filter paper folded with the fin-
> gers contribute sizable amounts of sodium. In handling glass stop-
> pered containers, one should cultivate the habit of inserting and
> withdrawing the stopper without giving it the customary twist, the
> abrading action of which releases sodium and potassium to the solu-
> tion (since found to be 40,000 particles/ml). New glassware often
> exhibits a surface contamination of soluble alkali, most of which
> can be removed by soaking the glassware for several days in dis-
> tilled water. Treatment of glass surfaces with silicon preparations
> is advisable. Glass stoppers, if fastened, should be held with rub-
> ber or polyethylene straps, never metal springs.
>
> Common filter paper may contain sodium and potassium, while
> acid-washed papers strongly absorb elements from trace solutions.

Quantitative Analysis Methods

There are many methods in the literature for quantitative analysis.
Only the three most commonly used will be explained.

The Calibration Curve Method. A series of standards are prepared and
their emission intensities plotted vs concentration. The unknown is then
determined by comparison with the calibration curve.

This is a good technique to use if you have several samples of the same kind, but it is time consuming if only a few samples are to be run. Unless simple samples are used, the solutions used to prepare the calibration curve must contain the same matrix elements. This is not always easy to do.

Solutions for flame emission, atomic absorption, and atomic fluorescence are usually in the part per million (ppm) of part per billion (ppb) region.

1 ppm = 1 mg/l = 1 μg/ml = a 1-g needle in a 1-ton haystack

1 ppb = 1 μg/l = 1 ng/ml = 1 drop of vermouth in a tank car of gin

The Dilution Method. This is a method that requires fewer standards than the previous method and which can be used if an interference is suspected.

Measure the unknown and then dilute it in half and measure it again. Repeat the process with a set of 2:1 standards. If there is no interference, the second reading in each case will be exactly one-half of the first reading. If it is not, then it can be corrected by taking twice the second reading minus one-half of the first reading.

Example calculation: A solution appeared to contain 68 ppm when measured by itself. However, it was known that the solution contained nearly 100 ppm. A dilution by two appeared to have a concentration of 41.5 ppm. The fact that 41.5 is not half of 68 indicates that an interference is present. To arrive at the correct value, take 2 x 41.5 - (1/2 of 68), which is 49. This is the corrected value of the 1/2-diluted solution, so the original must then be 2 x 49 or 98 ppm. (See Ref. 9.)

The Standard Addition (Spike) Method. Since matrix effects are common problems in all real samples and particularly so when using flame instruments, it is often convenient to use the standard addition method. The procedure is rather simple. Two solutions are required. The first solution contains an aliquot of the unknown, and the second solution contains an aliquot of the unknown plus a measured amount, but small volume, of a known (spike) solution of the element.

The increase in intensity of the second solution over the first solution is then caused by the added known. A linear relationship is assumed.

Cost Range

A perfectly satisfactory instrument can be obtained for about $5000, whereas the quality instruments would be in the $8000 to $10,000 range. Combination flame emission and atomic absorption equipment will run $15,000.

TABLE 3. Detection Limits by Flame Emission and Atomic Absorption[a,b]

Element	Wavelength (Å)	Flame Emission		Atomic Absorption	
		$N_2O-C_2H_2$	$Air-C_2H_2$	$N_2O-C_2H_2$	$Air-C_2H_2$
Ag	3280.7	0.02	--	--	0.005
Al	3961.5	0.005	--	0.1	--
	3092.8	--	--	--	--
As	1937.0	--	--	--	0.2
Au	2676.0	0.5	--	--	--
	2428.0	--	--	--	0.02
B	2496.8	--	--	--	--
Ba	5535.5	0.001	--	0.05	--
Be	4708.6(BeO)	0.2	--	--	--
	2348.6	--	--	0.002	--
Bi	2230.6	--	--	--	0.05
Ca	4226.7	0.0001	0.005	--	0.002
Cd	3261.1	2	--	--	--
	2288.0	--	--	--	0.005
Co	3453.5	0.05	--	--	--
	2407.2	--	--	--	0.005
Cr	4254.4	0.005	--	--	--
	3578.7	--	--	--	0.005
Cu	3274.0	0.01	--	--	--
	3247.5	--	--	--	0.005
Dy	4046.0	0.07	--	--	--
	4211.7	--	--	0.2	--
Er	4008.0	0.04	--	0.1	--
Eu	4594.0	0.0006	--	0.08	--
Fe	3719.9	0.05	--	--	--
	2483.3	--	--	--	0.005
Ga	4033.0	0.01	--	--	--
	2874.2	--	--	--	0.07
Gd	4401.9	2	--	4	--
	3684.1	--	--	--	--
Ge	2651.2	0.5	--	1	--
Hg	2536.5	--	--	--	0.5
Ho	4053.9	0.02	--	--	--
	4103.8	--	--	0.1	--

TABLE 3 (Continued)

Element	Wavelength (Å)	Flame Emission		Atomic Absorption	
		$N_2O-C_2H_2$	$Air-C_2H_2$	$N_2O-C_2H_2$	$Air-C_2H_2$
In	4511.3	0.002	--	--	--
	3039.4	--	--	--	0.05
Ir	3800.1	30	--	--	--
	2639.7	--	--	--	2
K	7664.9	--	0.0005	--	0.005
La	5501.3	8	--	--	--
	4418.2 (LaO)	0.1	--	--	--
	3927.6	--	--	8	--
Li	6707.8	0.00003	--	--	0.005
Lu	4518.6	1	--	--	--
	3312.1	--	--	50	--
Mg	2852.1	0.005	--	--	0.0003
Mn	4030.8	0.005	--	--	--
	2794.8	--	--	--	0.002
Mo	3903.0	0.1	--	--	--
	3132.6	--	--	--	0.03
Na	5890.0	--	0.0005	--	0.002
Nb	4058.9	1	--	3	--
Nd	2924.5	0.2	--	--	--
	4634.2	--	--	2	--
Ni	3414.8	0.03	--	--	--
	2320.0	--	--	--	0.005
Pb	4057.8	0.2	--	--	--
	2833.1	--	--	--	0.03
Pd	3634.7	0.05	--	--	--
	2476.4	--	--	--	0.02
Pr	4951.4	1	--	10	--
Pt	2659.5	2	--	--	0.1
Rb	7800.2	--	0.001	--	0.005
Re	3460.5	0.2	--	1.5	--
Rh	3692.4	0.02	--	--	--
	3434.9	--	--	--	0.03
Ru	3728.0	0.02	--	--	--
	3498.9	--	--	--	0.03

TABLE 3 (Continued)

Element	Wavelength (Å)	Flame Emission		Atomic Absorption	
		N_2O-C_2H_2	Air-C_2H_2	N_2O-C_2H_2	Air-C_2H_2
Sb	2175.8	--	--	--	0.1
Sc	4020.4	0.03	--	--	--
	3911.8	--	--	0.1	--
Se	1960.3	--	--	--	0.5
Si	2516.1	--	--	0.1	--
Sm	4760.3	0.2	--	--	--
	4296.7	--	--	2	--
Sn	2840.0	0.5	--	--	--
	2246.0	--	--	--	0.06
Sr	4607.3	0.0001	--	--	0.01
Ta	4812.8	5	--	--	--
	2714.7	--	--	5	--
Tb	4318.9	0.4	--	--	--
	4326.5	--	--	2	--
Te	2142.8	--	--	--	0.3
Ti	3998.6	0.2	--	--	--
	3642.7	--	--	0.1	--
Tl	5350.5	0.02	--	--	--
	2767.9	--	--	--	0.2
Tm	3717.9	0.02	--	--	--
	4105.8	--	--	1	--
V	4379.2	0.01	--	--	--
	3184.0	--	--	0.02	--
W	4008.8	0.5	--	--	3
Y	3620.9	0.4	--	3	--
	4077.4	--	--	0.3	--
Yb	3988.0	0.002	--	0.04	--
Zn	2138.6	--	--	--	0.002
Zr	3601.2	3	--	5	--

[a]From Ref. 10.

[b]In μg/ml in aqueous solution, measured in nitrous oxide-acetylene or air-acetylene premixed flames formed by 5- to 10-cm slot burners.

Advantages and Disadvantages

Table 3 is a comparison of flame emission and atomic absorption for 62 elements. Of these, flame emission is more sensitive in 35 cases. Comparisons of this type are dangerous because the nature of the sample the element is in is not considered nor are identical conditions always obtained. The important item is that flame emission is no longer limited to the alkalies and the alkaline earths but can be used for a wide variety of elements.

Some of the good and bad features of flame emission are presented below.

Good features:

1. Qualitative analysis is possible.
2. Quantitative analysis on several elements at once is possible.
3. The most sensitive technique for alkali metals.
4. Nonmetals can be determined by using band-head emissions.
5. Chemiluminescence can be used to increase sensitivity.
6. The operator has many ways to vary the instrument sensitivity.

Bad features:

1. Band emission may interfere.
2. Experimentally it takes a while to learn to do it right.
3. The sensitivity depends on the excitation potential.
4. Low stability.
5. Subject to spectral interference.
6. Dependent on flame temperature.
7. Low precision unless done by a skilled operator.

ATOMIC ABSORPTION

Atomic absorption spectroscopy is a process whereby a sample solution or solid is vaporized and the metals present converted to neutral atoms. The neutral atoms thus formed absorb radiation from an external source and the amount of this absorption is then measured.

The Need for Atomic Absorption

A detailed look at flame emission methods, particularly those of 20 years ago, indicated that it is really a very inefficient process. Figure 17 indicates those places in the process where significant losses in sensitivity result.

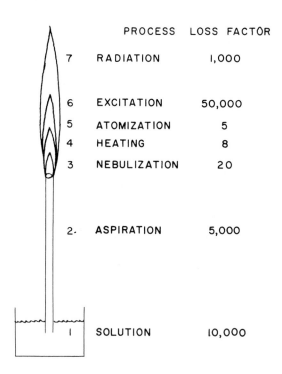

PROCESS	LOSS FACTOR
7 RADIATION	1,000
6 EXCITATION	50,000
5 ATOMIZATION	5
4 HEATING	8
3 NEBULIZATION	20
2. ASPIRATION	5,000
1 SOLUTION	10,000

FIG. 17. Sensitivity losses in the flame emission process.

At step 1 in Fig. 17 we find that a 100-ppm solution, which is a rather concentrated solution for this type of analysis, has resulted in a 10,000-fold dilution compared to the original solid.

At step 2 we find it takes about 10 liters of gas to aspirate 2 ml/min of solution, a further dilution of 5000. Only about 5% of the 2 ml of liquid is used because the drop size is too big to be useful; a further 20-fold loss occurs at step 3.

When the 10 liters of gas are heated to flame temperature, it expands to about 80 liters and results in another eightfold loss.

Neutral atoms are desired next, and this varies considerably. If we assume a 20% average conversion, then we have a fivefold loss.

The Boltzmann equation is used to determine how many of the neutral atoms become excited.

$$N_{ex} = N_g g \ e^{-\Delta E/kT} \tag{25}$$

where

N_{ex} = the number of neutral atoms excited.

N_g = the number of neutral atoms in the ground state.

g = statistical weight factor for the particular energy levels.

$-\Delta E$ = the energy to excite the atom.

k = Boltzmann constant, 1.38×10^{-16} erg-degree^{-1} molecule^{-1}.

T = flame temperature in Kelvin (K).

Because this is a very important equation in flame techniques, an example calculation will be given.

Example calculation: What is the N_{ex}/N_g ratio for a sodium system at 3000 K if g = 2 and the resonance line is at 589.6 nm? Remember, $\Delta E = h\nu$.

$$N_{ex} = 1(2) \exp\left[\frac{6.62 \times 10^{-27}\text{erg-sec}(3 \times 10^{10}\ \text{cm/sec})}{3 \times 10^3\ \text{deg}(1.38 \times 10^{16}\ \text{erg/deg})(5.896 \times 10^{-5}\ \text{cm})}\right]$$

$$N_{ex} = 1(2)\ e^{-8.14}$$

(Note: To do e on a slide rule, set the power on the D scale and read the answer off the appropriate LL scale. For + exponents, use the LL1, 2, and 3 scales and for - exponents, use the LL01, 02, and 03 scales. In this case, use the LL03 scale for numbers -1 to -10.)

$$N_{ex} = 1 \times 2 \times 0.000294$$

$$= 5.88 \times 10^{-4}$$

or 1 out of every 58,800 neutral atoms is excited. Notice that very few atoms are excited at any one time.

Step 7 has to do with the direction of the emission. Since the radiation can be emitted in all directions and we only measure over one small solid angle, another factor of 1000 or so is lost.

One begins to wonder if there is anything left to measure. In fact, we know that flame emission techniques, using what radiation is collected, are very sensitive in many cases. What could we do if we did not have these losses?

The first attempt at improvement was to place a reflecting mirror on the opposite side of the flame to decrease the radiation loss (step 7).

The Boltzmann equation gave a clue as to what might be tried. The smaller ΔE is, the more N_{ex} are formed. This is why neutral atoms are desired, because they have the smallest ΔE.

The temperature is another possibility. A large temperature value will also produce a larger N_{ex} as shown in Table 4.

TABLE 4. The Effect of Temperature on N_{ex}/N_g [a]

Line	g_g/g_{ex}	N_{ex}/N_g		
		2000 K	3000 K	4000 K
Na 589.6 nm	2	9.86×10^{-6}	5.88×10^{-4}	4.48×10^{-3}
Ca 852.1 nm	2	4.44×10^{-4}	7.24×10^{-3}	2.98×10^{-2}
Zn 213.9 nm	3	7.29×10^{-15}	5.58×10^{-10}	1.48×10^{-7}

[a] From Ref. 11.

The race was on to find the hottest flame, and O_2-C_2H_2 was found to be the most practical. Cyanogen $[(CN)_2]$-oxygen flames produce temperatures up to 5600° C and have enough energy to excite almost every element in the periodic table; however, cyanogen is very expensive, a small lecture bottle costing nearly $50.00, and it is quite toxic, behaving like cyanide. As a result, it is not used.

Something else needed to be done. Two places are worth investigating: one is the fact that only one out of 58,800 neutral sodium atoms is excited and the other is the flame itself. If we could just get rid of the flame and the solutions it required or if we could make the neutral atom excitation more efficient, the possibilities existed for a significant lowering of sensitivities.

Early attempts at eliminating the flame failed. In 1955, Walsh, in Australia, and Alkemade and Milatz, in Germany, found a way to improve the efficiency of exciting the neutral atoms. Over the years, Walsh's method has been more widely adapted.

In essence he asked the question, "Why do we only get 1 out of 58,000 neutral atoms of Na to become excited?" The reason is that we get the energy to excite the neutral atoms by collisions with the other atoms and molecules in the flame and unless the energy of the collision happens to match an energy transition within the atom or molecule, then no excitation takes place. Atoms are very particular; they must have exactly the right energy to become excited or nothing happens. This is borne out by the fact that in the reaction zone a metal atom will undergo 10^4 to 10^5 collisions in about 10^{-5} sec and yet only 1 out of 58,000 Na atoms at 3000 K has just the right combination. This ratio is even higher for most other elements.

What is needed is a way to provide energy of just the right amount. Walsh did this by applying an external source of energy and not relying upon

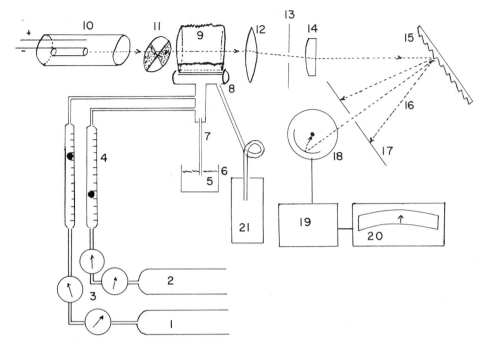

FIG. 18. The basic components of an atomic absorption spectrophotometer:

1. C_2H_2, N_2O, or H_2
2. Air
3. Pressure gauges
4. Flow meters
5. Sample solution
6. Sample holder
7. Capillary
8. Nebulizer
9. Slot flame
10. Hollow cathode
11. Chopper
12. Condensing lens
13. Entrance slits
14. Collimating lens
15. Diffraction grating
16. Diffracted beam
17. Exit slits
18. Phototube
19. Amplifier
20. Readout meter or recorder
21. Gas trap and waste

the flame. His source of energy was the hollow cathode lamp (see Fig. 19). The cathode of a hollow cathode lamp is made from the same metal as the element you want to measure. For example, a copper hollow cathode would be used to determine copper in a sample. Therefore the copper wavelengths emitted from the hollow cathode have the same energy as the energy required to excite the copper atoms in the sample, and a much more efficient excitation process is possible.

However, the radiation emitted from the excited atoms is not measured, but instead the energy from the hollow cathode absorbed by the atoms is measured (hence, atomic absorption).

Figure 18 is a diagram of the component parts of the instrument. Notice that all of the components are the same as flame emission with the addition of the hollow cathode, a chopper, and a different burner.

How Does the Hollow Cathode Work?

Figure 19 is a diagram of a hollow cathode tube. Electrons given off by the cathode accelerate toward the anode. Along the way they ionize argon atoms (sometimes neon) that are then attracted to the cathode. When the relatively large, highly accelerated argon atoms bang into the cathode, their energy is sufficient to knock several metal atoms off of the cathode surface. Some of these atoms are now in the excited state. When these excited atoms give off their energy, the radiation emitted is characteristic of the metal the cathode was made from. As a result, a copper hollow cathode will give off radiation that copper atoms in the flame can readily absorb and that almost no other element will be able to use. Therefore atomic absorption spectroscopy is almost completely free from spectral interference.

High Intensity Lamps. A recent improvement has been the high intensity lamp shown in Fig. 20. Normal lamps are based on an excitation process, and even though you have large quantities of neutral atoms, you can use only those that are excited. By using a hollow cathode you hope to increase the local concentration of neutral atoms, but you never get as many as you want. Then, too, self-absorption can be so intense that reversal occurs. If you simply increase the current, you increase the band width (Stark effect,

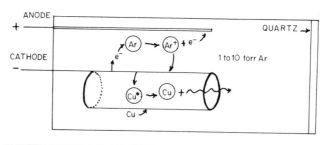

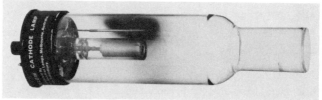

FIG. 19. Diagram of a hollow cathode lamp.

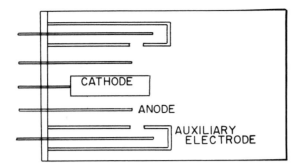

FIG. 20. Diagram of a high-intensity hollow cathode lamp.

discussed later), and this increase in current does not help over much of a range.

The excitation process in a hollow cathode lamp is really a two-step process, the production of ions to cause the sputtering and the sputtering process itself. A high intensity lamp employs two sets of electrodes which provide a high current for the first process and a second, separate, lower current for the second process.

This lower energy for the second process reduces the interference caused by excitation of the filler gas. The net result is that the intensity can be increased without increasing the band width, and you can use narrower slits and less gain in the amplifier. This means more sensitivity and less spectral interference.

Multiple Element Lamps. It would seem that a cathode made up of several elements would serve well for multiple element analyses. This has not worked as well as hoped. One of the difficulties is that the metals have different melting points, and the one with the lowest melting point boils off very fast when the current is increased to use the other elements. This also increases pressure broadening (discussed later). Those multiple lamps that work the best are those whose elements melt at nearly the same temperature. A "Gatling gun" arrangement seems to work fairly well in that the other cathodes can be warmed up while one is being used for the analysis.

Lamp Life. Hollow cathode lamps eventually wear out. A lamp usually lasts for about 500 hr.

The main reason the lamp wears out is that the filler gas is removed either due to entrapment by metal atoms or by absorption in the glass. Another cause is the loss of metal from the cathode. A third cause is leakage of air into the tube. This is noticed by the purple glow that

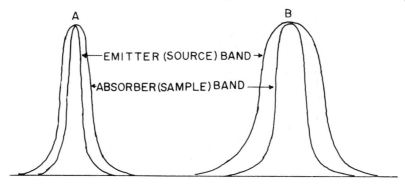

FIG. 21. Diagram showing good (A) and bad (B) absorption situations.

begins to appear. The last cause of importance is the slow oxidation of the cathode.

Why Use a Hollow Cathode?

In an absorption process you want a line source with a line width less than that of the absorber. This means that a larger fraction of the radiation emitted from the source is absorbed thereby permitting a more sensitive analysis to be obtained. This is illustrated in Fig. 21.

In the poor case we have a wide band width from the emitter (source), and the absorber (sample) has a narrow band width. This means the absorber can at best absorb only a fraction of the emitted radiation, and it will take a large concentration of metal to cause a detector response. In the good case, the emitter has a very narrow band width, maybe even narrower than the absorber. Now the absorbing metal can absorb nearly all of the emitted radiation, and it takes a very small concentration of metal to cause a detector response.

The poor case can be compared to weighing a ship and its captain, then weighing the ship and determining the captain's weight by difference. The subtraction of two large numbers to obtain a small difference is usually quite erratic. Atomic absorption lines are about 0.01 Å wide, so the source will have to provide very narrow lines. The hollow cathode lamp is one of the best devices known for providing a narrow line source. The following section will explain why this is so.

Line Broadening

From Fig. 21 we can see that the width of the line is quite important if we are to have a sensitive measurement. The line width associated with the atoms in the flame is difficult to control further, so they become the reference and then attempts are made to adjust the source line so it is as narrow as possible by comparison. There are four main factors contributing to line width: the natural width, Doppler broadening, Lorentz or pressure broadening, and the Stark effect. These are described below.

Natural Line Width. If the ground state of an atom was an exact energy and the excited state was an exact energy, then the difference would be an exact value and the line would be infinitely narrow. However, the Heisenburg uncertainty principle permits a small change in energy because neither the energy of the ground state nor of the excited state can be measured with infinite accuracy.

Natural line widths are of the order 10^{-3} to 10^{-5} Å and are considered to be negligible.

A line obtained by passing energy through two parallel slits has an intensity profile similar to that shown in Fig. 22.

The atom in the flame therefore has a narrow line width naturally until other factors broaden it. Since the hollow cathode lamp contains the same kinds of atoms, the lines from a hollow cathode also have a narrow width initially.

Doppler Broadening. This broadening is due to molecular motion. The velocity of the molecular motion is added or subtracted from the velocity of the emitted radiation, depending upon the relative motion of the atom at the time of the emission. This is shown in Fig. 23.

Doppler broadening depends on the mass of the atom and the temperature, but a value of about 10^{-1} to 10^{-2} Å is normal for flames. In a flame, with a definite velocity in one direction, there is a tendency to have less broadening than if the gas flow were absent. If the source is to match this,

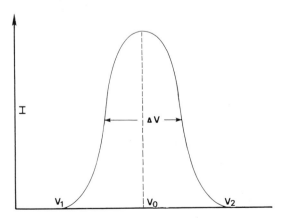

FIG. 22. Diagram showing a line intensity profile.

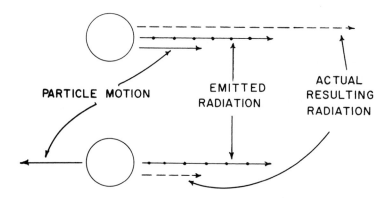

FIG. 23. The Doppler Effect.

then something must take the place of the gas flow. This is the hollow
cathode. The electrical field established by the hollow cathode tends to
restrict the sideways motion of the sputtered atoms so that the Doppler
broadening is comparable to that of the flame.

Lorentz or Pressure Broadening. Lorentz broadening occurs when an atom
is struck by another atom just as it is ready to emit its radiation. Since
the probability of such collisions increase as the gas pressure increases,
this is usually called pressure broadening. For normal temperatures, the
time it takes for a collision is about 10^{-13} sec. This means that if the
period for a visible region wave is about 10^{-15} sec, then about 100 vibra-
tions can occur within the atom or molecule during the collision. This
alters the energy and broadens the line. Pressure broadening is about the
same as Doppler broadening, about 10^{-1} to 10^{-2} Å.

The pressure within the flame can be quite high over small local areas,
but since it burns at atmospheric pressure, this can be used as the pressure
for comparison. The pressure within the hollow cathode lamp is usually between 1 and 10 torr.

The Stark Effect. If ions or electrons are present in the radiation
source, their strong electric fields may interact with the atom during collision or even near collisions. These local fields are continuously changing
and their interaction with the electric field of the atom gives rise to line
broadening. These outside electric fields can come from electrons, ions,
dipoles, and even quadrupoles. This is one of the problems that the high
intensity lamp helps to reduce. There are 10^{11} to 10^{13} electrons/cm^3 in a
normal flame. A hollow cathode lamp operates at 5 to 10 mA, and if all of
this current were due to electrons, then it would amount to 10^{13} electrons,

which is as much if not more than in the flame. However, by proper design, the main concentration of electrons is outside of the hollow cathode, so the Stark effect is actually less than in the flame.

The magnitude of the Stark effect is about 10^{-1} to 10^{-2} Å, the same as Doppler and pressure broadening.

Nebulizer Burners

Originally the nebulizer burners used for atomic absorption were the same as those used in flame emission. In an attempt to provide a longer path for the absorption of radiation, several burners were placed in a row. This arrangement was difficult to handle because it was hard to get two or three burners to burn the same and they were very noisy, the three-burner combination making it almost necessary to wear ear plugs.

A second method was to put mirrors around a single flame and pass the beam through the flame several times as shown in Fig. 24. This had some beneficial effect but not nearly what was expected. The reason for this apparent failure is shown in Fig. 25. Notice that there is a certain region in the flame that has the highest concentration of the neutral atoms and unless you measure there, you get decreased sensitivity. This region is usually different for each metal, and as a result most burners have a height adjustment on their mounting frames.

The current solution to the problem is to use "slot burners" such as the Lundegardh (Fig. 26), the Boling double or triple slot (Fig. 27), or the grooved N_2O (Fig. 28). All of these are laminar flow, premixed types. They burn quietly and provide a long flame path for radiation to be absorbed.

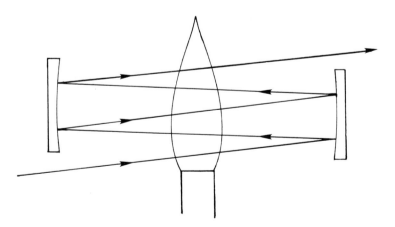

FIG. 24. The use of mirrors to increase sensitivity.

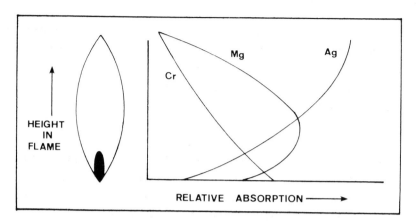

FIG. 25. Flame profile of some element concentrations [12].

Lundegardh Type. The slot is about 10 cm long and 1 mm wide. Either
a barrier plate or the fuel jet is used to separate the large droplets coming
out of the capillary. These large droplets drain away into a water bucket.
(Note: There is a loop in the drain line which should be filled with water
to prevent acetylene from escaping into the room.) Since the large droplets
have been removed, the gas flow is very smooth and the flame burns quietly.
The flame is also more reproducible and there are definite zones in it where

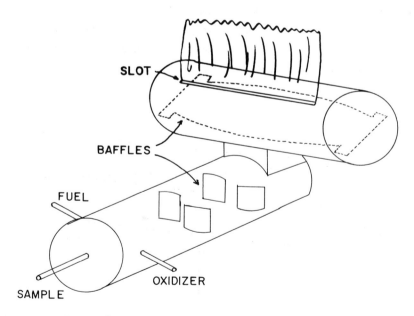

FIG. 26. Lundegardh-type burner nebulizer.

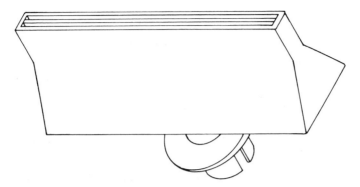

FIG. 27. The Boling triple-slot burner head.

measurements should be made. This correct height has to be determined for
each element, but a place to start is about 2 mm above the first cone.

A slightly fuel-rich flame is desired. This is obtained by first
getting an orange to yellow flame and then turning back the air until the
yellow just disappears.

The wires on the ends of the burner are flashback safety wires. If
the burner should flashback, the ends of the burner will blow out. These
wires keep the ends from flying around and maybe hitting someone.

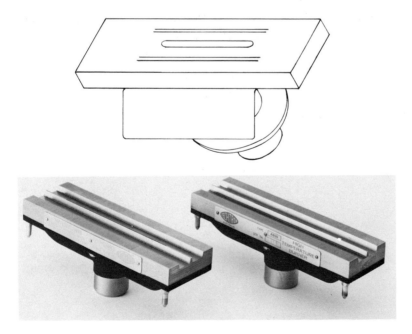

FIG. 28. Nitrous oxide burner head.

Flashback is a problem with slot burners. Drafts of air from people walking by can be enough to disrupt the gas flow and cause a flashback. A dirty slot is another cause of flashback as is too low a gas flow. Because O_2-C_2H_2 has such a high burning velocity, it is seldom used, but air-C_2H_2 works quite well with slot burners.

A piece of cardboard is usually used to clean out the slot. A razor blade can be used, but care should be used or the slot will be nicked. A dirty slot can be detected easily by looking at the flame and noticing any streaking in it. The carbon deposits also tend to glow and increase the flame background.

Boling Type. The triple-slot burner has a definite advantage over the single-slot type. The two outside slots tend to interact with the surrounding air and provide a shield for the inner slot. Measurements are then made primarily through the center slot. This arrangement also drastically reduces the danger of flashback, and because the center flame is protected, it is easier to reproduce measurements and more sensitivity is available due to a somewhat higher temperature and less compound formation from the oxygen in the surrounding air.

Nitrous Oxide Type. The use of nitrous oxide as an oxidizer was discovered by John Willis in 1965. This type of burner usually has a 5-cm slot because a 10-cm slot flashes back too easily. The early types were found to build up large carbon deposits at the edge of the slot. The remedy for this was to place two grooves on the burner head (see detail in Fig. 29) so the air could get to the carbon and burn it away.

Carbon deposits and "soot" contain polyacetylenes up to about $C_{10}H_2$ and hydrocarbons up to $C_{12}H_8$.

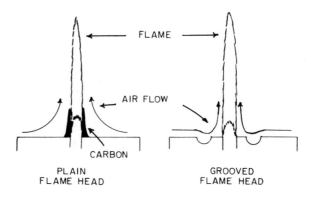

FIG. 29. Detail for reducing carbon deposits.

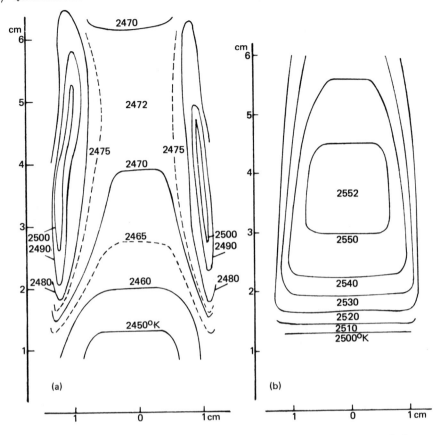

FIG. 30. Flame profiles, (a) rich, (b) stoichiometric [1].

The burner head is very heavy so that it will not warp at the high temperatures it reaches.

Figure 30 is a temperature profile of a premixed air-acetylene flame.

Flameless Atomic Absorption

Referring back to Fig. 17, we can see that other ways to improve atomic absorption would be either to use solid samples rather than dilute solutions or to get rid of the flame.

One early attempt to use solids was to mix the sample with gunpowder and form a pellet. When the pellet flashed, there was a sudden release of atoms into the beam. The difficulty with this technique was and is that gunpowder contains too many trace contaminants and the background blanks are too high for ppb analyses except for Au and Ag.

Volatile Vapors. A method that has found extensive usage, although being limited originally to mercury but now being extended to arsenic and

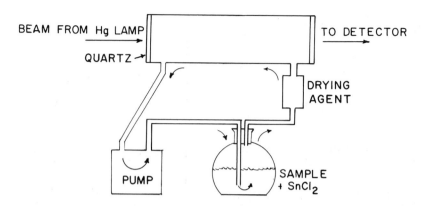

FIG. 31. Diagram of the apparatus used to determine mercury by flameless atomic absorption spectroscopy.

selenium, was developed in Canada. Originally it was a method to determine Hg in ores, but it became quite popular in this country by being used to determine Hg in all types of fish. Figure 31 shows the apparatus needed. The Hg-in-fish procedure will be used to explain how this technique works.

A Typical Analysis. Five grams of ground-up fish are placed in a 250-ml round-bottom flask and 20 ml of 7 $\underline{N}$ HNO$_3$, 25 ml of 18 $\underline{N}$ H$_2$SO$_4$, and 1 ml of 2% NaVO$_3$ are added. A Snyder condenser is added and the sample digested 1 hr. Twenty milliliters of HNO$_3$-HClO$_4$ (1:1) is added and heated to white fumes. The condenser is washed and allowed to drain into the flask. The flask is removed and the sample transferred to a 100-ml volumetric flask, stoppered, and taken to the atomic absorption instrument.

The instrument has been modified as follows. An Hg lamp at 3 mA is used as the source and the slot burner has been removed and replaced with a glass tube with quartz end windows. The wavelength of the monochromator is set at 2537 Å, the slits at 160 μm.

A pump with a capacity of about 2000 ml/min is used. Anhydrone [Mg(ClO$_4$)$_2$·2H$_2$O] is used as the drying agent. A 25-ml aliquot of the sample is added to a 150-ml Florence flask. This is diluted to 100 ml with dilute HNO$_3$-H$_2$SO$_4$ solution. Twenty milliliters of reducing solution is added to the flask which is immediately stoppered. The Sn^{2+} reduces the Hg^{2+} to Hg, which has a vapor pressure of about 2 × 10^{-3} torr at 25° C. As an air bubble passes through the solution it has zero initial Hg concentration and by the second law of thermodynamics (high concentration goes to low concentration), Hg from the solution goes into the air bubble. This wet bubble is passed up through the anhydrone to dry it, thus reducing detector noise. The dry Hg vapor then passes through the cell where it absorbs part of the beam, the amount being recorded.

This is a very sensitive technique. The author used a germicidal lamp, a fish aquarium pump, and an old Beckman DU and obtained Hg in pond water to a few parts per billion.

Arsenic and selenium have been determined by a similar technique. Here the sample is placed in a flask containing Zn. Acid is added, and the hydrogen formed reacts with the As or Se to form volatile AsH_3 or H_2Se which is then passed through the cell in a similar manner. This is much harder to reproduce than the Hg method.

The Tantalum Strip Technique. The tantalum strip (Fig. 32) eliminates the flame completely and can be used with several elements. A three-stage process is usually involved, but only 5 to 50 µl samples are required. The sample is placed in the middle of the strip and an Ar-H_2 gas mixture passed over the strip. The absence of O_2 is necessary to prevent the Ta from becoming brittle, and the H_2 provides a good reducing atmosphere for producing neutral atoms. The first step, drying, is done by passing a low current (5-10 A) for a few seconds through the strip. If the sample contains organic material, then a second step, ashing, is usually done. This is necessary because the carbon particles are thrown up into the beam and produce a noisy signal. Increased current (10-15 A) can be used, but sometimes a drop of HNO_3-$HClO_4$ (1:1) is added first. After the smoke has been swept out, the third step, atomization, is carried out by raising the current to 60-80 A for about 5 sec.

The strip lasts for about 100 determinations. The advantages are the very small samples required, little sample preparation, and high sensitivities can be obtained, comparable with but not quite as good as those shown in Table 5.

The Carbon Rod Furnace. In 1961 the Russian, L'vov, actually produced the forerunner of what is now known as the carbon rod atomizer. He used a hollowed-out carbon rod to hold the sample. This carbon rod was about the size of a piece of chalk, and he heated it with an induction furnace. In 1967, Massmann used electric heating, which was more convenient although a bit less sensitive. Figure 33 is a diagram of the Perkin-Elmer apparatus, and Fig. 34 is a diagram of the Varian-aerograph system.

The ends of the rod are connected to electrical terminals and from 2 to 12 V and 0 to 500 A are applied. The furnace can be brought to white

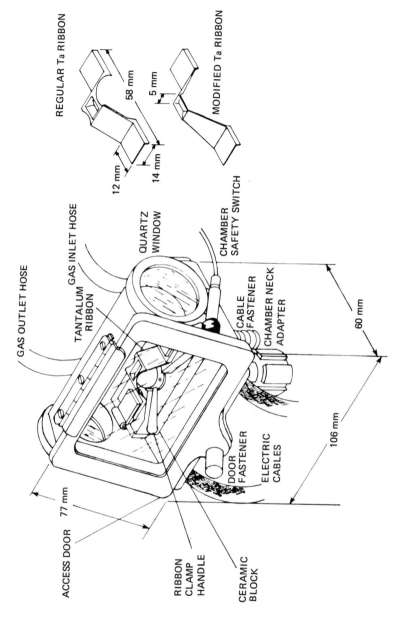

FIG. 32. The tantalum strip apparatus [13].

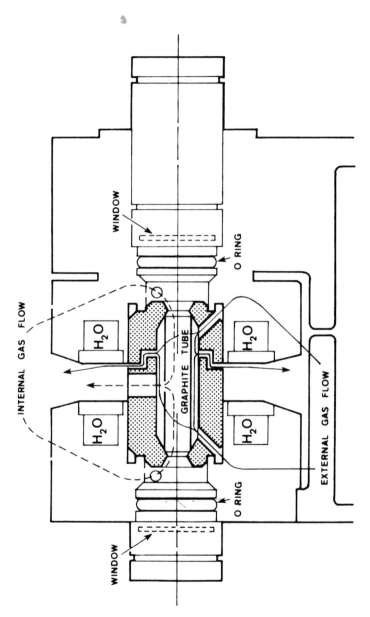

FIG. 33. The Perkin-Elmer carbon rod furnace. (Courtesy of Perkin-Elmer Corp., Norwalk, Conn.)

TABLE 5. Carbon Rod Sensitivities[a]

Element	Absolute Grams	Concentration in 5-μl Sample (ng/ml)	Element	Absolute Grams	Concentration in 5-μl Sample (ng/ml)
Ag	2×10^{-13}	0.04	Li	5×10^{-12}	1.0
Al	3×10^{-11}	6.0	Mg	6×10^{-14}	0.012
As	1×10^{-10}	20	Mn	5×10^{-13}	0.1
Au	1×10^{-11}	2.0	Mo	4×10^{-11}	8.0
Be	9×10^{-13}	0.18	Na	1×10^{-13}	0.02
Bi	7×10^{-12}	1.4	Ni	1×10^{-11}	2.0
Ca	3×10^{-13}	0.06	Pb	5×10^{-12}	1.0
Cd	1×10^{-13}	0.02	Pd	2×10^{-10}	40
Co	6×10^{-12}	1.2	Pt	2×10^{-10}	40
Cr	5×10^{-12}	1.0	Rb	6×10^{-12}	1.2
Cs	2×10^{-11}	4.0	Sb	3×10^{-11}	6.0
Cu	7×10^{-12}	1.4	Se	1×10^{-10}	20
Eu	1×10^{-10}	20	Sn	6×10^{-11}	12
Fe	3×10^{-12}	0.6	Sr	5×10^{-12}	1.0
Ga	2×10^{-11}	0.4	Ti	3×10^{-12}	0.6
Hg	1×10^{-10}	20	V	1×10^{-10}	20
K	9×10^{-13}	0.18	Zn	8×10^{-14}	0.016

[a]Courtesy of Varian Aerograph, Palo Alto, California.

heat within 2 sec. Argon is used to sweep out O_2 which would cause the carbon to burn, and cooling water is necessary to keep the rest of the apparatus from getting too hot. The sample is added by a syringe into the top hole. The advantage is that sensitivities like those shown in Table 5 can be achieved. The main disadvantage is that the rod absorbs the sample before the solvent can be evaporated and this causes a slow release of the sample atoms and a bit lower sensitivity. Coating the rod with kerosene or wax, as is done with graphite electrodes for emission spectroscopy, does not seem to work well. Reproducibility has always been a problem. It was found that the end windows fogged up due to the direction of the air flow. Therefore the Perkin-Elmer system has the Ar flow to the center and effectively shields the end windows.

In order to overcome the absorption by the rod, to make an overall cooler system, and to confine the sample atoms into an even smaller space, the arrangement shown in Fig. 34 is used.

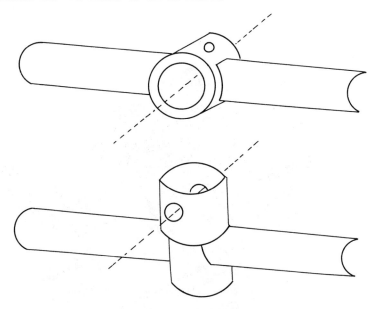

FIG. 34. The Varian carbon rod atomizers: top, rod type; bottom, cup type. (Courtesy of Varian-Techtron Co., Palo Alto, California.)

A ceramic center piece about 1 cm in diameter is spring loaded between two carbon rods which make electrical contact. The ceramic does not absorb like the Massmann furnace, yet carries enough current to get hot very quickly. A normal sample is 2-5 μl with 20 μl being placed in the cup. Figure 35 is a photograph of the Varian carbon rod atomizer, Model 63.

Table 5 is a compilation of the sensitivities for several elements. The results are read out in weight rather than concentration because a dry sample is used.

Figures 36 to 38 show the results of three applications of this technique. Figure 36 is a measure of vanadium in crude oil. One gram of oil is dissolved in 10 ml of xylene and a 5-μl sample is used. Notice how the recorder deflects during the drying step, the ashing step, and finally the atomization step.

Figure 37 is obtained by passing 50 ml of the sample air through the cup. Figure 38 is a determination of Ni in dried orchard leaves.

A Typical Analysis. This is the procedure for determining Fe in serum as presented by Glenn et al. [14].

Argon (14 liters/min) mixed with H_2 (2.6 liters/min) was the sweep gas. Standard Fe solutions of from 10 to 250 μl/ml were prepared with deionized

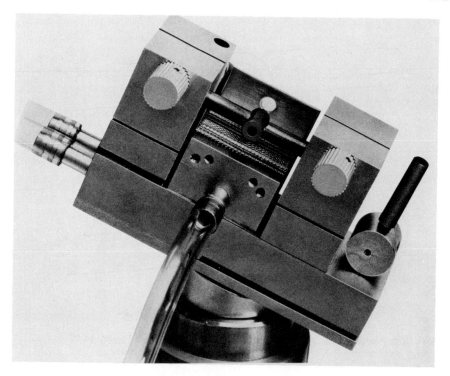

FIG. 35. The Varian Aerograph Model 63 carbon rod furnace. (Courtesy of Varian-Techtron Co., Palo Alto, California.)

water and stored in the plastic bottles. The wavelength of 284.3 nm from a Fe hollow cathode was used, and the sample was added with a 10-μl syringe. One μl of sample was placed in the cavity of the graphite rod. The sample was dried for 20 sec at 200° C (20 A), ashed 30 sec at 400° C (40 A), and then atomized for 3 sec at 1920° C (125 A). The rod was allowed to cool for 30 sec before application of another sample. One hundred fifty to 200 determinations could be done before a new rod was needed.

Choppers

If a flame is used for an atomic absorption measurement, the flame will produce emission just as in flame emission techniques. This emitted radiation will add to the radiation coming from the hollow cathode lamp and produce a low result because there appears to be less radiation absorbed. In order to correct for this, the beam from the hollow cathode is chopped, that is, it is periodically interrupted by a rotating sector wheel or else

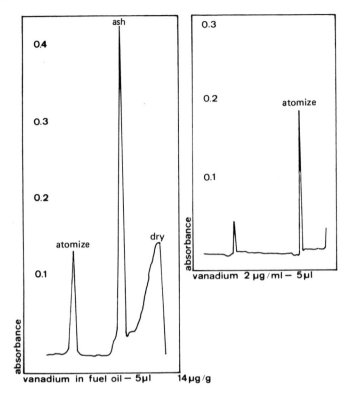

FIG. 36. Vanadium in Basra crude oil. (Courtesy of Varian-Techtron Co., Palo Alto, California.)

interrupted electrically within the lamp itself. This means that the lamp radiation is effectively alternating current, while the radiation emitted from the flame is direct current. The detector amplifier is designed to separate these different signals and amplify only that from the lamp.

Double-Beam Operation

Double-beam operation in ordinary spectroscopy is a technique used to correct for all absorptions not related to the sample such as solvent effects, sample cells, reagents, and power fluctuations. This is desirable because then the signal measured is due only to the sample. The technique is to pass one beam through the entire system including the sample and to pass a second beam through a duplicate system with the sample missing. The two beams are compared, and the difference is due only to the sample.

Double-beam operation has been tried with atomic absorption but has been only partially successful. Figure 39 shows one arrangement for double-

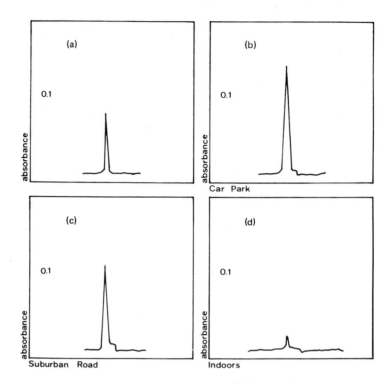

FIG. 37. Lead in air suspended particles: (a) aqueous lead, 5×10^{-10} g;
(b) car park, 9.3×10^{-10} g, 18.6 µg/m³; (c) suburban road, 6.9×10^{-10} g,
13.8 µg/m³; (d) indoors, 0.99×10^{-10} g, 1.98 µg/m³. (Courtesy of Varian-
Techtron Co., Palo Alto, California.)

beam operation. The reasons for this difficulty are that either two flames
are necessary, which cannot be maintained exactly the same, or the sample
flow into one flame must be interrupted periodically, and this has not been
done successfully. As a result, we have partial double-beam operation,
correcting for everything except the flame. This is actually better than
first expected because the greatest source of fluctuations occurs in the
lamp and these are then balanced out.

     Hydrogen Gas Corrections. Hydrogen is present in most hollow cathode
metals because it is used to reduce many metal oxides to the pure metal.
This produces a strong continuous background in the ultraviolet region, reduces the excitation energy and reduces the lamp stability. This is noticed
by a flattening of the sample calibration curve. Therefore an H_2 or D_2 lamp
is sometimes used in a second beam.

     Filler Gas Corrections. The filler gas in the hollow cathode is usually
either Ar or Ne. Helium is not satisfactory because it is too light for
good bombardment of the cathode and it produces spark lines.

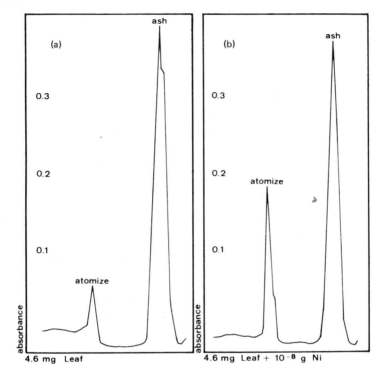

FIG. 38. Nickel in orchard leaves: (a) leaf, 4.6 mg, 6.25 x 10^{-9} g, 1.35 µg/g of leaf; (b) 4.6 mg leaf + 1 x 10^{-8} g Ni. (Courtesy of Varian-Techtron Co., Palo Alto, California.)

Argon gives the best results in most cases because it is heavier and therefore more efficient in the sputtering of the metal off of the cathode. It appears to last longer in the lamp, but the lines it produces from the cathode are less intense than those of Ne.

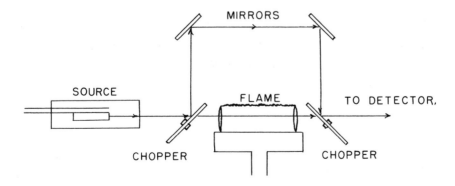

FIG. 39. A double-beam arrangement for atomic absorption.

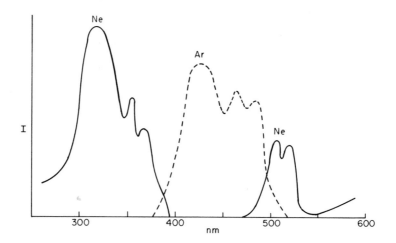

FIG. 40. General areas in which Ar and Ne have background spectra.

Neon produces less background in the main working region (Fig. 40), but it is removed from the tube much faster than Ar. Ne is usually used for Pb, Fe, and Ni.

Experimental Procedures

There are certain techniques that have been developed during the years that atomic absorption spectroscopy has been in operation, and these should be followed if accurate and reproducible results are desired. Several of these are briefly mentioned below.

Solutions.

1. Stock solutions should be from 500 to 10,000 ppm and diluted as needed.

2. Label the stock bottle caps also because the contamination of dilute solutions is easy.

3. Never pipet directly from a stock bottle. Always shake the stock bottle to mix the drops condensed on the sidewalls, pour a small amount into a clean beaker, rinse the pipet two or three times with this solution, and then pipet your sample.

4. Avoid glass and metal containers, and if the sample is of a biological nature, then a sterile bottle is required for storage.

5. Use distilled-deionized water for all standards and other solutions. The alkalies and alkaline earths may require double or triple distillation treatment.

6. If trace organics are a problem, treat the distilled water with $KMnO_4$. This will also remove morpholine, which is often added to prevent corrosion of the steam lines that transport the steam used to provide most of the distilled water.

7. If the sample is dissolved in an organic solvent in a large beaker, cover the top of the beaker with a split watch glass during aspiration or the vapors will get up into the flame and produce noise in the detector signal.

General Items

1. Clean glassware with HCl (1:1) and rinse three to four times with distilled-deionized water. Avoid dichromate cleaning solution, alcoholic KOH, or soap if possible, but if necessary rinse many times.

2. Silica gel is preferred for desiccators.

3. Hg, As, and Se are lost in preliminary sample handling if the temperatures exceed $500°$ C; Hg is lost at much lower temperatures.

4. If the solution is high in salts, dilute the solution rather than use a less sensitive line.

5. A dirty capillary from the sample solution is detected by noticing that the standards drift to a lower value on repeated trials.

6. A burning-out lamp is indicated by the fact that high concentrations can no longer be put on scale.

7. Always shut off the fuel first (you will have fewer flashbacks).

8. The optimum range is usually 10-100 times the sensitivity.

9. Atmospheric absorption interferes with the halogens, As, Se, and P.

10. To test for an electronic problem: if the meter is steady when on a line and goes off scale if you put your hand in the beam, your problem is not electronic.

General Safety

1. Always wear safety glasses because a large amount of UV radiation comes from the flame.

2. If you must poke around inside of the instrument, stick one hand in your pocket so you do not short-circuit yourself.

TABLE 6. Recommended Safe Limits for Several Compounds[a]

Compound	mg/m^3	Compound	mg/m^3
U	0.05	Fe	1.5
PH_3	0.07	HF	2
AsH_3	0.1	Mn	5
Cr_2O_3	0.1	Zn	5
Hg	0.1	HCl	7
Se	0.1	Mg	15
Te	0.1	HOAc	25
Cd	0.1	HNO_3	25
Pb	0.2	CO	110
Sb	0.5	CCl_4	315
As	0.5	$CHCl_3$	487
Ba	0.5	Gasoline	2000
H_2SO_4	1	CO_2	9000

[a]From Ref. 15.

3. A small fume hood should be placed over the flame. N_2O flames are known to be a problem since nitrous oxide is an anesthetic. However, the combustion products and the solvents can be toxic if several samples are being determined and long exposures are possible. Table 6 lists several of those compounds that are commonly used and their recommended safe limits.

Interferences

An _interference_ is any process that changes the normal measurement. Books can and have been written about interferences. More time and money are spent on removing interferences than on any other phase of metal analyses. It is one thing to determine Pb in distilled water and an entirely different problem to determine Pb in paint or milk. This is the one subject that has been known to make grown men cry.

There are three major types of interference: spectral, chemical, and physical. The simplest and safest way to counteract most interferences is to _always run a known control sample along with your unknown_. This has been found by experience to compensate for interferences that cannot be corrected for any other way or else would require too much time to do.

Spectral Interferences. These are caused by having the energy levels (emission and absorption lines) of one element, ion, or molecule overlapping the energy levels of the element being determined. This is a very serious problem in flame emission and requires narrow slits and a very good monochromator to minimize. Atomic absorption has almost no spectral interference because of the hollow cathode source. This is one of the prime reasons why atomic absorption is often favored over flame emission.

Chemical Interferences. This interference is caused by the presence or absence of a chemical reaction. For example, the sample compounds may not dissociate in the flame (a lack of a chemical reaction), or it may react with another element or radical and produce radiation, a process called chemiluminescence. The most common problem, however, is having a chemical reaction take place such as the time-honored phosphate interference with calcium. Here the calcium and phosphate react to form a compound which is difficult to handle in the flame. This causes low calcium results.

Three basic approaches have been used to remove this type of interference and can be applied to almost any other metal in some form or another. The calcium phosphate system will be used as an example.

More insoluble compound formation: Lanthanum is added to the system. This metal forms a more insoluble compound with phosphate than does calcium so the calcium is set free.

Ion exchange resins: The sample is passed through an anion exchange column, usually in the OH^- form, and the phosphate is replaced with OH^-.

Chelation: In this case the metal ion, Ca^{2+}, is chelated with ethylene diaminetetraacetic acid (EDTA). This protects the Ca^{2+} until the EDTA is burned away in the flame, and the Ca^{2+} can be reduced to the metal before it has a chance to react further.

Both flame emission and atomic absorption are susceptible to chemical interferences. The use of the N_2O-C_2H_2 flame has helped reduce chemical interferences but has not eliminated them.

Physical Interferences. These involve altering the physical processes involved in the entire measurement. This includes such things as solution viscosity, salt concentration, drop size, or surface tension. The carbon rod furnace eliminates many of these interferences.

Remember, always run a known control sample along with your unknown!

Example calculation: A sample of baby food was found to contain 2.0 ppm of Zn. A 1.0-ppm Zn spike was added by the standard addition method and 2.7 ppm Zn obtained. What is the percent recovery in this analysis and what is the concentration of Zn in the baby food?

1. The percent recovery is

$$\frac{0.7 \text{ ppm found} \times 100}{1.0 \text{ ppm added}} = 70\% \text{ recovery}$$

It is not

$$\frac{2.7 \text{ ppm found} \times 100}{3.0 \text{ ppm added}} = 90\% \text{ recovery}$$

The reason is that the 2.0 ppm originally found was not yet corrected for the recovery, and that could be established only by adding the known spike.

2. The actual amount of Zn present. Two ppm is 70% of the true value; therefore the true value is

$$\frac{2.0 \text{ ppm}}{0.7} = 2.8 \text{ ppm Zn}$$

Advantages and Disadvantages

One of the first questions usually asked about an instrument is how sensitive is it or what are its detection limits. Many people use these terms interchangeably by mistake, and it makes quite a difference what you really mean. Figure 41 illustrates the difference.

<u>Sensitivity</u> is the concentration (usually in ppm) required to produce a 1% change in absorption. <u>Detection limit</u> is the concentration required to produce a signal-to-noise ratio of 2. In Fig. 41, both systems have the same sensitivity, but the left one has a far better detection limit.

Some of the advantages of atomic absorption compared to flame emission spectroscopy listed by Munoz are as follows:

1. More sensitive for many transition elements

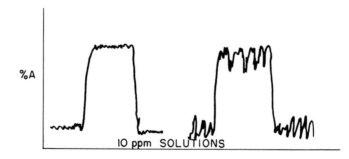

FIG. 41. The difference between sensitivity and detection limits.

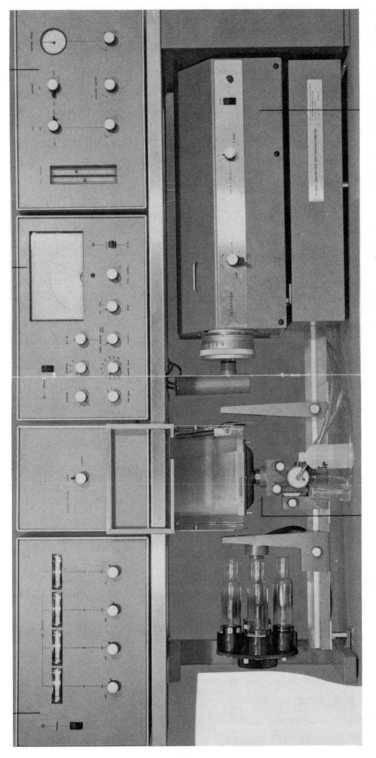

FIG. 42. A Varian-Techtron Model AA-5 Atomic Absorption Spectrophotometer. (Courtesy of Varian-Techtron Co., Walnut Creek, California.)

2. Less interelement interferences

3. Generally uses only resonance lines

4. Very easy experimentally to operate the instrument

5. Independent of excitation potential, therefore more sensitive for elements of high excitation potential

6. High stability

7. Almost free from spectral interference

8. High sensitivity and precision and less dependent on flame temperature

Some of the disadvantages are the following:

1. Cannot do qualitative analysis

2. Only one element at a time for quantitative analysis

3. Best absorption lines for some elements lie in the far UV and you get atmospheric interference

4. Less flexibility for varying instrument sensitivity

Cost Range

Atomic absorption instruments range from about $5000 to $25,000, the range depending on the monochromator, the readout advice, single or double beam, and the burner options. Figure 42 shows one of the better instruments.

ATOMIC FLUORESCENCE SPECTROSCOPY

Atomic fluorescence spectroscopy is a process in which atoms in a flame are excited by the absorption of external radiation, and the fluorescent radiation emitted during deactivation is measured at right angles to the source. Figure 43 is a diagram of the basic components. Notice that the components are quite similar to atomic absorption and flame emission instruments. The burner is changed, usually to produce a circular flame, and the source is usually an electrodeless discharge lamp (EDL). Other than that, the components are the same.

The basic concept of atomic fluorescence is not new. It was used by astronomers in the early 1900s. Fluorescence from flames was first reported in 1924. In 1962, Alkemade suggested the possible use of atomic fluorescence as an analytical technique. Winefordner in the United States has pioneered

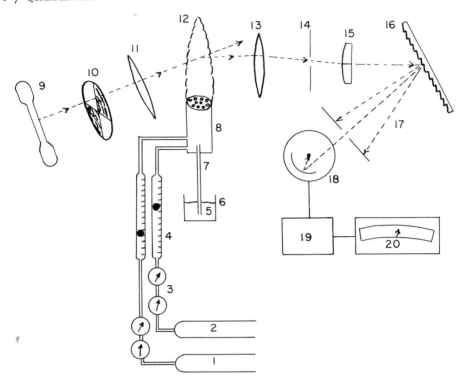

FIG. 43. Diagram of the components of an atomic fluorescence instrument.

1. Fuel, H_2 or C_2H_2
2. Oxidizer, O_2
3. Pressure gauges
4. Flow meters
5. Sample solution
6. Sample holder
7. Capillary
8. Cicular burner
9. Electrodeless discharge lamp
10. Chopper
11. Lens
12. Flame
13. Lens
14. Entrance slits
15. Collimating lens
16. Diffraction grating
17. Diffracted beam
18. Phototube detector
19. Amplifier
20. Readout meter or recorder

the development of this technique, and most of the following material was obtained from his papers.

The Fluorescence Principle

Atomic fluorescence is basically the same as molecular fluorescence with which many of you are already familiar. Figure 44 will be used to help explain how fluorescence occurs.

Consider an atom having an electron in a ground state (1). Radiation from an external source transfers its energy to the electron and raises it to an excited state (2). This takes about 10^{-15} sec. The electron may

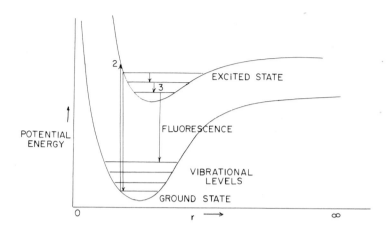

FIG. 44. Energy diagram for a fluorescence process.

lose its energy immediately by dropping back to 1, a process called <u>resonance</u>
<u>fluorescence</u>. The electron may lose its energy by collision with other atoms
and drop back to 1 without giving off any radiation. However, a few atoms
will follow the fluorescence path in that the electron will lose part of its
energy by collision, dropping back to 3, a process that requires about 10^{-12}
sec. The electron will stay at 3 for 10^{-8} to 10^{-4} sec and then return to 4.
The radiation given off during this last step is called <u>fluorescence radia-</u>
<u>tion</u>. Its energy is less than the exciting energy under these circumstances.
If, as sometimes occurs, the excited atom is further excited by collision with
another atom before it deactivates, then the fluorescent radiation is higher
in energy than the excitation source and we have <u>sensitized fluorescence</u>.

    Since an atom that has been excited can emit its radiation in any di-
rection when it deactivates, it is possible to measure this radiation at
right angles to the source radiation and not have to compensate or correct
for the high intensity of the source. Once before, we mentioned the analogy
of measuring the ship and the captain to determine the weight of the captain.
By measuring at right angles, we measure the weight of the captain directly.

    <u>Fluorescence Intensities</u>. Table 7 will give you some indication of why
fluorescence techniques have taken a bit of time to develop. The amount of
radiation that is fluorescent is only a small percentage of the total source
radiation.

    These low intensities have a tremendous influence on the type of source
that can be used, and only sources of extremely high initial intensities
can be used for trace analysis.

TABLE 7. Some Fluorescence Intensities at 90 deg to the Source Based on a
100-ppm Solution

Metal	% of Source Intensity
Zn	0.008
Cd	0.009
Hg	0.003

Sources

Three types of sources have been used: hollow cathodes, which have
been discussed earlier, continuous sources such as the xenon arc, which has
a high intensity, and electrodeless discharge lamps.

Hollow Cathode Lamps. These were among the first sources tried but are
not the source of choice in many cases at this time. Atomic line widths are
not as important in atomic fluorescence, so the narrow-line hollow cathode
with its corresponding low intensity is not usually used.

Continuous Sources. A xenon arc is an example of a continuous source.
This is about a 150-W arc. This source can induce fluorescence in Cu, Ag,
Au, Pb, Bi, Zn, Cd, Ca, Ba, Ga, Ni, Mg, and Tl.

Electrodeless Discharge Lamps. These were originally single-element
lamps designed to do the same thing as a hollow cathode, but they have a
much higher intensity. Table 7 shows why a high initial intensity is desired. Now multielement lamps are available. Figure 45 is a diagram of an
electrodeless discharge lamp (EDL).

An easily volatile metal salt of the element whose radiation is desired, usually the iodide, is placed in a quartz cavity. This cavity is
small (9 mm x 5 mm) and is evacuated to a few torr. This salt is vaporized
and excited by passing energy in the microwave region (2450 MHz at 120 W is
one combination) into the cavity. The radiation emitted is quite intense,
has reasonably narrow lines, and loses little of its power by self-absorption.

Multielement discharge lamps (for example, Ag, Cu, Pb, Mn, and Sn as
the iodides) have been prepared. In general, the detection limit when using
these multielement sources is about a factor of 10 poorer than with single-
element sources.

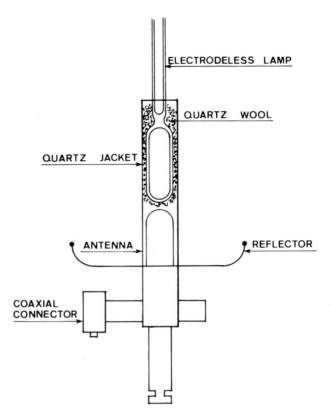

FIG. 45. Diagram of a microwave induced electrodeless discharge lamp [16].

Nebulizer Burners

Circular Burners. The arrangement that produces the highest intensity
is a circular, turbulent-flow, total consumption-type burner. These burners
give the highest sensitivities, are insensitive to the nebulizing gas, and
are free of flashbacks. Figure 46 is a diagram of one such burner.

The secondary reaction zone should be avoided because H_2 appears to
quench the fluorescence in this region. This can be corrected somewhat by
adding Ar, producing a 10-fold increase in signal, although the signal is
quite noisy.

Ultrasonic Nebulization. The droplets present in the normal flames
scatter the source radiation thus causing a sizable error. In order to
minimize this, organic solvents have been used since the droplets produced
are much smaller. Figure 47 shows how serious this scattering problem
can be.

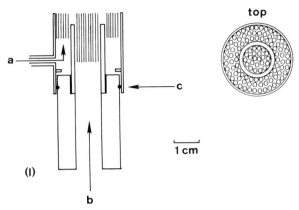

FIG. 46. Circular burner head, cross section and top view. (Courtesy of
Perkin-Elmer Co., Norwalk, Connecticut.)

The use of organic solvents reduces scattering but does not eliminate
it. At the current time the use of ultrasonic nebulizers seems to offer
the best method for reducing scattering. There are a few additional benefits that accrue from the use of an ultrasonic nebulizer and these will be
mentioned shortly.

Figures 48 and 49 show two ultrasonic nebulizers. Figure 48 is of an
older design, but it is easier to understand how it operates, so you can
then understand how the more involved systems function. The sample solution
is slowly dropped onto a plate vibrating at an ultrasonic frequency. The

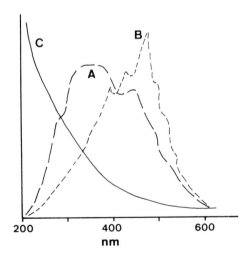

FIG. 47. The effect of scattering on the flame: A, scattered curve (uncorrected); B, spectral response curve; C, scattering curve (corrected).

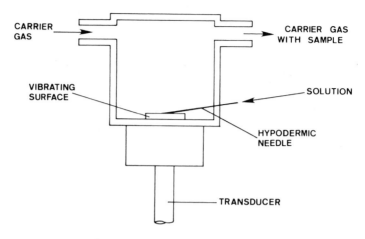

FIG. 48. An ultrasonic nebulizer [17].

plate shown in Fig. 48 is capable of nebulizing 0.72 ml of water a minute
with 70% of the particles having a diameter of 0.8 to 1.0 μm. This compares
with a regular turbulent-flow burner that has about 30% of the droplets
greater than 20 μm in diameter. A frequency greater than 500 kHz is necessary if 1-5 ml of solution is to be nebulized per minute, with droplets in

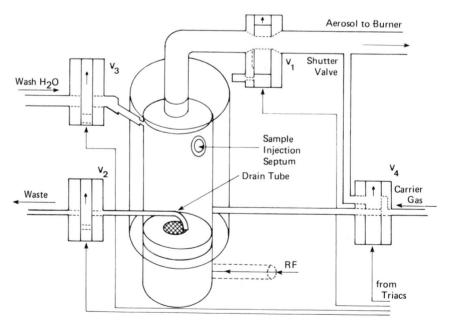

FIG. 49. An ultrasonic nebulizer for an automated system [18].

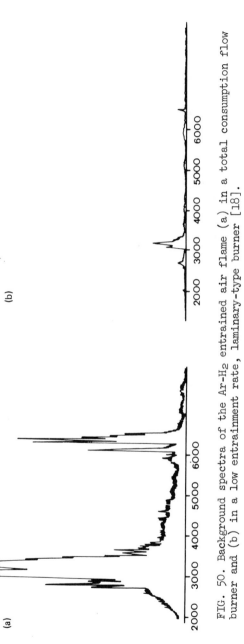

FIG. 50. Background spectra of the Ar-H₂ entrained air flame (a) in a total consumption flow burner and (b) in a low entrainment rate, laminary-type burner [18].

the 5-μ range. This nebulizer when used for flame emission spectroscopy produced intensities two to three times greater than the normal burners.

The apparatus shown in Fig. 49 provides an increase in atomic fluorescence of about 100-fold. This is due to three major factors: 1. The scattering is sharply reduced. 2. The smaller droplets produce a much more efficient desolvation which increases the atomic concentration in the flame. 3. A lower temperature can be used which means the background noise is much less. Figure 50 shows a comparison of the background noise for two different flame systems.

Comparison of Various Techniques

Table 8 shows a comparison of the various techniques discussed thus far. An electrodeless discharge lamp was used for the atomic fluorescence measurements. Remember, comparisons of this type are dangerous since different samples and conditions are used for each instrument. Therefore, Table 8 will give you a fair idea of what can be done but should be viewed with caution.

TABLE 8. Comparison of Atomic Fluorescence, Atomic Absorption, and Atomic Emission Techniques[a]

Metal	Atomic Fluorescence (ppm)	Atomic Absorption (from Perkin-Elmer Co.) (ppm)	Atomic Emission (Koirtyohann) (ppm)
Ag	0.0001	0.005	0.02
Au	0.2	0.2	0.5
Be[a]	2	0.003	0.2
Bi	0.7	0.05	9
Ca	0.02	0.002	0.0001
Cd	0.00001	0.005	0.9
Co	0.1	0.005	0.03
Cr	10	0.005	0.003
Cu	0.005	0.005	0.01
Fe	0.25	0.005	0.03
Ga	1.0	0.07	0.01
Ge	10	1.0	0.5
Hf[a]	3	15	--
Hg	0.1	0.5	20
In	0.1	0.05	0.005

TABLE 8 (Continued)

Metal	Atomic Fluorescence (ppm)	Atomic Absorption (from Perkin-Elmer Co.) (ppm)	Atomic Emission (Koirtyohann) (ppm)
Mg	0.008	0.0003	0.004
Mo[a]	2	0.03	0.3
Ni	0.04	0.005	0.03
Pb	0.5	0.03	0.3
Sb	0.4	0.1	1.5
Sc	10	0.1	0.03
Se	0.4	0.5	--
Sn	0.03	0.001	30
Te	0.5	0.3	30
Ti[a]	6	0.1	0.2
Tl	0.008	0.025	0.002
U[a]	5	30	30
Zn	0.00004	0.002	100
Zr[a]	4	5	3

[a]Requires an N_2O-C_2H_2 flame.

Advantages and Disadvantages

The main advantages are that a simple spectrum is obtained which means that less expensive monochromators can be used; if a circular flame is used, several source lamps can be placed simultaneously around the flame, and as a result several elements can be determined at once.

The main disadvantage is that not all elements can be made to fluoresce, and electrodeless discharge lamps are still rather expensive.

Winefordner has stated his belief that "when as many hours of research time have been spent developing atomic fluorescence as have been spent on atomic adsorption...atomic fluorescence will be the technique of choice." This remains to be seen, but for those elements that fluoresce, this technique seems to work quite well. For the moment however, most instruments have been built by the individual investigators.

A Typical Analysis

The example given is the determination of calcium, copper, magnesium, manganese, potassium, and zinc in soil extracts. This work was done by

Dagnall et al. [19]. Once the sample is ready to measure, it requires only 16 sec to determine all six elements.

Ten grams of each of the 13 air-dried soils were shaken with 100 ml of 1 $\underline{M}$ ammonium acetate solution at room temperature for about 2 hr on an automatic shaker. The solution was then filtered and the extract diluted as required. The soil extracts were diluted both 10- and 100-fold with distilled water, and the extracts at both dilutions were made to contain 1500 μg/ml strontium and 250 μg/ml sodium in a similar fashion to the standards to insure that interferences and ionization effects were negligible. All six elements were determined in each of the three dilutions of the extract (concentrated extract, 10-, and 100-fold dilutions) in order to insure that measurement for each element could be made at a concentration on the linear portion of the calibration graph for that element. Tables 9 to 11 illustrate the results that were obtained and how they compare with atomic absorption analysis.

TABLE 9. Detection and Upper Concentration Limit of the Atomic Fluorescence and Atomic Emission Spectrophotometric Determinations

Element	Wavelength (nm)	Detection Limits (μg/ml)	Upper Concentration Limit (μg/ml)
Calcium	422.7	0.007	5
Copper	324.8	0.01	4
Magnesium	285.2	0.004	4
Manganese	279.5	0.01	4
Potassium[a]	766.5	0.007	2
Zinc	213.9	0.007	5

[a]Flame atomic emission.

TABLE 10. Precision of Atomic Fluorescence Signals. Relative Standard Deviation (%)

| Element | Concentration (μg/ml) | | | |
	5	1	0.5	0.25
Calcium	0.5	1.9	3.2	4.3
Copper	0.9	6.5	6.8	3.4
Magnesium	0.2	1.0	1.4	2.4

TABLE 10 (Continued)

Element	Concentration (μg/ml)			
	5	1	0.5	0.25
Manganese	0.7	4.0	8.8	11.0
Potassium[a]	0.3	0.9	1.7	4.3
Zinc	0.5	4.5	3.2	3.4

[a]Flame atomic emission.

TABLE 11. Determination of Elements in Ammonium Acetate Soil Extracts

Soil	Technique[a]	Concentration in Soil (ppm)					
		Ca	Cu	K[b]	Mg	Mn	Zn
1	AA	320	0.6	180	86	12.9	2.39
	AF	316	0.5	180	82	12.2	2.42
2	AA	1380	0.3	167	52	5.1	0.72
	AF	1510	0.5	160	46	4.3	0.8
3	AA	1100	0.2	187	81	6.0	1.14
	AF	1081	0.3	180	75	5.6	1.4
4	AA	980	0.4	167	100	7.7	1.7
	AF	999	0.5	150	102	7.0	1.7
5	AA	1190	0.2	134	97	6.4	0.43
	AF	1199	0.3	130	90	5.5	0.32
6	AA	2200	0.6	167	314	1.0	0.89
	AF	2380	0.7	160	311	1.05	1.0
7	AA	1500	0.3	243	85	6.4	1.31
	AF	1520	0.4	230	78	5.6	1.30
8	AA	1460	0.3	165	96	12.8	1.97
	AF	1450	0.3	170	89	11.3	2.07
9	AA	1500	0.3	250	85	6.4	1.31
	AF	1520	0.4	250	78	5.6	1.3
10	AA	1420	0.3	168	117	28.8	0.9
	AF	1478	0.5	160	115	28.6	1.1
11	AA	900	0.5	153	24	1.2	0.75
	AF	980	0.5	150	23.3	1.85	0.73
12	AA	1630	0.6	193	112	10.2	1.14
	AF	1840	0.5	190	111	9.5	1.25

TABLE 11 (Continued)

Soil	Technique[a]	Concentration in Soil (ppm)					
		Ca	Cu	K[b]	Mg	Mn	Zn
13	AA	1940	0.1	168	75	17.5	0.76
	AF	1950	0.4	160	68	16.3	1.0

[a]AA, atomic absorption; AF, atomic fluorescence.

[b]Flame atomic emission.

ARC EMISSION SPECTROSCOPY

Emission spectroscopy is the application of spectral line intensities to determine atomic concentrations. What this means is that sample atoms are excited by the energy from an arc, spark, plasma jet, or discharge tube; the excited atoms then emit radiation as they revert to the ground state, and this emitted radiation is separated by a monochromator, the wavelengths determining which elements are present and the intensity determining how much of each is present. Figure 51 is a diagram of the components of an emission spectrograph.

This technique has certain advantages over flame emission, atomic absorption, and atomic fluorescence because it is capable of detecting not only all of the known elements but also large numbers of them at the same time. For example, Kniseley has determined 30 elements in either blood or oil samples down to the ppm region in most cases and the ppb region in several cases in 2 min with ±5% error. True, he used the latest equipment, which will be discussed at the end of this section, but there are many applications where instruments of lesser quality can be quite useful.

The principal difference between emission spectroscopy and flame emission is that the source produces temperatures from 6000 to 10,000 K compared to the 2500 to 3000 K for flame emission, and this additional energy is sufficient to excite all of the known elements. Of the 105 elements, about 90 have been examined by emission spectroscopy, of which nearly 70 are in the routine category, the nonmetals and gases requiring special methods and the very high atomic number elements being so scarce that no spectra have been obtained.

With normal equipment this is a technique for materials present from 1% to 0.001%. With specialized equipment, it is possible to go as low as 0.0000001% in favorable cases.

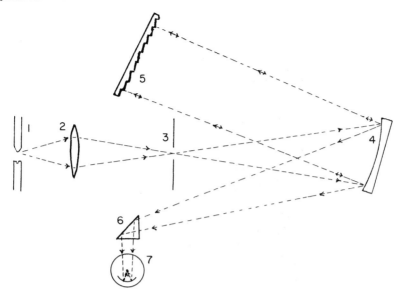

FIG. 51. Components of an emission spectrograph.

1. Source   5. Reflection grating
2. Condensing lens   6. Total reflection prism
3. Entrance slits   7. Detector, phototubes, or photo-
4. Collimating mirror   graphic

Qualitative analysis (finding what is there) is relatively easy, while
quantitative analysis (how much) is laborious unless good equipment is
available.

Types of Spectra

Spectra are generally divided into three types: line, band, and continuous (Fig. 52).

Line spectra are produced by a single transition within an atom or
molecule. The spectrum has the shape of a narrow line because the emitted
radiation is passed through a closely spaced (10- to 50-μm) vertical slit.
Slits are preferred over other shapes because they allow separation of energies that are closer together.

Band spectra are obtained from molecules. When atoms are combined to
form molecules, several energy levels are formed, many of which are very
close to each other. Actually, each energy level may produce a line, but
with most instruments these lines are not well separated and are so close
together that they appear to be a band.

A continuous spectrum is on the same order as the band spectrum except
that a continuous spectrum covers the entire region being observed. In

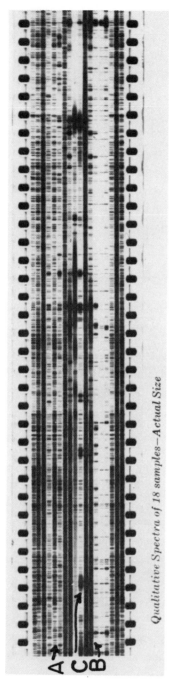

Qualitative Spectra of 18 samples—Actual Size

FIG. 52. Demonstration of line (A), continuous (B), and band spectra, (C). A qualitative spectrum of 18 samples, actual size. (Courtesy of Applied Research Labs., Glendale, California.)

emission spectroscopy, it is formed by the hot carbon electrodes and causes
a general darkening of the background. Such a spectrum can usually be removed by readjusting the position of the electrodes.

Sources

Sources for emission spectroscopy consist of arcs, sparks, discharge
tubes, and plasma jets.

The Direct Current Arc. The direct current (dc) arc is the most common
source and is probably the best source for qualitative work. Figure 53 shows
the process involved in exciting spectra with a direct current arc.

Electrons are emitted by the cathode and strike the anode (A to B) with
such force that they heat the anode, causing it to give off positive ions
(B to C). These ions migrate toward the cathode as a large positive space
charge. Electrons coming from A are not quickly accelerated because of the
nearness of the positive charges, and the energy of these electrons is sufficient to produce ionic spectra as well as neutral atom spectra, the latter
being about 10 to 20 times greater than the D region. In the D region, the
electrons have enough energy to produce neutral atom spectra. This is the
region generally used because it is more reproducible, although it is not

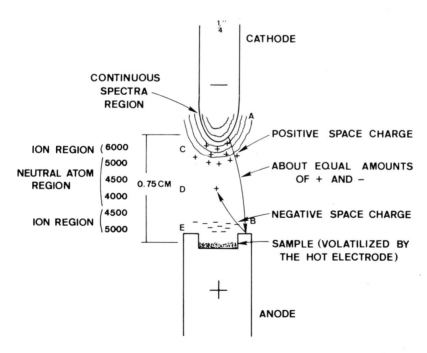

FIG. 53. Diagram of the direct current arc process.

satisfactory for trace amounts of elements. Using 1/4-in. carbon electrodes
spaced about 1/8 in. apart, a current of about 6 A is obtained when 150 V
are applied. These electrodes get quite hot and should not be looked at
directly unless dark glasses are used. The UV radiation given off can
damage your eyes unless they are protected.

A disadvantage of the dc arc is its poor reproducibility because the
arc wanders around the electrode. In addition, only neutral atom spectra
are produced in quantity. The advantages include (1) simplicity of operation
and low cost, (2) production of an abundant number of lines, and (3) efficiency for rapid qualitative analysis down to the ppm range.

The Alternating Current Spark. The high-voltage alternating current
(ac) spark is a more sophisticated source. The real difference between an
arc and a spark is that the arc is started once and continues to discharge,
while the spark must be initiated at every cycle just like the spark plug
in your car. The ac spark usually occurs in two forms: a low-frequency
(60 c/sec), low-voltage (2000-4000 V) form, and a high-frequency (kc/sec),
high-voltage (10,000-100,000 V) form. Both types are steadier than the direct current arc and are preferred for quantitative work. The high-frequency spark can be used for the analysis of metal film on other metals and
for biological samples.

The spark is steadier because every time it is activated, it can strike
a new spot, and local fractional distillation of the components is avoided.
Fewer lines are produced because, in spite of the higher initial voltage
required to create the spark, the working voltage is considerably less.

The high-voltage, high-frequency spark can produce temperatures as high
as 10,000 K yet the electrode remains fairly cold. Upon impact of a particle
accelerated by 10,000 V, there is a tremendously fast transfer of energy
into the sample in a very small area. Even if the sample is a highly conducting metal, it will not be able to conduct this heat energy away sufficiently fast and as a result there is a rapid temperature build up (up to
10,000 K), but in a very small area. This effectively causes a minute portion of the sample to "explode" into the spark to be ionized or excited.
Nearly all of the heat energy is therefore dissipated, and the remaining
sample does not get hot.

Discharge Tubes. Discharge tubes are used to obtain spectra of gases.
The gas is placed inside of a glass tube, with a quartz window to pass the
UV, the pressure is reduced to a few torr, and 2000 to 5000 V are applied
across the electrodes. The electrons passing between the electrodes strike

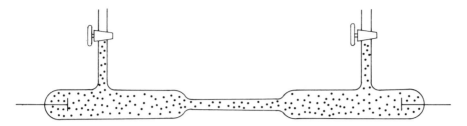

FIG. 54. Diagram of a gas discharge tube.

the gas molecules and excite them. When they return to the ground state
they give off their spectrum. Such a tube is shown in Fig. 54.

Plasma Jets. A plasma is a flame or electrical discharge that has an
unusually high concentration (> 1%) of positive and negative ions present.
These jets can be made to have very high temperatures, from a few thousand
degrees to 50,000 K with about 10,000 K the range for emission spectroscopy.
Figures 55 and 56 are a diagram and a photograph of the most common low-
frequency type of plasma jet, and Fig. 57 is a diagram of an improved high-
frequency plasma system.

Plasma formation: The following material was taken in abstract form
from a preprint article by V. A. Fassel and R. N. Kniseley [20]. Refer to
Figs. 57 to 59.

> Place a quartz tube about 2.5 cm in diameter inside a coil
> connected to a high frequency generator operating typically in the
> 4 to 50 MHz range at power levels of 2 to 5 Kw. Pass Ar through
> the tube. The plasma is started by using a Tesla coil to generate
> the first free electrons.
>   Let us now examine the course of events leading to the forma-
> tion of the plasma. The high frequency currents flowing in the
> induction coil generate oscillating magnetic fields whose lines of
> force are axially oriented inside the quartz tube and follow ellip-
> tical closed paths outside the coil as shown [in Fig. 58]. The
> induced axial magnetic fields in turn induce the seed electrons
> and ions to flow in closed annular paths inside the quartz tube
> space. This flow of electrons - the eddy current - is analogous
> in behavior to the current flow in a short circuited secondary of
> a transformer. The radio frequency field is an alternating field
> and therefore the induced magnetic fields are varying in both di-
> rection and strength. This causes the electrons to be accelerated
> each half cycle. The accelerated electrons and ions meet resis-
> tance to their flow, Joule or ohmic heating is a natural conse-
> quence, and additional ionization occurs. The steps just discussed
> lead to the almost instantaneous formation of a plasma. The over-
> all appearance is a three zone flame; the inner core, very intense,
> brilliant white and nontransparent, a second cone about 1 to 3 cm
> above the induction coil and which is bright but somewhat trans-
> parent, and the tail flame which is barely visible until sample is

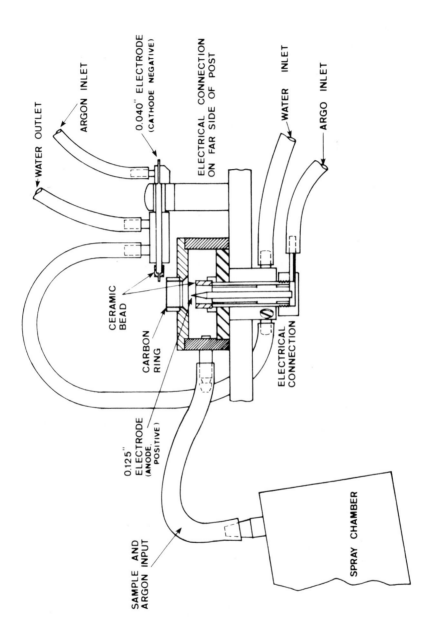

WATER OUTLET

ARGON INLET

0.040" ELECTRODE
(CATHODE NEGATIVE)

ELECTRICAL CONNECTION
ON FAR SIDE OF POST

WATER INLET

ARGO INLET

CERAMIC
BEAD

CARBON
RING

ELECTRICAL
CONNECTION

0.125"
ELECTRODE
(ANODE,
POSITIVE)

SAMPLE AND
ARGON INPUT

SPRAY CHAMBER

FIG. 55. Construction of the argon plasma device. (Courtesy of American Laboratory, August 1971.)

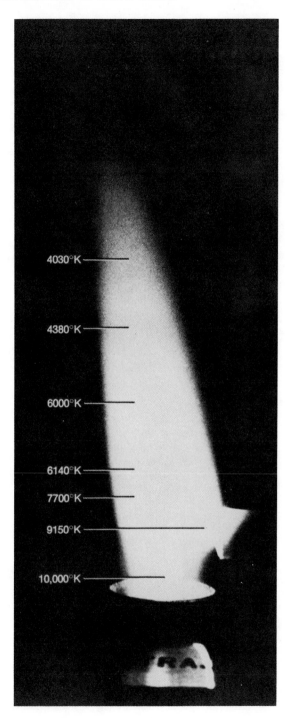

FIG. 56. Temperature profile of the plasma flame.   (Courtesy of American
Laboratory, August 1971.)

added to the plasma. The second region is used for analytical work.

Thermal isolation of the plasma:

The plasma formed in this way attains a gas temperature of the 9000 to 10,000° K range. At these temperatures the plasma must be thermally isolated lest the quartz tube melt under sustained operation. This isolation is achieved by Reed's vortex stabilization technique [Fig. 59] which utilizes a flow of argon introduced tangentially. This figure also shows the complete assembly of concentric tubes and argon flow patterns for sustaining the plasma after it has formed. The tangential flow of argon, which is typically in the 10 l/min range, streams upward tangentially, cooling the inside walls of the outermost quartz tube and keeping the plasma away from the wall. The plasma itself is anchored near the exit end of the concentric tube arrangement.

In addition to the vortex stabilization flow of Ar, there is another lower velocity flow of about 1 l/min that transports the sample either as an aerosol, a powder, or a thermally generated vapor to the plasma.

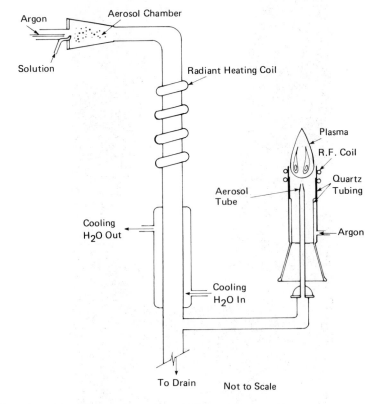

FIG. 57. Schematic diagram of the plasma jet and sample introduction system [21].

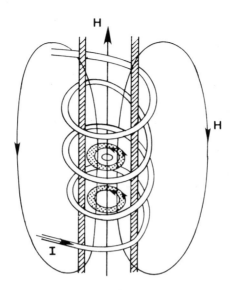

FIG. 58. Magnetic fields and eddy currents generated by an induction coil
[20].

Sample introduction: Because of the high temperatures of the plasma
and the resulting sharp temperature gradient, it has been difficult to get
the sample actually into the flame, and for several years this was a major
drawback to using this technique. It did no good to produce a theoretically
desirable hot source if the sample could not be injected into it. As a result the detection limits were never as low as believed possible. This is
shown in Fig. 60 on the left. The sample simply went around outside of the
plasma and little reacted. Fassel and Kniseley found that if the frequency
of the induction coil was increased to about 30 MHz, then the plasma became
doughnut shaped (Fig. 60 right) and the sample could be injected into the
center of the doughnut. This was still not into the 9000 to 10,000 K region, but it was into a 7000 K region which is about twice that of a normal
hot flame. The net result was a general lowering of the detection limits
by two or three orders of magnitude, and emission spectroscopy was taken
from the ppm region into the ppb region, now of considerably more value in
solving current problems.

Advantages and disadvantages: According to Kniseley,

typical residence times of the sample in the plasma before the
observation height is reached is in the 2.5 m sec range. The
combination of high temperatures and relatively long residence
times should lead to complete solute vaporization and a high, if

not total, degree of atomization of the analyte species in the core of the plasma. Once the free atoms are formed they occur in a chemically inert environment, as opposed to the violently reactive surroundings in combustion flames. Thus their lifetime, on the average, should be longer than in flames.

The plasma system described above possesses other unique advantages. First, after the free atoms are formed, they flow upstream in a narrow cylindrical radiating channel so it is easier to use all of the available radiation. Second, at the normal height of observation, the central axial channel containing the relatively high number density of analyte free atoms has a rather uniform temperature profile with very few low temperature atoms surrounding it. Thus self absorption is held to a minimum. This means that with good detectors, calibration curves covering

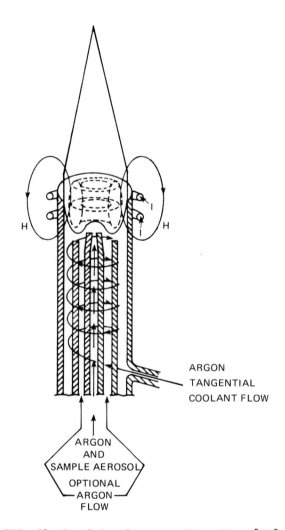

ARGON
TANGENTIAL
COOLANT FLOW

ARGON
AND
SAMPLE AEROSOL

OPTIONAL
ARGON
FLOW

FIG. 59. Complete plasma configuration [20].

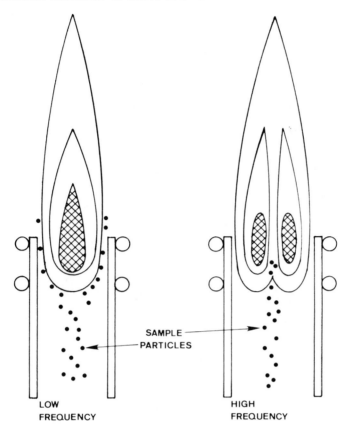

FIG. 60. Sample particle paths for different plasma shapes [20].

at least five orders of magnitude are possible thus eliminating
the usual multiple dilutions required previously.

   The other advantages of these plasmas worthy of note are
(a) no electrodes are used, hence contamination from the electrodes normally used in other plasmas or arcs is eliminated; and
(b) the plasma operates on non-explosive noble gases, hence the
systems can be used in locations where combustibles are not allowed.

Monochromators

Prisms and gratings are the monochromators used with emission spectrographs with reflectance gratings now being almost universally preferred.

   One of the important items to consider in a grating is the resolving
power. This is the ability to clearly distinguish two adjacent lines in a
spectrum. The equation for doing this is

$$R = \frac{\lambda}{\Delta\lambda}$$

where

R = resolving power = nN

n = order of the spectra

N = number of lines on the grating actually being illuminated

λ = average wavelength of the lines involved

Δλ = difference between these lines

Example calculation: What is the resolving power of a grating that has 40 lines/mm if 20 mm are illuminated in a first-order spectrum?

$$R = nN \tag{26}$$
$$= 1 \times 40 \times 20$$
$$= 800$$

Example calculation: Is a spectrograph with a resolution of 800 capable of resolving the 4731- and 4739-Å lines of selenium?

$$R = \frac{\lambda}{\Delta\lambda} = \frac{4735}{4739 - 4731} = 592$$

Since the R of the instrument is 800, it is quite capable of resolving these two lines. A high-resolution grating will have from 50,000 to 70,000 lines per inch.

Detectors

The two major types of detectors are (1) photographic plates or film and (2) phototubes. An instrument that uses photographic detection is called a spectrograph, while an instrument that uses a phototube is called a spectrophotometer.

Photographic Plates. Photographic plates are usually used for research applications or for the analysis of nonroutine samples; 4-in. × 10-in. plates are common or 35-mm film is used. Figure 52 is a photo of spectra on 35-mm photographic film. The type of emulsion to specify is spectrum analysis no. 1.

Phototubes. If repetitive analyses of similar samples are to be done, such as a large number of Al or steel alloys, then the phototube is preferred.

For example, suppose an Al sample is to be examined. It consists primarily of Al with a dozen or so other elements in trace amounts, but the concentration of each one is critical to the properties of the alloy. Suppose you obtained a photographic film of the spectra of the Al and each of

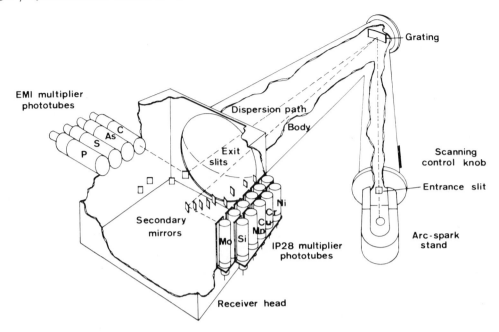

FIG. 61. A quantometer: the Quantovac. (Courtesy of Applied Research Labs, Glendale, California.)

the elements suspected. Then you made a metal plate the same size and after locating an intense line for each element, cut a slot in the plate at that place for each element, then placed a phototube behind each slot as in Fig. 61. Since Al is always present and in large concentrations, use it for an internal standard. Make the alloy sample the anode and a carbon rod the cathode. Start the spark and collect the emitted radiation on each phototube. Suppose that you set it so that when the phototube detecting Al reaches 1000 arbitrary units the instrument automatically shuts off. Now suppose Cu read 5 units, which from a previously obtained calibration curve you determine equals 0.05% Cu. Each element can be done in this same manner at the same time. Such an instrument is called a quantometer. By applying a vacuum of about 15 torr and flushing the arc-spark stand with Ar to remove the absorption due to O_2 below 1900 Å, the elements P, S, As, C, Hg, and Si can also be determined.

The instrument shown in Fig. 61 can determine 15 elements in a steel sample in 2 min within 3-5%.

Mountings

Prism Mountings. There are many different ways to arrange the components of an emission spectrograph and these arrangements are called mountings.

Figures 62 and 63 show the two most common prism mountings, the <u>Cornu</u> and the <u>Littrow</u>. Prism mountings suffer from being nonlinear in dispersion.

The Cornu mounting is usually used for qualitative work since the range from 2100 Å to 7000 Å is covered on one 10-in. plate.

The Littrow mounting requires only one lens, one piece of quartz, and takes up half the space for the equivalent resolution of the Cornu mounting. The large Littrow covers the range 2000 to 8000 Å on three 10-in. plates.

<u>Grating Mountings</u>. Figures 64 and 65 show some of the grating mountings, the <u>Wadsworth</u> and <u>Czerny-Turner</u>. Both have linear dispersion and are <u>stigmatic</u>. Stigmatic means that both the horizontal and vertical components of the spectral line are in focus in the same place. Older models of grating spectrographs using curved gratings had astigmatism in that the line was not in focus from top to bottom but was from side to side. Since line widths are narrow, being in focus from top to bottom is of more importance for quantitative work. As a result, corrections had to be made when using astigmatic systems.

Each element has its own pattern of lines, a few of which are shown in Fig. 66. (Impurity lines are marked.) By comparing the position of the lines in the unknown with known spectra, the elements present can be identi-

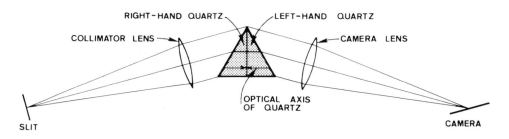

FIG. 62. Schematic diagram of a Cornu mounting.

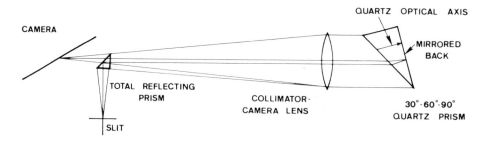

FIG. 63. Schematic diagram of a Littrow mounting.

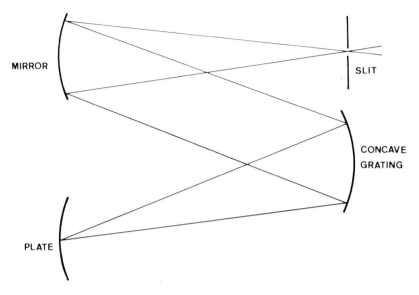

FIG. 64. Schematic diagram of the Wadsworth mounting.

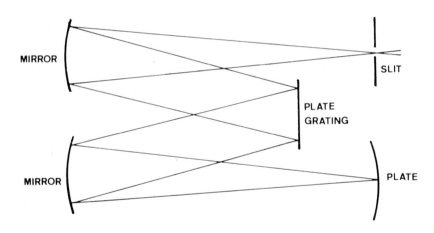

FIG. 65. Schematic diagram of the Czerny-Turner mounting.

fied. A general rule of thumb is that at least three lines must match before
a positive identification can be made.

To facilitate this comparison a powder has been prepared containing 50
elements, each in sufficient concentration so that only about 7 lines of
each element appear. This is done to simplify the spectra as well as the
identification. This powder is called "Raies Ultimes" or RU powder. A
portion of such a spectrum is shown in Fig. 67. Iron has lines that cover

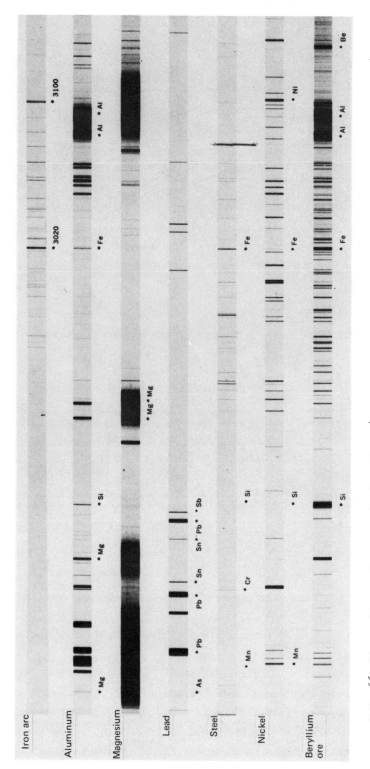

FIG. 66. Line patterns for several elements. (Courtesy of Jarrell-Ash Co., Newtonville, Massachusetts.)

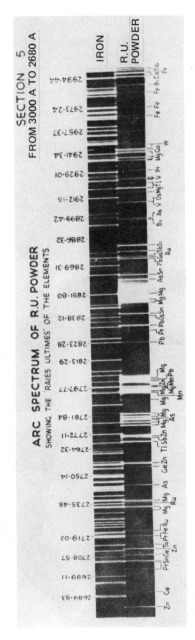

FIG. 67. Arc spectrum of RU powder from 2680 to 3000 Å. (Courtesy of Jarrell-Ash Co., Newton-ville, Mass.) (Prepared by Research Laboratories, The General Electric Co. Ltd., Wembley, England; published by Hilger & Watts Ltd., Hilger Division, London NW.)

the entire region observed and is used as a reference spectrum to locate the lines of other elements.

The 50 elements are Li, Na, Rb, K, Cs, Cu, Ag, Au, Be, Mg, Ca, Sr, Ba, Zn, Cd, Hg, B, Sc, Y, La, Al, In, Tl, C, Si, Ge, Sn, Pb, Ti, Zr, P, As, Sb, V, Nb, Ta, Cr, Mo, W, Mn, Fe, Co, Ni, Ru, Rh, Pd, Os, Ir, Pt, and Bi.

Quantitative Analysis

The intensity of the lines as they appear on a photographic plate is proportional to the concentration over narrow concentration ranges. The exact details of relating the exposure to concentration and this in turn to blackness are beyond this presentation. However, in general, the blackness of the lines is proportional to the concentration, and this blackness is measured with an instrument called a <u>densitometer</u>. A densitometer is essentially a very good UV spectrophotometer tilted 90 deg. One of the most recent designs is shown in Figs. 68 and 69.

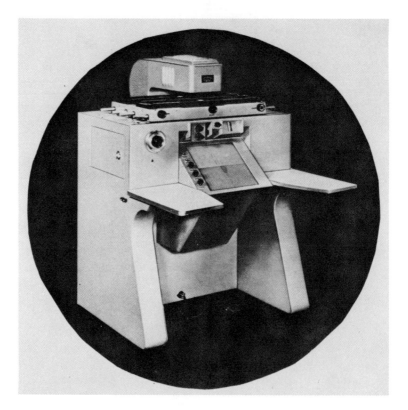

FIG. 68. A photograph of the JAco comparator microphotometer. (Courtesy of Jarrell-Ash Co., Newtonville, Mass.)

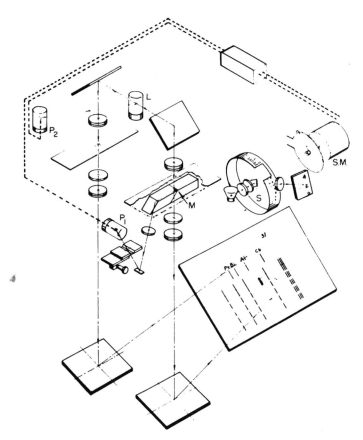

FIG. 69. The optical arrangement of the JAco microphotometer. (Courtesy of Jarrell-Ash Co., Newtonville, Mass.)

Comparison of Techniques

Table 12 compares the detection limits for several different spectroscopic techniques. Attempts were made to put them on a common basis. However, these data represent the best that can be obtained under ideal conditions.

TABLE 12. Comparison of Experimentally Determined Detection Limits in μg/ml or ppm[a]

Element	High-Frequency Plasma (μg/ml)	Atomic Absorption	Atomic Fluorescence	Flame Emission
Ag	0.004	0.005	0.0001	0.008
Al	0.002	0.03	0.005	0.005

TABLE 12 (Continued)

Element	High-Frequency Plasma (μg/ml)	Atomic Absorption	Atomic Fluorescence	Flame Emission
As	0.04	0.1	0.1	50
Au	0.04	0.02	0.05	4
B	0.005	6	--	30
Ba	0.0001	0.05	--	0.002
Be	0.0005	0.002	0.01	0.1
Bi	0.05	0.05	0.05	2
Ca	0.00007	0.001	0.000001	0.0001
Cd	0.002	0.001	0.00001	0.8
Ce	0.007	--	0.5	10
Co	0.003	0.005	0.005	0.03
Cr	0.001	0.003	0.004	0.004
Cu	0.001	0.002	0.001	0.01
Dy	0.004	0.2	0.3	0.05
Er	0.001	0.1	0.5	0.04
Eu	0.001	0.04	0.02	0.0005
Fe	0.005	0.005	0.008	0.03
Ga	0.014	0.07	0.01	0.01
Gd	0.007	4	0.08	2
Ge	0.15	1	20	0.5
Hf	0.01	8	100	20
Hg	0.2	0.5	0.02	40
Ho	0.01	0.1	0.1	0.02
In	0.03	0.05	0.002	0.003
La	0.003	2	--	2
Lu	0.008	3	3	0.2
Mg	0.0007	0.0001	0.001	0.005
Mn	0.0007	0.002	0.002	0.005
Mo	0.005	0.03	0.06	0.1
Na	0.002	0.002	--	0.0001
Nb	0.01	1	1	0.06
Nd	0.05	2	2	0.2
Ni	0.006	0.005	0.003	0.02
P	0.04	--	--	--
Pb	0.008	0.01	0.01	0.1
Pd	0.007	0.03	--	0.05

TABLE 12 (Continued)

Element	High-Frequency Plasma (µg/ml)	Atomic Absorption	Atomic Fluorescence	Flame Emission
Pr	0.06	10	1	0.07
Pt	0.08	0.1	--	2
Rh	0.003	0.03	0.1	0.02
Sb	0.2	0.1	0.05	0.6
Sc	0.003	0.1	0.01	0.01
Se	0.03	0.1	0.04	100
Sm	0.02	2	0.1	0.1
Si	0.01	0.1	--	5
Sn	0.3	0.02	0.05	0.3
Sr	0.00002	0.01	0.01	0.0002
Ta	0.07	5	--	20
Tb	0.2	2	0.5	0.03
Te	0.08	0.1	0.05	200
Th	0.003	--	--	200
Ti	0.003	0.09	0.1	0.2
Tl	0.2	0.03	0.008	0.02
Tm	0.007	0.2	0.1	0.02
U	0.03	--	--	10
V	0.006	0.02	0.07	0.01
W	0.002	3	--	0.5
Y	0.0002	0.1	--	0.04
Yb	0.0009	0.04	0.01	0.002
Zn	0.002	0.002	0.00002	50
Zr	0.005	5	--	10

[a]From Ref. 20.

A Typical Analysis

The typical analysis will be to determine the trace elements in a sample of horse blood using the plasma source. This procedure is reported in detail in Ref. 21. Notice that only 25 µl of sample is necessary. Table 13 shows the experimental facilities and operating conditions.

Figure 70 shows a schematic diagram of the microliter-sample handling system. A short piece of gum rubber or Tygon tubing (1.18 mm i.d.) is attached to the polyethylene sample uptake tubing (0.77 mm i.d. x 1.23 mm o.d.)

TABLE 13. Experimental Facilities and Operating Conditions

Nebulizer	Pneumatic type described by Kniseley et al. [21].
Plasma power supply	Lepel High-Frequency Laboratories Model t-2.5-1-MC2-J-B generator, with attached tuning and coupling unit, 2.5 kW, frequency set to ~30 MHz. The load coil was two turns of 5-mm o.d. copper tubing, i.d. of coil was 27 mm.
Gas flows	Argon used throughout with 10 liters/min through the coolant tube and 1.1 liters/min through the aerosol tube. No "plasma gas" flow was used. Gas flow system described by Kniseley et al. [21].
Spectrometer	Hilger-Engis Model 1000, 1-m Czerny-Turner mounting scanning spectrometer, with grating (1200 rulings/mm) blazed for 500.0 nm. Reciprocal linear dispersion of 8 nm/mm in first order.
Slits and order	Both entrance and exit slits were 25 μm wide, 4 mm long, and straight-edged. First-order spectra were used throughout.
Detector electronics	The photocurrent from an EMI 6225B phototube was amplified with a Keithley Model 410 picoammeter and recorded with a Leeds and Northrup Speedomax recorder. Time constant was ~3 sec.
Average sample nebulization rate	3.3 ml/min

from the pneumatic nebulizer (Fig. 57). A simple pressure or pinch clamp is placed around the length of larger tubing to control the sample flow.

1. The sample uptake tube is filled with blank solution by opening the clamp and allowing normal nebulizing action.

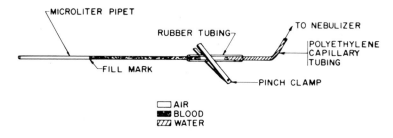

FIG. 70. Microliter sample injection system [21].

2. The flow is stopped by closing the clamp, and a small air bubble is then
   introduced by removing the tubing from the solution and momentarily opening the clamp.

3. The microliter pipet containing the sample is inserted into the open end
   of the rubber tubing with the extra volume end (above the calibration
   mark) open to the atmosphere; in this way an air bubble is left in the
   extra volume end.

4. The end of the pipet is then placed in a beaker containing the blank
   solution and the clamp is opened to allow nebulization to proceed.

   In this procedure, the air bubbles separate the sample solution from
the blank solution, causing the sample aerosol to travel through the plasma
as a separate cloud.

   Glass disposable microsampling pipets (Corning No. 7099-S, 25 µl) were
used for sampling. Table 14 shows the results obtained.

   Costs

   The costs of emission spectrographs vary considerably. It is possible
to get a small student-type apparatus for detecting about a dozen elements
for about $1500. The next step up, using film is about $4000. From there
on it depends on all of the combinations desired, but an excellent photographic plate detector spectrograph with densitometer can be obtained for
about $45,000 to $50,000. If phototube detectors and a computer readout
device are desired for multiple element analysis, then the cost becomes
more like $70,000 to $80,000.

TABLE 14. Typical Analytical Results Obtained from 25-µl Aliquots of Horse
Blood and Serum

Element	Found (mg/l)	Normal (mg/l)
Al	0.20	0.2
Ca	110	101
Cu	1.4	0.7-1.6
Fe	450	420-280
Mg	20	21
Mn	0.070	0.04

NEUTRON ACTIVATION ANALYSIS

Neutron activation analysis is a technique in which nonradioactive elements are made radioactive by the interaction of their nuclei with highly energetic charged particles (protons, deuterons, alpha particles) by neutrons or by energetic photons. When the radioactive atoms decay, their decay products, alpha particles, beta particles, or gamma rays are detected. The amount of the element present is proportional to the intensity of the emission. For example, suppose you wanted to determine traces of arsenic in cigarette paper. A neutron from a source strikes an atom of ^{75}As to produce ^{76}As and a gamma ray. The gamma ray is then detected.

$$^{75}_{33}As + ^{1}_{0}n \rightarrow ^{76}_{33}As + ^{0}_{0}\nu \tag{27}$$

Table 15 shows the general regions of the detection limits for several of the elements. As you will see later, these can vary considerably.

TABLE 15. Detection Limits for Activation Analysis

Detection Sensitivity (g)	Element	Detection Sensitivity (g)	Element
10^{-11}	Europium	10^{-9}	Praseodymium
	Dysprosium		Vanadium
10^{-10}			Ytterbium
	Manganese	10^{-8}	
	Indium		Aluminum
	Samarium		Cobalt
	Holmium		Chlorine
	Lutetium		Zinc
	Rhenium		Potassium
	Iridium		Phosphorus
10^{-9}			Germanium
	Arsenic		Selenium
	Bromine		Barium
	Iodine		Cesium
	Gold		Cadmium
	Uranium		Erbium
	Tungsten		Gadolinium
	Tantalum		Hafnium
	Terbium		Osmium
	Copper		Rubidium
	Gallium		Yttrium
	Sodium		Thorium
	Scandium	10^{-7}	
	Lanthanum		Cerium
	Palladium		Chromium
	Antimony		Mercury
	Thulium		Platinum

TABLE 15 (Continued)

Detection Sensitivity (g)	Element	Detection Sensitivity (g)	Element
10^{-7}	Thallium Silver Tin Tellurium Molybdenum Neodymium Strontium Ruthenium Zirconium	10^{-6}	Magnesium Sulfur Iron Titanium Nickel Calcium Niobium Silicon Bismuth

The Units of Measurement

The units of measurement for radioactive decay are shown in Table 16. The unit may be modified as micro (μ), milli (m), or mega (M), e.g., micro-curie (μCi).

Characteristics of the Different Radiations

Radioactivity is a general term applied to the emission of high-energy particles and electromagnetic radiation emanating from the unstable and excited nuclei of atoms. The following are brief descriptions of those radiations of most concern in this chapter.

Alpha particles are helium nuclei (2 protons and 2 neutrons) moving at high speeds. They are doubly positive charged and have an energy range of about 5 to 9 MeV. All alpha particles from a given isotope have the same energy and nearly identical penetration ranges.

Beta particles are distinguishable from simple electrons only by the fact that they originate in the nucleus and are usually moving at great

TABLE 16. Units of Radioactivity Measurement

Name	Symbol	Magnitude
Curie	Ci	3.7×10^{10} disintegrations/sec
Rutherford	rd	1.0×10^{6} disintegrations/sec
Roentgen	r	1.6×10^{12} ion pairs/g of air
Specific activity		Disintegrations/g/sec

speed. They are negatively charged and have typical energies of from 0 to 4 MeV.

Gamma rays originate in the nucleus which has been left in an excited state because of some previous disintegration or interaction. The fact that gamma rays have discrete energies is evidence that the nucleus exists in various energy levels. Later on you will see how advantage is taken of this fact to identify the different elements present.

Neutrons are neutral particles having energy ranges of from 0 to 10 KeV.

Basic Components

Figure 71 shows the basic components required for activation analysis. A source is used to activate the sample. If the sample's half-life is short, then the sample is transferred to the detector by a pneumatic tube in just a few seconds. The radiation desired is detected, amplified, and then transferred to some sort of readout device. This may be as simple as reading the meter needle on a Geiger-Muller counter, or it may involve separating the energies from the various transitions and either visually observing them on an oscilloscope or plotting them out for computer analysis.

The production of radioactive atoms is complicated by the fact that they decay continuously. It is like trying to fill a bucket with water if there is a hole in the bucket. If there is a small hole in the bucket and you have a fast means of adding water, then you can fill the bucket; otherwise, you seem to wage a losing battle. The same effect occurs with activation analysis. If the desired element decays slowly, then it requires only a low-level source to make a sample sufficiently radioactive for analysis; however, if the element decays rapidly, then a high-level (and usually correspondingly expensive) source must be available.

Sources. There are four general types of neutron sources which are being used for neutron activation analysis:

1. Nuclear reactors, like a Triga reactor, which produces thermal neutron fluxes of 10^{11} to 10^{15} neutrons/cm^2/sec.

2. Neutron generators, like the Van de Graaff and Cockcroft-Walton generators, having thermal fluxes of 10^8 to 10^{13} neutrons/cm^2/sec.

3. Isotopic sources, like a polonium-beryllium powder, in which neutrons are generated from the target by bombardment by alpha particles from the source. These have thermal fluxes of 10^4 to 10^9 neutrons/cm^2/sec.

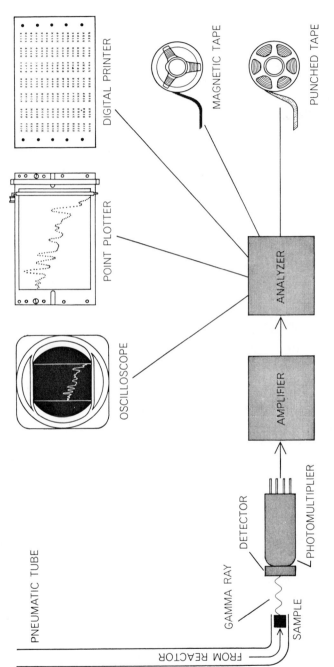

FIG. 71. Schematic diagram of the components necessary for neutron activation analysis [22].

4. A direct neutron source, like californium-252, which emits neutrons directly. Its thermal flux is 10^7 neutrons/cm^2/sec.

The neutrons generated by these sources are far too energetic to interact efficiently with target nuclei to produce gamma rays which can be detected. Remember, you are not trying to split a nucleus but merely trying to raise it to an excited state. Therefore the neutrons must be slowed down or moderated. Hydrogen is the best moderator, but water, heavy water, beryllium, or graphite (all light atomic number elements) can be used. A neutron that has been slowed sufficiently is called a thermal neutron, and at 20°C this means it has an energy of 0.025 eV and is traveling about 2200 m/sec. This requires about 5.7 cm of H_2O, 11.0 cm of D_2O, 9.9 in. of Be, or 18.7 in. of graphite.

Nuclear reactors: Nuclear reactors are major installations costing hundreds of thousands of dollars. They use ^{235}U most commonly. A general equation for the production of neutrons in such a reactor is

$$^{235}_{92}U + {}^1_0n(\text{thermal}) \rightarrow X + Y + \nu{}^1_0n \tag{28}$$

ν is 2.5 for ^{235}U and 2.9 for ^{239}Pu. These neutrons have an energy range of from about 0.1 to 20 MeV and there can be as many as 10^{15} thermal neutrons produced per cm^2 per second. This number of neutrons is necessary if ppb analyses are desired. Because of the high cost of the facility, less expensive methods for the production of neutrons are desired and several are available that produce enough thermal neutrons to permit ppm analyses to be made. Figure 72 is a diagram of a nuclear reactor.

Neutron generators: Neutron generators produce neutrons by accelerating a beam of particles, usually deuterons, to about 500 keV energy and allowing them to strike a target (deuterium or tritium). The target then releases neutrons which are used to bombard the sample. There are many types of neutron generators such as the Cockcroft-Walton, Van de Graaff, cyclotron, linear accelerators, betatron, syncrotron, etc. We will limit this discussion primarily to the Cockcroft-Walton and the Van de Graaff types. Their main difference is how they produce the original ions to be accelerated. The Cockcroft-Walton instrument uses a highly charged transformer (up to 800,000 V), while the Van de Graaff generator uses a moving belt to generate high voltages. This can be easily demonstrated in most parts of the country by walking on a wool or nylon carpet during times of low humidity and then touching someone to give him a shock. A jump of the spark of 1/4 in., which is not unusual, is about 6000 V. Van de Graaff

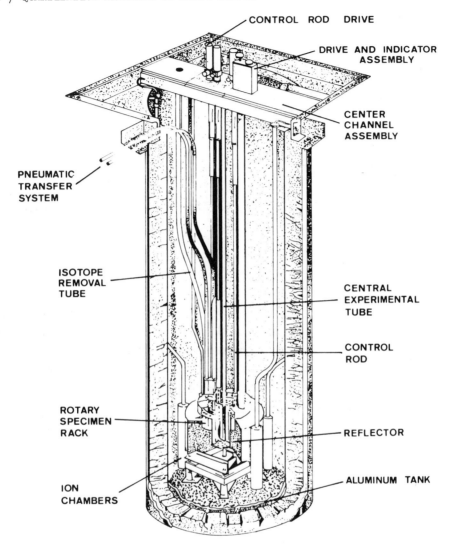

FIG. 72. Cross section of a Triga Mark I reactor. (Courtesy of Kansas State University, Department of Nuclear Engineering.)

generators can build up potentials of over a million volts. Figure 73 is a diagram of the basic idea of the neutron generator.

The neutron generator is maintained at a low pressure and deuterium gas is admitted at a controlled rate into the ion source where it is ionized. The ions produced are directed, by the application of a suitable electric field, into the accelerating section, where they are accelerated up to an energy equivalent to the potential drop across the accelerating

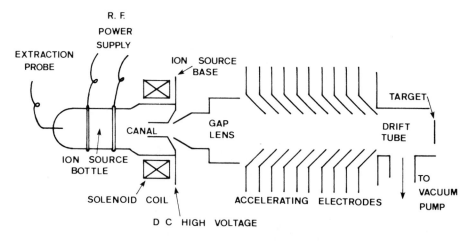

FIG. 73. Schematic of a pumped neutron generator [23].

section for singly charged ions. After passage through a potential free
section, called the <u>drift tube</u>, the accelerated ions strike a suitable target, resulting in the generation of high-energy neutrons. Deuterium atoms
are preferred particles because it requires only 2 MeV for them to split
into a neutron and a proton, a process which produces 16 MeV of energy,
leaving a net of 14 MeV. Alpha particles on the other hand, while they have
2 neutrons, require 28 MeV to split yet produce only 32 MeV, leaving a net
of 4 MeV. Four such systems employed in the Van de Graaff or Cockcroft-
Walton generators are shown in Eqs. (29)-(32) (^{2}H = deuterium, D, and ^{3}H =
tritium, T).

$$^2H + D_2O \text{ (ice)} = {}^3He + {}^1n \tag{29}$$

$$^2H + T_2O \text{ (ice)} = {}^4He + {}^1n \tag{30}$$

$$^2H + {}^7Li = {}^8Be + {}^1n \tag{31}$$

$$^2H + {}^9Be = {}^{10}B + {}^1n \tag{32}$$

The cost of an average system would be about $25,000 for the generator
plus an additional $15,000 for the multichannel analyzer and the detector.

<u>Isotopic neutron sources</u>: In this case a radioactive isotope that re-
leases alpha particles is placed next to a target element. When the target
is bombarded with these alpha particles the target emits neutrons which are
then used to bombard and activate the sample.

Several of the most commonly used alpha particle emitting isotopes are
^{210}Po, ^{214}Am, ^{222}Ac, ^{226}Ra, ^{228}Th, and ^{239}Pu. The alpha particles emitted

from these sources have energies of 4-6 MeV and as a result only light elements are capable of interacting. Beryllium is a common target with B, Li
and F also being used but producing lower neutron yields. For example, Po
is encapsulated together with Be powder and the following reactions take
place:

$$^{210}Po \to \alpha \tag{33}$$

$$\alpha + {}^{9}Be \to {}^{12}C + {}^{1}_{0}n \ (4 \ MeV) \tag{34}$$

Table 17 shows a few other systems and the fluxes they can produce.

These are obviously low-level sources and are not good for trace analysis. However they are quite good when you have large amounts of sample
because they are relatively inexpensive and require considerably less in
the way of shielding and other safety precautions.

Direct neutron source: A direct neutron source is an isotope that
produces neutrons without going through an intermediate step such as bombarding a target. Californium-252 has been found to be an excellent direct
neutron source. It is an intense neutron emitter. It produces 2.3×10^9
n/sec/mg, yet it decays slowly enough for practical use, having a half-life
of 2.65 years. Moreover, the energy distribution of ^{252}Cf neutrons is
essentially below the threshold energies of a number of reactions that cause
interferences and are present when reactors or neutron generators are used.
The energy range is from about 0.1 to 6.1 MeV, and the material is easy to
work with to build sources since 1 mg generates only 0.04 W of heat.

The usual amount sold or rented is 100 µCi at \$10.00/µg. There is a
\$1250 charge for shipping or for encapsulating it if you desire.

According to Dr. G. T. Seaborg, former chairman of the Atomic Energy
Commission (AEC), "^{252}Cf has two characteristics that make it especially

TABLE 17. Isotopic Neutron Sources

Alpha Emitter	Half-life	Target	Neutron Flux $(n/cm^2/sec)$
Ac-222	22 y	Be	1.5×10^7
Po-210	138 d	Be	2.5×10^6
		B	5×10^5
		Li	4×10^4

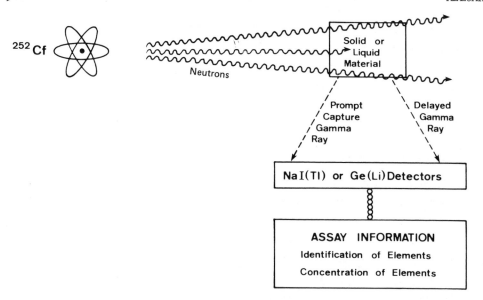

FIG. 74. Neutron activation analysis with ^{252}Cf [24].

valuable. It lasts a long time compared with other isotopes, therefore it can be shipped and still have activity left. Second, the isotope emits a prodigious quantity of neutrons. A tiny quantity of Cf, just a curie of it weighing 2 mg, emits almost as many neutrons/cm^2 as a reactor. It is for this reason that ^{252}Cf has been called a hip-pocket reactor."

Figure 74 illustrates neutron activation analysis with ^{252}Cf.

Detectors. When a sample atom is irradiated by neutrons from one of the sources just discussed and itself becomes radioactive, it may decay by several pathways, producing a number of particles and/or rays. Gamma rays are of the most interest for analytical work because each element has a gamma ray spectrum just like each organic compound has an infrared spectrum. We usually have several different elements present in our samples, so we not only need a means of detecting the emitted radiation but we need some means of determining from which element it came. This section explains just two of the many methods currently used to detect gamma rays. The next section on analyzers will explain how the gamma ray spectrum is obtained.

The two types of detectors discussed are the crystal scintillation counter of which the NaI(Tl) crystal will serve as the example, and the semiconductor detector, with the Ge(Li) serving as the example. (Note: The Ge(Li) detector is often referred to as a "jelly" detector and the Si(Li) detector as a "silly" detector.)

The scintillation counter is more efficient and is easier to maintain than the semiconductor detectors, but the semiconductor detectors have about a 10-fold better resolution, as can be seen in Fig. 82.

Crystal scintillation counters: The basic principle behind the operation of the scintillation counter is that an energetic particle incident upon a luminescent material (a phosphor) excites the material; the photons which are created in the process of de-excitation are collected at the photocathode of the photomultiplier tube where the photons cause the ejection of electrons. The electrons ejected from the photocathode are then caused to impinge upon other electrodes, each approximately 100 V higher in potential. There are about 10 of these electrodes, called dynodes, in the photomultiplier tube. In the acceleration from dynode to dynode, more electrons are formed (ejected), and therefore a large amplification may be obtained so that a measurable pulse is observed at the output.

It would be expected that the greater the energy of the incident particle, the greater the number of electrons which would be produced. This indicates that the scintillation counter could be used to obtain the energy of the particle. In the scintillation counter, advantage is not taken of the proportional properties; however, the scintillation spectrometer, which will be discussed later, uses these proportional characteristics of the scintillation process to good advantage.

Figure 75 shows a diagram of one type of crystal scintillation counter.

NaI(Tl) detectors are available in sizes from very small to very large; the most common crystal size is 3 in. in diameter by 3 in. high. Well detectors are also available, i.e., with a hole or cavity in the center of the crystal into which a sample can be placed. The well detector configuration increases the counting efficiency.

The two spectrometric characteristics of major interest with NaI(Tl) detectors are counting efficiency and energy resolution. Counting efficiency is the fraction of the gamma rays of interest counted by the detectors as compared to the total number of gamma rays emitted by the sample. High-efficiency detection systems are especially useful for ^{252}Cf applications where large or high-activity samples may not be available. The absolute counting efficiency for gamma rays from a ^{252}Cf point source located 1 cm away from a 3-in. x 3-in. NaI(Tl) detector ranges from ~35% at 100-keV gamma ray energy to ~15% at 2 MeV.

The resolution of an NaI(Tl) detector is generally specified as "full width at half maximum" (FWHM) and is measured in percent. FWHM is the width

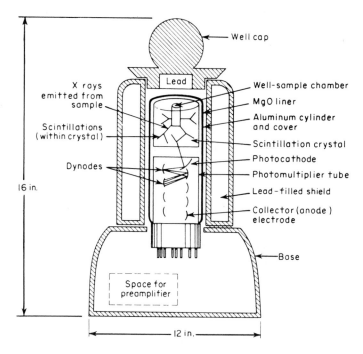

FIG. 75. Crystal scintillation counter [25].

of the observed gamma ray peak at one-half of its maximum height. The resolution of a good 3-in. x 3-in. detector will be 7 to 8% at 663 keV.

NaI(Tl) detectors are available integrally mounted to a photomultiplier tube and hermetically sealed in a light-tight, moisture-proof container. Such a detector is a fairly rugged device suitable for field use; in the 3-in. x 3-in. size, the detector sells for about $1000.

Semiconductor detectors: Germanium, a semiconducting material, can be made sensitive to gamma radiation by placing small amounts of an impurity, such as lithium, into the germanium crystal structure. When a gamma ray interacts in the crystal, an electrical charge is produced. The charge is collected and amplified to produce a voltage pulse whose height is proportional to the amount of energy deposited in the crystal by the gamma ray.

A single crystal of semiconductor material such as Si or Ge will not make a suitable counter because of the dc current in the crystal. Random variations of this current may produce pulses similar to the radiation-induced pulses. To reduce this current a p-n junction in reverse bias is used (see Fig. 76).

In thermal equilibrium, the conduction electrons contributed by the donor atoms (the impurity atoms in an n-type semiconductor) predominate in the n region. Here the conduction electrons neutralize the space charge of the donor atoms. Similarly, the holes contributed by the acceptor atoms (the impurity atoms in the p-type semiconductor) neutralize the space charge of the acceptor atoms in the p region. In addition, at the junction between the two regions, diffusion allows electrons to move into the p region and holes into the n region. In this process the electrons leave behind positively charged donor ions and the holes leave negatively charged acceptor ions. These ions are fixed and form a double layer. The electric field of the double layer essentially prevents further diffusion across the junction. In reverse bias, the holes accumulate closer to the negative electrode and the electrons to the positive electrode. The region in the middle is practically free of charge and is, therefore, called the <u>depletion region</u>. Because of the concentration of the charges close to the electrodes, the potential drop is essentially confined to the depletion region. Consequently, if radiation enters the depletion space, electron-hole pairs, which are

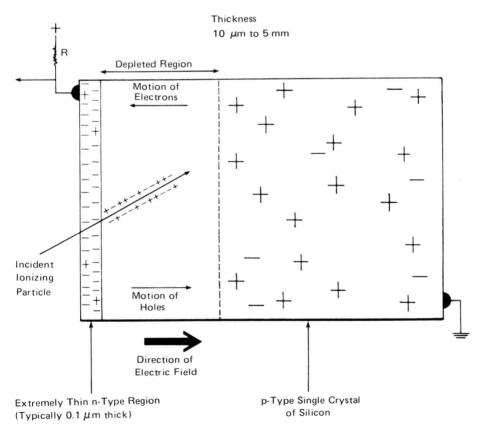

FIG. 76. Schematic diagram of a p-n junction counter [26].

subjected to practically no potential difference, will rarely be collected
at the electrodes. Therefore, the sensitive area of the counter is the depletion region. The ultimate maximum in width depends upon the effective
purity of the material and upon the breakdown voltage of the junction. For
example, a p-type silicon base material of 10,000 ohm-cm resistivity has
about 4×10^{12} acceptors/cm^3. At a reverse bias of 500 V, a width of 0.7
mm results.

Reverse biased p-n or n-p junctions are used as nuclear detectors.
The schematic diagram of such a detector is shown in Fig. 76. The n layer
is made extremely thin, typically 0.1 μm, so that the energy loss in this
layer is very small. Most detectors currently in use are of three different
types, and they are discussed below.

Diffused junction detector: This type is often produced by diffusing
a high concentration of donor impurities into a p-type material. Silicon
is usually used as the base material. Single crystals of high resistance
are sliced into 1-mm pieces. Then phosphorus is diffused into one surface
of these slices. A common method is to coat one side with phosphorus pentoxide dissolved in glycol and to heat the slice at 800° C in dry nitrogen
for 1/2 hr. The phosphorus diffuses into the base material while the glycol
leaves the base material covered with a black residual deposit. After diffusion, proper electric connections are made to the p and n sides. A typical counter arrangement is shown in Fig. 77.

Special care is taken to reduce deterioration of the crystal and to
minimize surface current, as distinct from volume current produced by
electron-hole pairs. The metal container is filled with nitrogen or sometimes maintained under vacuum. Diffusion counters have also been prepared
by diffusing acceptors, such as boron and gallium, into n-type silicon
crystals.

Barrier layer detectors: If n-type silicon is exposed to air, the
surface layer oxidizes. The oxidized layer has the characteristics of a
p layer. Since the layer is very thin, the junction is very close to the
surface. Hence energy losses by the radiation outside the active volume
is minimal. Since the oxidized layer is not conducting, a thin gold coating
of about 40 μg/cm^2 is applied to the surface, and electric connection is
made to this layer. Connection to the back side is made through a nonrec-
tifying metal contact. Surface barrier Si detectors can be operated at
room temperature.

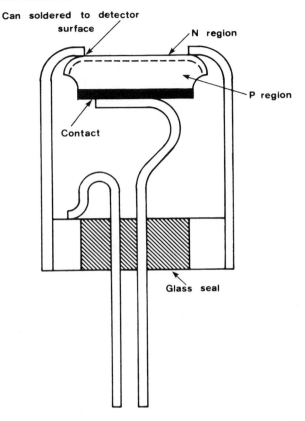

FIG. 77. Encapsulated diffused junction detector [26].

Lithium-drifted detectors: Lithium is a donor atom. It does not go
into substitutional sites as do other donor atoms such as phosphorus. Instead, it enters interstitial sites. The diffusion coefficient is about
10^7 higher than that for phosphorus and therefore, deep diffused junctions
can be prepared. Diffusion is usually achieved in two steps. First, lithium
is coated on single crystals and diffused into them by heating. In the second step the sample is heated and strong reverse bias is applied. This
helps the lithium atoms to diffuse deeper into the crystal. There are three
regions: the p region, the n region, and an intrinsic region. The last
region results from the compensation or neutralization of the p-type impurities by the lithium atoms. The intrinsic region constitutes the active
volume of the detector. This type of drifted detector is also known as an
n-i-p device. Lithium drift devices can be prepared in both germanium and
silicon crystals.

Some spectrometric characteristics of major interest with Ge(Li) detectors are counting efficiency and energy resolution. The counting efficiency of a Ge(Li) detector depends principally on its active volume. Detectors are available with active volumes as large as 100 cm^3. Efficiency is generally specified by comparing the counting efficiency of the Ge(Li) detector to that of a 3-in. x 3-in. NaI(Tl) detector. Detectors with efficiencies as high as 15% at 1.33 MeV [as compared to a 3-in. x 3-in. NaI(Tl) detector with a source-to-detector distance of 25 cm] are now available.

The resolution of Ge(Li) detectors is specified as keV FWHM. A typical high-efficiency detector may have a resolution of a 2- to 3-keV FWHM at 1.33 MeV; this resolution is a factor of 10 to 15 times better than that obtained with an NaI(Tl) detector.

Germanium(lithium) semiconducting detectors must be stored and operated at low temperatures, usually liquid nitrogen temperature, because of the high mobility of the lithium ions in germanium at room temperature. This cooling requirement decreases the portability of Ge(Li) detectors. Nevertheless, Ge(Li) detectors have been used in rugged environments and for field operation.

The cost of a Ge(Li) detector depends on the quality and use of the detector. A high-resolution, low-energy photon detector may cost $4000 to $8000. A high-efficiency (15%) detector may cost $15,000 to $20,000. Detectors with intermediate efficiency (5%) and good resolution (2.5 keV) may cost $5000 to $10,000.

Analyzers

Method of operation: Gamma ray spectrometry differs only in the addition of a differential pulse height analyzer to the gamma ray counter, enabling one to determine the number of pulses of any given energy as a function of that energy. Any pulse which is larger than the potential on the grid of the first tube will cause that tube to operate, and the pulse will be counted in the scintillation counter. In the scintillation spectrometer, a second discriminator is used to form a window. Thus, if the pulse is larger than the first grid potential, it will be counted, providing it is smaller than the second discriminator setting. This is illustrated in Fig. 78. If the pulse is not large enough or if it cuts both discriminators, it will be counted. In practice, it is fairly common to tie the two discriminators together, with the window, ΔE, set at some given value. Then the channel level may be varied through the energy region selected, as shown in Fig. 79. Note that ΔE is constant, but the channel is being varied. In

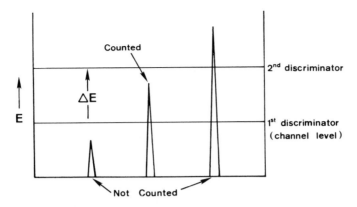

FIG. 78. Function of grid potential in scintillation spectrometry.

a multichannel analyzer several hundred channels operate at once rather than
moving one over a range.

When the channel level is at 1, three counts will be recorded; at 2,
two counts will be recorded; at 3, one count will be recorded; at 4, two
counts will be recorded; etc. Thus, one obtains the spectrum shown in Fig.
80.

Inspection and comparison will show how similar this is to the ultraviolet, visible, and infrared spectra. In absorption spectrophotometry, several
energy levels in the molecule will absorb radiation, each level being measured to obtain an absorption spectrum. Here, an atom is giving off several
energies, and we are examining each energy to see how much is present, obtaining a spectrum. Figure 81 shows the scintillation spectra of iodine-131
and iron-59 obtained by using a single-channel analyzer and a sodium iodide
(Tl) crystal. Actually, those data should be shown in the form of histo-
grams, but the simpler method of drawing a continuous curve has been followed. Only when the window becomes infinitely smaller would the solid
curved line be proper.

The peaks observed are due to the gamma energy (photopeak) or scattering
(Compton). Also, in some cases one can see annihilation radiation when an
x-ray is annihilated and an electron and positron are formed. This shows
up at a peak at 0.51 MeV. From the knowledge of gamma energies involved,
one can do much to construct an energy-level decay scheme for the radio-
nuclide being analyzed.

When counting a sample which may have two or more radioisotopes present,
one may count under one peak only to obtain the radiation from that particular isotope. For example, in Fig. 81, if the window is set to count from a

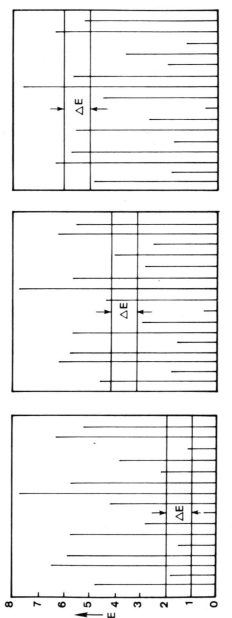

FIG. 79. The use of discriminators in obtaining differential spectra.

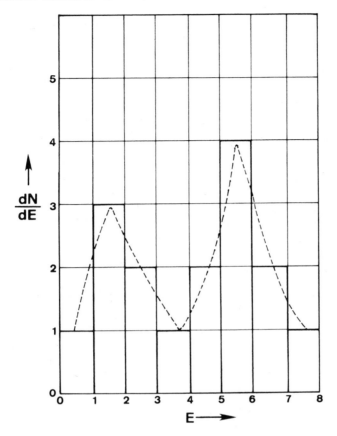

FIG. 80. Differential spectrum obtained from Fig. 79.

span of 0.14 MeV and the channel level is adjusted to 1.04 MeV, the 1.1-MeV
photopeak of iron-59 may be easily counted and no contribution from iodine-
131 will be made to the count rate.

Comparison of spectra: The spectra of a sample counted by both a 3-in.
x 3-in. NaI(Tl) detector and an intermediate-efficiency Ge(Li) detector are
shown in Fig. 82. Even though the Ge(Li) detector is much less efficient
than the NaI(Tl) detector, the higher resolution of the Ge(Li) detector
allows the gamma ray peaks from many elements to be observed and measured
quantitatively.

Detector costs: The costs of these detectors with some of their peripheral equipment are shown in Table 18.

Gamma ray spectroscopy components: Figure 83 is a schematic diagram
of the components necessary to operate a detection system for gamma rays
and qualitatively identifies the elements present. The block diagram in

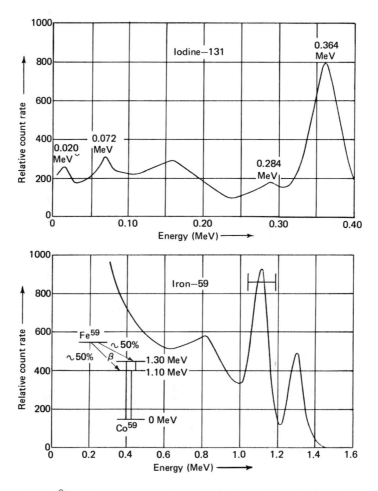

FIG. 81. The gamma spectra of iodine-131 and iron-59.

Fig. 83 shows the various parts of the scintillation apparatus. The crystal
(often thallium-activated sodium iodide) is mounted in an aluminum can and
is seated on the photomultiplier. A thin layer of silicone oil is often
used between the crystal and the photomultiplier tube to obtain more efficient light collection. High voltage is supplied to the tube from a very
stable power supply. The voltage is approximately 1000 V, allowing for a
differential of about 100 V between each of the dynodes. The pulses collected on the anode are then sent to the grid of the first tube in the preamplifier, usually a cathode follower. Then the pulses are passed on to
the linear amplifier, amplified, and passed on to the pulse-height analyzer.
A scaler will count the number of pulses and an oscilloscope will display
the gamma ray spectrum visually.

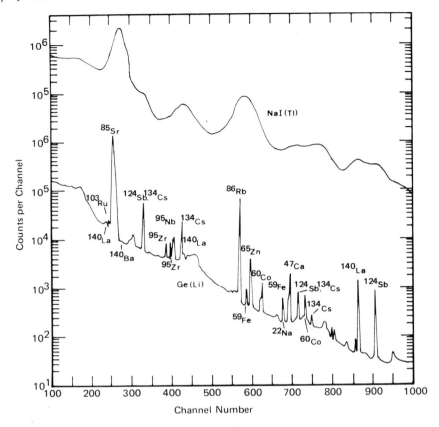

FIG. 82. Gamma ray spectra of neutron-activated sea water taken with NaI(Tl) and Ge(Li) detectors [27].

TABLE 18. Costs of Various Detector Systems[a]

Detector	Peripheral Equipment	Approximate Cost ($)
NaI(Tl)		1,000
NaI(Tl)	Amplifier-Discriminator-Counter	2,000
NaI(Tl)	Amplifier, Single Channel Analyzer, Counter	3,000
NaI(Tl)	Multichannel Pulse Height Analyzer	10,000
2NaI(Tl)	Multidimensional Pulse Height Analyzer	25,000
Ge(Li)		7,000
Ge(Li)	Amplifier, Single Channel Analyzer, Counter	9,000
Ge(Li)	Multichannel Pulse Height Analyzer	25,000
Ge(Li)	Compton Suppression System	40,000

[a]From Ref. 27.

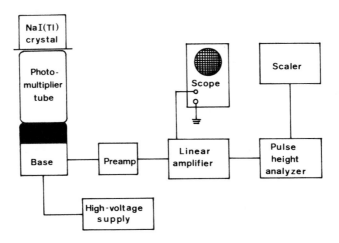

FIG. 83. Block diagram of a scintillation spectrometer.

Radioactive Decay

The radioactive decay obeys a statistical law identical with that encountered in monomolecular and first-order chemical kinetics and in optical
absorption phenomena. Such a law states that the rate of decay is proportional to the total number of radioactive atoms present. Often it is un-
necessary and even unrealistic to study the decay of specific numbers of
atoms because the atoms decay faster than the counting device can keep up.
Therefore we have two terms, the disintegration rate, which is the actual
number of atoms disintegrating, and the count rate, which is the number the
detector actually counts.

The equation commonly used to calculate the activity after the sample
has had a period in which to decay is

$$A = A_0 \exp\left(\frac{-0.693t}{t_{1/2}}\right) \tag{35}$$

where

t = time

$t_{1/2}$ = time for 1/2 of the radioactive atoms to decay

A_0 = initial count rate

A = count rate at time t

Example calculation: A sample of ^{92}Mo ($t_{1/2}$ = 10.1 d) used in a trace element feeding study was shipped with an original activity of 50 μCi. It arrived after a delay in shipment 9 days later. What is its current activity and what is this activity in disintegrations per minute?

$$A = 50 \exp(-0.693 \times \frac{9}{10.1})$$

$$= 50 \exp(-0.617)$$

$$= 50 \times 0.539$$

$$= 26.9 \text{ μCi}$$

Recall that

$$1 \text{ Ci} = 3.7 \times 10^{10} \text{ dps}$$

or

$$1 \text{ Ci} = 2.2 \times 10^{12} \text{ dpm}$$

and

$$1 \text{ μCi} = 2.2 \times 10^{6} \text{ dpm}$$

therefore

$$A = 26.9 \times 2.2 \times 10^{6} \text{ dpm}$$

$$= 5.04 \times 10^{7} \text{ dpm}$$

Production of Radioactive Atoms

The half-life of the radioisotope being produced in a nuclear transformation has a definite bearing on the total time over which one can efficiently produce transmutations. The rate of decay depends only upon the number of radioactive atoms present; as one produces transmutations, the rate of decay of the produced isotope will gradually increase. The number of radioactive atoms will stop increasing when their rate of decay is equal to their rate of production. For an irradiation time $t = t_{1/2}$, 50% saturation is reached; for $t = 2t_{1/2}$, 75% saturation; and for $t = 5t_{1/2}$, 97% saturation. Thus bombardment times greater than four or five half-lives of the radioisotopes being produced give little further increase in activity.

The general equation used to determine how many radioactive atoms you can produce is

$$\frac{-dN^*}{dt} = \Phi\sigma_{act}N_t[1 - \exp(\frac{-0.693t}{t_{1/2}})] \tag{36}$$

where

$-dN^*/dt$ = number of radioactive atoms produced/sec

N_t = number of target atoms

Φ = neutron flux on the target nuclei

σ_{act} = nuclear cross section for the activation (this is in barns,
     1 barn = 10^{-24} cm^2)

t = time since activation

$t_{1/2}$ = half-life of the decaying radioactive atoms

There are two extremes to this equation which are quite useful because they can simplify the equation.

Case 1: When $t \ggg t_{1/2}$,

$$\frac{-dN^*}{dt} = \Phi\sigma_{act}N_t t_{1/2} \tag{37}$$

Case 2: When $t_{1/2} \ggg t$,

$$\frac{-dN^*}{dt} = 0.693\Phi\sigma_{act}N_t t_{1/2} \tag{38}$$

Sensitivity Calculations

Whenever you consider using neutron activation analysis, you wonder if it will work on your sample. Few people have their own sources and detection equipment and must borrow them. Before you design a major research effort it would be wise to make a few calculations to see if you have a chance of success with the equipment you have available. The following example calculation is designed to show you the basic calculations you can make if you know some basic facts about your sample and about the nuclear equipment available.

Example calculations: It has been reported that about 4 µg of toxaphene (68% Cl) is required to kill an alfalfa weevil in the early fall or spring when its fat content is low. Suppose you want to verify this by activation analysis and perhaps extend this to other pesticides. Within a short driving distance there is a ^{252}Cf source with a flux of 5 x 10^8 neutrons/cm^2/sec and

they have a gamma ray detector with a 20% efficiency. From a handbook you
find that ^{37}Cl is possibly a good choice since it forms ^{38}Cl with a half-
life of 37 min plus a gamma ray. Chlorine-36 is not a good choice because
it has a half-life of 3×10^5 years, which would mean that you would have
to irradiate it for a very long time to produce a reasonable count rate.
Chlorine-37 occurs naturally as 24.6% of the isotope abundance. It has a
cross section of 0.56 barns. Let us assume that all of the Cl is from the
toxaphene and that with a 37-min half-life we can easily irradiate for 5
half-lives. Therefore,

$\Phi = 5 \times 10^8$ neutrons/cm^2/sec

$t = 5 \times 37$ min $= 185$ min

$t_{1/2} = 37$ min

$\sigma_{act} = 0.56 \times 10^{-24}$ cm^2

$$N_t = \frac{wt_{Cl} \times 6.02 \times 10^{23} \times \text{abundance}}{\text{atomic wt Cl}}$$

$$= \frac{4 \times 10^{-6} \text{ g} \times 0.68 \times 6.02 \times 10^{23} \text{ atoms/mole} \times 0.246}{35.45 \text{ g/mole}}$$

$$= 1.13 \times 10^{16} \text{ atoms}$$

$$\frac{-dN^*}{dt} = 5 \times 10^8 \times 0.56 \times 10^{-24} \times 1.13 \times 10^{16}[1 - \exp(-0.693 \times \frac{185}{37})]$$

$$= 31.6(1 - 0.03)$$

$$= 30.6 \text{ dis/sec/weevil, or } 1836 \text{ dis/min}$$

The counter was 20% efficient, which would give 367 counts/min. Background varies, but with good shielding a value of 10-20 counts/min is normal.
The net result is that this method could be used, but it is marginal. You
probably should use more than one weevil at a time.

Advantages of Activation Analysis

There are several advantages which the use of activation analysis has
over other techniques. Some of these are

1. You can "see" an otherwise invisible sample.

2. A wide range of concentrations can be covered from a 100% sample down
   to a few ppb if the source is adequate.

3. Almost any size or shape of the sample is permitted.

4. The nature of the surrounding material has little effect, although it must sometimes be corrected for.

5. It is nondestructive.

X-RAY FLUORESCENCE

X-ray fluorescence is a technique in which x-rays are used to bombard a sample, producing secondary x-rays characteristic of the elements in the sample. These secondary x-rays are separated and detected and in this manner both qualitative and quantitative analyses can be made.

This is a technique that can be used to detect several elements simultaneously but usually requires the presence of at least one part per 10,000 to be detected. Recent improvements in detectors have pushed this limit down to 10 ppm for some elements, but this is still not what is considered a low-level technique. Figure 84 is a diagram of an x-ray fluorescence instrument.

There are several different analytical x-ray techniques: diffraction, absorption, emission, fluorescence, and the closely related electron probe and ion probe. We will discuss two types of x-ray fluorescence, and x-ray diffraction only to the extent it is used in fluorescence. We will end with small sections on the electron probe and the ion probe.

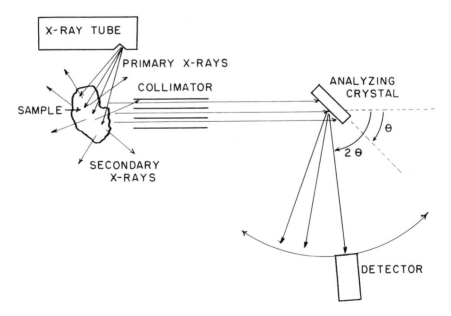

FIG. 84. Flat crystal reflection type of x-ray fluorometer.

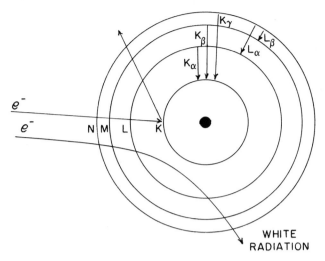

FIG. 85. Schematic representation of electronic transitions which produce characteristic x-ray spectra.

Production of X-rays

Figure 85 is a schematic representation of the production of x-rays. High-energy electrons or gamma rays are directed to the target atoms. Most of these electrons will be repelled by the electrons of the atoms, thereby losing some of their energy and producing a continuous radiation called white radiation or Bremstralung (braking radiation) like that shown in Fig. 86. However, only about 0.01 to 0.1% of the impinging electrons will get through the electron shield and have sufficient energy to interact with an inner shell electron to eject it from the inner shell. Suppose the

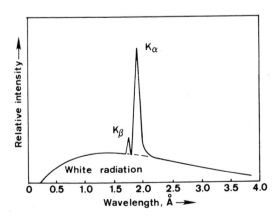

FIG. 86. X-ray emission from an iron target, 50 kV.

ejected electron was from the K shell. This is a choice position because
it is closest to the positive nucleus and has the lowest potential energy.
Therefore electrons from the surrounding L, M, N, etc., shells can and do
fill the vacancy. If an electron from an L shell fills the K vacancy, the
energy released produces an x-ray, and it is called K_α. If the vacancy is
filled by an M electron, the x-ray produced is a K_β. Since the L-shell
electrons are closest, they are most likely to fill the vacancy, and as you
can see in Fig. 86 they produce the highest intensity. The K_β are more
energetic x-rays but are less likely to be formed, in fact only about 15%
as often.

If an electron goes from the L shell to the K shell to produce a K_α
x-ray, what happens to the L shell vacancy? This can be filled in the same
manner as the K shell only with M, N, O, etc., shell electrons, producing
L_α, L_β, etc., x-rays. This process can in principle continue for several
steps. However, eventually you get to the place where the energy differences are no longer in the x-ray region (soft x-rays), and you find that
the original bombarding electrons fill the vacancies and stop the process.

Since each element has its own arrangement of electrons and protons,
the energies between the K, L, M, N, etc., shells are different for each
element and as a result the x-rays produced in this manner are characteristic of the target element.

Components of the X-ray Fluorescence Spectrometer

Sources. The source is normally the x-rays from a heavy element such
as Mo or W. Figure 87 is a diagram of a commercial x-ray tube. The electrons are accelerated from the cathode to the anode by the application of

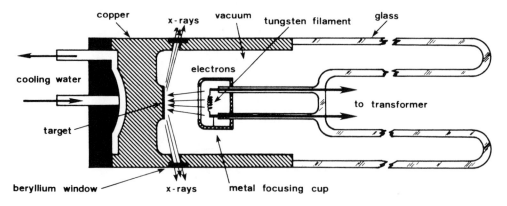

FIG. 87. Diagram of a commercial x-ray tube [28].

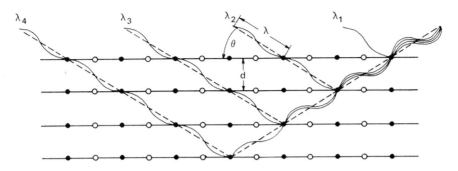

FIG. 88. The x-ray diffraction process.

from 30,000 to 50,000 V. When they strike the target metal, x-rays are
produced (2-50 mA) which are directed through Be windows to the sample.
The tube gets quite hot and must be cooled. This requires about 30 gal of
H_2O/hr.

Recently, gamma ray sources have been introduced for use in "portable"
x-ray units.

Collimators. The secondary x-rays generated within the sample are
emitted in all directions. It is imperative that at least a portion of
these go in a known direction so that the detector can function properly.
The x-ray beam must therefore be collimated. This is done by using either
a bundle of small-diameter (0.5-mm) nickel tubes a few centimeters in length
or several closely spaced metal plates.

Sometimes two collimators are used, one between the sample and the
analyzer crystal and the second, not as precise, between the crystal and
the detector.

Analyzers. The combination of the analyzer crystal, detector, and
angle measurement apparatus is called a goniometer and is one of the most
expensive components in the x-ray instrument.

In order to understand how a goniometer functions, it is necessary to
know something about x-ray diffraction.

One of the properties of x-rays is that they travel in straight lines
and they are very penetrating. In addition, as electromagnetic radiation,
x-rays may be diffracted. In the case of x-rays, the right order of spacings for diffraction exists in crystals where the atomic or ionic distances
are of the order of a few angstroms.

When an x-ray strikes a layer of atoms in a crystal, it can be diffracted as shown in Fig. 88. If another x-ray (λ_2) strikes the layer below

the first layer and the total distance it travels is an even number of wavelengths behind the first wavelength λ_1, then λ_2 can add to λ_1 since they are both in phase. If this is repeated for several layers, the emerging x-ray beam is strong enough to be detected by a photographic film or other x-ray detector.

This occurs only if λ and d are just right. Sir Lawrence Bragg and his son were the first to show how these variables were interrelated.

$$n\lambda = 2d \sin \theta \tag{39}$$

where

λ = the incident wavelength

d = spacing between atom layers

θ = angle of incidence

n = order of the radiation

We know d, and if θ is measured, then λ, the characteristic x-rays, and therefore the elements present in the sample can be determined. Since the angle θ depends on the wavelength, the analyzer crystal must be rotated to determine the various elements. As the crystal rotates through an angle θ, the detector must rotate through an angle 2θ.

The Bragg equation places some severe restrictions on d. As a result, a variety of different spacings must be available if all elements are to be examined with maximum sensitivity. Table 19 lists several crystal materials and the lowest atomic number element that can be determined.

TABLE 19. Selected Analyzing Crystals

Material	2nd Spacing ($\overset{\circ}{A}$)	K_α	L_α
LiF	4.028	K(19)	In(49)
NaCl	5.039	S(16)	Mo(42)
Quartz	8.50	Si(14)	Rb(37)
Ethylene diamine tartrate (EDDT)	8.808	Al(13)	Br(35)
Calcium sulfate	15.12	Na(11)	Ni(28)
Mica	19.8	F(9)	Mn(25)
Potassium acid phthalate (KAP)	26.0	O(8)	V(23)
Half K salt of cyclohexane, 1,2-di acid	31.2		
Tetradecano amide	54		

TABLE 19 (Continued)

Material	2nd Spacing (Å)	K_α	L_α
Dioctadecylterephthalate	84		
Dioctadecyladipate	90		

The reflectivity of the last four materials in Table 19 is extremely high, which means that the detection limits for the lighter elements can be lowered. Those materials are still being evaluated.

The use of oriented soap films that can be made easily into curved surfaces is a recent innovation that permits d values from 25 to 100 Å and allows lower atomic number elements to be examined.

Detectors. Detectors are usually the thallium-activated NaI scintillation counter or the Ge(Li) detector. They were discussed in detail in the section on radioactivity.

It should be noted that whereas the characteristic spectrum of an x-ray tube has superimposed on it the white radiation, the fluorescent spectrum does not have this disadvantage. This is shown in Fig. 89.

Nondispersive X-ray Units

Recent advances in electronics have permitted the construction of pulse height analyzers with sufficient accuracy to make it possible to collect the emitted x-rays from an irradiated sample and separate them without using a

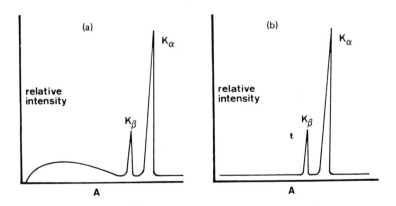

FIG. 89. (a) Chromium target at 50 kV, and (b) chromium excited by x-rays from a W tube (fluorescence) operated at 50 kV.

dispersing crystal. A radioactive isotope is used for the source which makes
this type of x-ray fluorescence unit "portable."

The Applied Research Laboratories Model N940 nondispersive analyzer will
be used as an example of this type of instrument. The schematic diagram of
the components is shown in Fig. 90, and a photograph is presented in Fig. 91.
This unit weighs about 150 lb and is in effect portable.

A spectrum is obtained by exciting the sample with an isotope x-ray
source; it is then analyzed by an energy-responsive proportional counter,
usually referred to as a detector. The use of a nondispersive system allows
a close-coupled source/detector geometry which eliminates the need for vacuum or helium purged paths.

Detector pulses, after amplification, are fed to a pulse-height analyzer (PHA) for effective element separation, then to a counter, and a four-
digit light-emitting diode (LED) display output. When the atomic numbers
of the wanted elements are very close together, one or more easily changed
filters can be inserted to give further physical discrimination.

SYSTEM SCHEMATIC

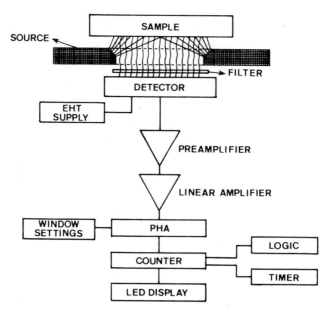

FIG. 90. Schematic diagram of a nondispersive x-ray unit. (Courtesy of
Applied Research Laboratories, Sunland, California.)

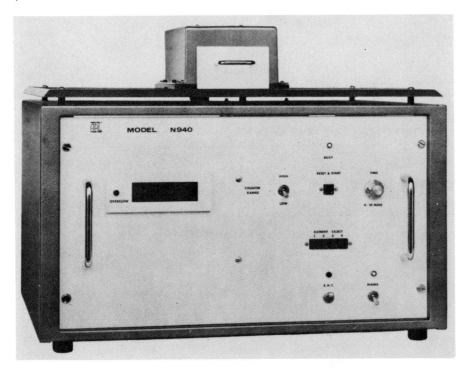

FIG. 91. Photograph of the ARL Model N940 nondispersive x-ray analyzer. (Courtesy of Applied Research Laboratories, Sunland, California.)

The x-ray analysis times are relatively short, often only a few seconds, and since the method is nondestructive, it is possible to obtain many repeat measurements from the same sample. An electronic timer for determination of the analysis period is provided.

Sources. The sources are annular in shape so that the excited radiation from the sample passes through the center of the source to the detector. This arrangement permits extremely close coupling with a path length of less than 10 mm and gives adequate sensitivity for light elements. Details of each source are given in Table 20. Solid, liquid, and powder samples are equally acceptable, the maximum sample size being approximately 50-mm diameter x 45 mm high. Polythene sample holders, specially designed for liquid and powder samples, are available. As there is no vacuum differential, extremely thin windows can be used; a 6-μm thickness of Mylar film is typical.

Detectors. A very high detection efficiency is provided by the gas-filled Exatron proportional detector used. These detectors produce output

TABLE 20. Sources for Nondispersive X-ray Units[a]

Type	Typical Activity (mCi)	Half-life (years)
Fe-55	20	2.7
Am-241	3	470
Pu-238	30	86

[a]Courtesy of Applied Research Laboratories, Sunland, California.

TABLE 21. Element Coverage of Alternative Source/Detector Combinations[a]

K Spectra   Si P S Cl K Ca Sc Ti V Cr Mn Fe Co Ni Cu Zn-As-Sr-Mo-Ag-Sn-Ba

L Spectra   Sr___Mo___Sn_____Ba_____W_____Pb_U

```
        ┌─────────────────────────┐
        │  Fe⁵⁵ - Neon Exatron    │
        └─────────────────────────┘

              ┌──────────────────┐
              │  Fe⁵⁵ - Argon    │
              │     Exatron      │
              └──────────────────┘

                  ┌─────────────────────────────────┐
                  │   Pu²³⁸ - Xenon Exatron         │
                  └─────────────────────────────────┘

                                    ┌──────────────────┐
                                    │  Am²⁴¹ - Xenon   │
                                    │     Exatron      │
                                    └──────────────────┘
```

[a]Courtesy of Applied Research Laboratories, Sunland, California.

pulses proportional in amplitude to the energy of the x-ray that produces
the pulse. The detector is placed to receive as much of the fluorescent
radiation as possible, and its output thus consists of a train of pulses
whose heights are related to the energies of the incoming x-rays. The three
types of detector available differ by reason of their gas fillings: neon,
argon, or xenon. Table 21 shows the various detector/source combinations
used in this instrument and the element range covered.

The gas-type detectors mentioned here were not discussed previously.
We will discuss two types, (1) the Geiger-Muller counter, because people
have heard of it and it illustrates the principles involved, and (2) the
proportional counter.

Geiger-Muller Counters: The Geiger-Muller tube, hereafter referred to
as a GM tube, is shown schematically in Fig. 92. The GM tube is very sensitive to alpha and beta particles (98% efficient) compared to gamma rays
(2% efficient). The GM counter is relatively cheap and simple to operate,
but it does not discriminate between types of radiation (alpha, beta, or
gamma), and it has a finite lifetime. It is steadily being replaced by
proportional and scintillation counters.

Suppose a ray of radiation comes through the mica window and strikes
an argon atom. The argon atom is ionized to produce a positive argon ion
and an electron. The positive ion moves toward the cathode about 1000 times
more slowly than the electron moves toward the anode. The electron, attracted by the high potential of the anode, is rapidly accelerated. In fact,
it has sufficient energy so that if it collides with an argon atom, another
ion and electron can be produced. Now two electrons are accelerating toward
the anode. These can produce a geometric progression of additional ions and
electrons. The net result, the "Townsend avalanche," is that thousands of
electrons reach the anode. When these electrons reach the anode, a small
current is produced, and this pulse signal is measured. In addition, some
of the electrons striking the anode may have enough energy to knock other
electrons from the anode and in turn can knock still other electrons loose.
This is known as the photon spread. When this reaches the end of the anode,
the voltage and current are so high that the wire may be destroyed, necessi-
tating the use of a glass bead to provide a larger surface area, thereby
decreasing the charge.

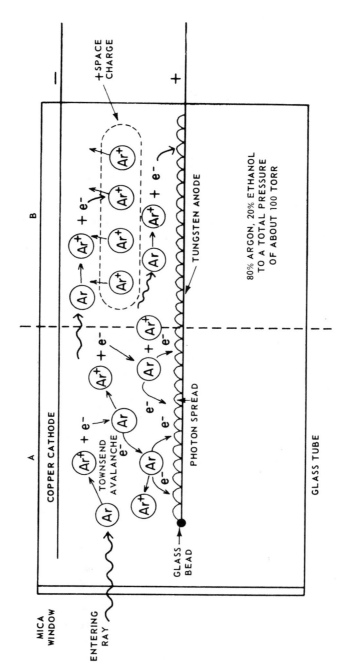

FIG. 92. Schematic drawing of a Geiger-Müller tube.

The total time it takes for this signal to build up is known as the
rise time, t_r, and is usually 2 to 5 µsec.

During this sequence of events the positive ions are slowly moving toward the cathode as a positive space charge. If they strike the cathode
with their full energy, then more photoelectrons will be generated — in fact,
more than the tube can handle. The net result is that the counter will
"burn out" if something is not done to dissipate this energy. Molecules,
which have many energy levels, are used for this purpose, ethanol being the
most common. The ionized argon atoms will transfer their energy to the
ethanol molecules. The ethanol molecules may then form ions or free radicals, but the energy is now spread out, and since the cathode has very little
affinity for them, no photoelectrons are produced. Since there is a limit
to the amount of "quenching gas" which can be added to this type of counter,
the counter will work only as long as quenching gas is present and will
then burn out.

Next, let us consider what happens if a second ray of radiation enters
the counter before the first ray has completed its reaction. (See section
B of Fig. 92.) If the ray ionized an argon atom at a point between the
cathode and the positive space charge, then the electron produced will not
"see" the anode but will recombine with an argon ion. The net result is
that a ray of radiation entered the counter but was not counted, and the
counter was then "dead."

Now consider a ray entering the counter between the positive space
charge and the anode. The electron produced will see the anode and be attracted to it. However, it does not have as much room to operate in as did
the first ray and therefore not as large a Townsend avalanche can be formed.
The result is that the pulse formed will be weak, compared to the original
pulse, and may not be detected. Again, the counter is dead. Dead times
(t_d) vary, but usually are between 80 and 100 µsec. This does not mean that
after 100 µsec the counter is completely ready to go again. It means only
that the next signal produced can be detected. Its amplitude will be weak.
The time it takes for the counter to recover completely is known as the
recovery time (t_{rec}) and varies from 200 to 350 µsec. The counter dead
time affects the counting rate and introduces an error into measurements.

Proportional counters: Geiger-Muller tubes are limited to about 15,000
c/min because of their long dead time. If the voltage applied to the anode

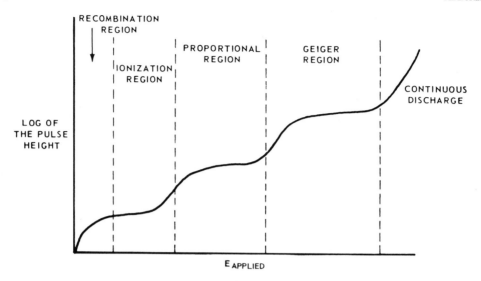

FIG. 93. Regions of pulse counting.

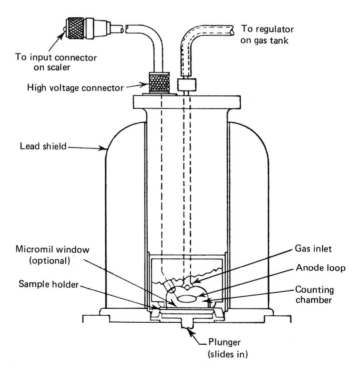

FIG. 94. A schematic of a flow through proportional counter. (Courtesy of Nuclear-Chicago Corp.)

of a GM tube is reduced to the point where it can collect electrons but not
form the photon spread, then the output pulse is proportional to the energy
of the initial ionization since the number of secondary electrons now depends upon the number of primary ion pairs produced initially. A device
operated in this manner is called a <u>proportional counter</u>. Figure 93 shows
the proportional region. The dead times are very short, of the order of
1 μsec, and therefore proportional counters can count up to 200,000 c/min.
The pulse signal is much weaker than with the GM tube, requiring a much
better amplification system. As a result, a proportional counter cannot be
made by simply lowering the anode voltage of a GM counter. Figure 94 shows
a schematic of a flow-through proportional counter.

Proportional counters can operate at atmospheric pressures, making it
possible to add quenching gas continuously. Since this can be endless, a
proportional counter can count indefinitely. They are very good for alpha
and beta particles, and because of their ionization efficiency, alpha particles are easily distinguished from beta particles.

The Electron Microprobe

One of the disadvantages of the x-ray fluorescence instrument is that
a large volume of sample is irradiated which makes it difficult to examine
small portions of a given sample. For example, suppose you desired to look
at the chemical composition of the grain boundaries in a piece of metal or
you wanted to have some idea as to where the Pb was in a liver cell. Normal
x-ray fluorescence source tubes can be focused to about 100 μm at best. This
area is too large to visualize the 1 μm^3 desired. Either a better method
for focusing x-rays is needed or a different source must be found. The
electron probe provides a different source. Electrons can be focused easier
than x-rays, and since we already know that high-speed electrons can generate
x-rays, then electrons seem to be a good choice. The electron probe is
really x-ray fluorescence with an exceptionally good means of focusing
electrons as the source. A cutaway view of one such commercial instrument
is shown in Fig. 95.

Because the x-ray source in the sample is essentially now a point source
(1 μm^3), the x-rays emitted are few and diverge widely. If collimators were
used, too much radiation would be lost. Therefore curved crystals are used
to collect the emitted radiation and focus it on the detector.

Using the electron probe, quantitative analysis may be made on less
than 1 μg of material, with the limit of detectability about 0.1%, and all

Model 400 Schematic

1. Cathode Z Axis Translator
2. Cathode Assembly
3. Grid Cup
4. Anode Plate
5. Beam Shield
6. Auxiliary Lens
7. Aperture Selector
8. Beam Scanning Deflection Plates
9. Stigmator
10. Electrostatic Beam Shield
11. Objective Lens
12. Light Microscope Objective
13. Differential Electron Detector
14. Specimen Holder
15. X-Ray Spectrometer
    (One Of Three Shown)
16. Diffracting Crystal Shown At
    Intermediate 2 Theta Angle
17. Proportional Detector Shown At
    Intermediate 2 Theta Angle
18. Diffracting Crystal Shown At
    High 2 Theta Angle
19. Proportional Detector Shown At
    High 2 Theta Angle
20. Column Alignment Translators
21. Monocular Viewing Or Camera Adapter
22. Oblique Illumination And Polarized
    Light Controls
23. Microscope Objective Translator
24. Specimen Stage Controls

    a. Microscope Field Rotation
    b. Focus
    c. Search And Specimen Selector
    d. Search
    e. f. g. Fine Controls
    h. Traverse

LOCUS OF
ROWLAND
CIRCLE CENTER

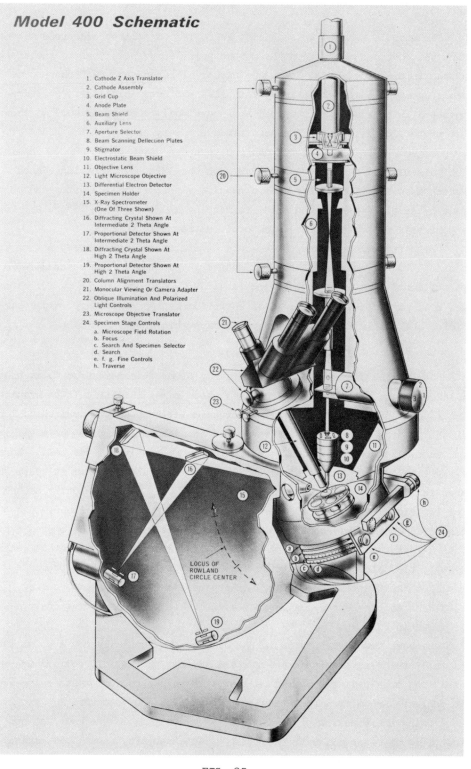

FIG. 95

of the elements above atomic number 11 can be detected. This method has tremendous potential for determining the whereabouts of trace metals in plant and animal tissue, but it costs in the neighborhood of $100,000.

The Ion Microprobe

The ion microprobe is a lot like the electron microprobe except that ions are generated in the sample rather than x-rays and a mass spectrometer is used as the detector rather than x-ray fluorescence (Fig. 96).

According to Bayard,

A spot of ions about 1 μm in diameter is formed on the sample surface with an ion source focused by two electrostatic lenses. The primary ions, either a reactive gas such as F^- or a heavy inert gas such as Ar^+, react with the sample and sputter off secondary ions. These secondary ions are collected by a high angular aperture mass spectrometer and analyzed to determine both the elements and isotopes present in the sample volume, typically 1-5 μm in diameter by only a few monolayers thick.

The source of ions is a duoplasmatron, a device using axially symmetric electrostatic and magnetic fields to move electrons and the gas which is being ionized in fairly long spiral paths through the device. Because of the long path length, the chance of an ionizing collision is high, and practically any gas, even air, can be used to give a high brightness source of either positive or negative ions; shifting rapidly from nitrogen to oxygen ions is also possible. The duoplasmatron will produce doubly ionized species and, in some cases, ionized molecular fragments. Since it is desirable to have only one type of ion interacting with the sample, a $90°$ bend electromagnet is used as a primary mass filter at the entrance to the electrostatic lens column. The magnetic field is adjusted so that only the desired type of ion is deflected more or less, depending on their mass-to-charge ratio.

As mentioned previously, two electrostatic lenses successively demagnify the source and focus the ion beam. It is unfortunate that electrostatic lenses must be used since magnetic lenses of equivalent demagnifying power have a much lower spherical aberration, the factor which limits the formation of ion spots less than 1 μm in diameter with ion currents high enough to be useful. Since, however, conventional axially symmetric electromagnetic lenses are weak focusing devices, utilizing only second-order focusing by fringe fields, they cannot handle the mass of the ions in the beam, and electrostatic lenses must be used instead. Even a H^+ ion, that is, a proton, weighs 1836 times as much as an electron, so that it is no wonder that the magnetic lenses used in the electron microprobe do not work, for example, on Ar^+ ions. In the future, there is the possibility of using strong, focusing, asymmetric magnetic

FIG. 95. Cutaway view of an electron probe instrument. (Courtesy of Materials Analysis Co., Palo Alto, California.)

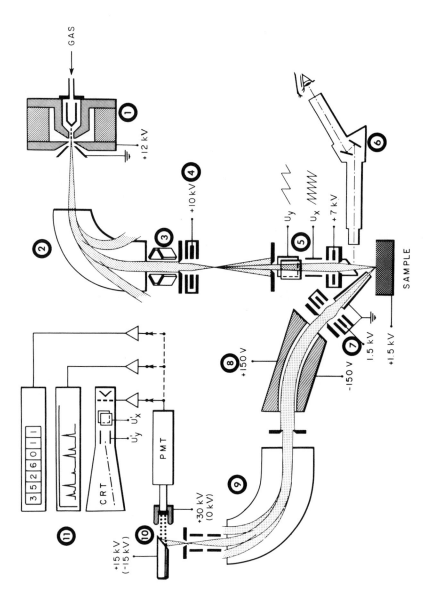

FIG. 96. An ion microprobe mass analyzer: 1. Duoplasmatron ion source. 2. Primary mass filter which allows one species of ion into the optical column. 3. Alignment deflector plates. 4. First electrostatic condenser lens. 5. Second electrostatic condenser lens and beam scanning deflector plates. 6. Optical microscope to view sample during analysis. 7. Lens to extract ions from sample. 8. Electrostatic velocity sector of analytical mass spectrometer. 9. Magnetic mass analyzer of spectrometer. 10. Ion detector and photomultiplier tube. 11. Readout electronics (oscilloscope, strip chart recorder, and scaler). (Courtesy of American Laboratory, April 1971.)

lenses such as quadrupoles or octopoles and achieving spot sizes of less than 0.1 μm with useful currents.

In addition to the electrostatic lenses, the ion optical column has a beam-scanning system that consists of electrostatic deflection plate sets which allow the beam to move an x-y raster on the sample in synchronism with the spot on a cathode-ray tube. The net result is an ability to build an image of the sample surface, showing the location of any chosen ion species. The resolution, on the order of 1 μm, is the same as the spot size.

The mass spectrometer performs two functions. First its electrostatic sector sorts the ions on the basis of velocity and brings most of them to a similar speed. Next, its magnetic sector sorts the ions on the basis of mass-to-charge [m/e] ratio. Only those ions having a discrete, selected m/e are passed through the exit slit to the detector. It is a simple matter to vary the magnetic field strength and thereby scan the entire mass range from 1 to 300 in less than 30 sec. An electrostatic lens increases the angular aperture of the system. Between 4 and 10% of the ions escaping the sample are collected by the spectrometer.

Table 22 shows the detection limits obtained during the analysis of a sample of "pure silicon."

The important thing to remember is the very small sample size required. This is more dramatically shown in Fig. 97, which compares several techniques. While the ion microprobe will detect a few ppb within a given sample, only about 10^{-19} g of the element desired need be present, which means a sample size of 10^{-10} g!

SPARK SOURCE MASS SPECTROMETRY

Mass spectrometry has long been useful in the identification and determination of the composition of mixtures, particularly those organic in nature. Techniques are now available to use a mass spectrometer directly as a detector for inorganic compounds.

This new technique is called spark source mass spectroscopy. It is basically the same as conventional mass spectroscopy except that a high-temperature source, a spark like that employed in emission spectroscopy, is used and a double focusing analyzer is usually required. It has three major advantages:

1. It can be used with alloys.

TABLE 22. Elemental Detection Limits in Pure Silicon[a,b]

Isotope Measured	Detection Limit
$^7Li^+$	0.012
$^{11}B^+$	0.025
$^{12}C^+$	0.050
$^{23}Na^+$	0.012
$^{24}Mg^+$	0.015
$^{27}Al^+$	0.012
$^{35}Cl^+$	0.100
$^{40}Ca^+$	0.011
$^{48}Ti^+$	0.015
$^{54}Fe^+$	0.207
$^{65}Cu^+$	0.019
$^{88}Sr^+$	0.013
$^{90}Zr^+$	0.022
$^{98}Mo^+$	0.048
$^{202}Hg^+$	0.056
$^{208}Pb^+$	0.024

[a] Values in ppm atomic; integration time, 10 sec.
[b] Courtesy of Materials Analysis Lab., Palo Alto, California.

2. It is nonselective with regard to sensitivity.

3. It is highly sensitive.

The basic ideas of mass spectroscopy is to produce ions (only positive ions will be discussed here) by bombarding molecules with high-energy electrons, then accelerating these ions in a definite direction so that they can be separated according to their mass or velocity. The separated ions are then detected and their intensity measured.

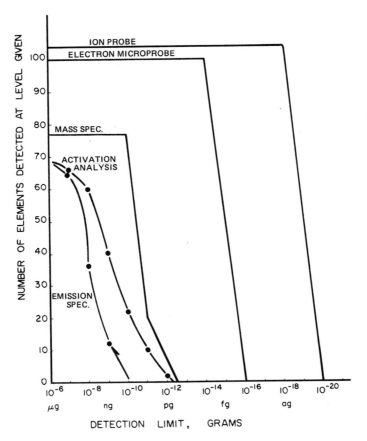

FIG. 97. Detection limits (g) for several analytical techniques [29].

There are several types of mass spectrometers available commercially. One of these, a single-focusing electromagnetic type, is shown in Fig. 98. Figure 96 shows a double-focusing mass spectrometer.

Each spectrometer has three major components: the ion source, the analyzer, and the detector.

The purpose of the ion source is to convert the sample or a portion of the sample into ions. Most mass spectrometers are designed to utilize only the positive ions produced. Figure 99 is a diagram of a conventional ion source used for organic compounds.

Electrons emitted from the filament are accelerated between E_1 and E_2 by a potential of about 70 V. When an electron strikes a molecule M, pos-

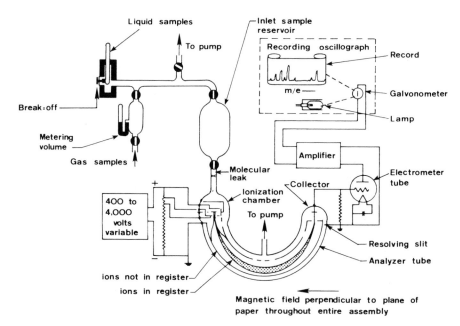

FIG. 98. Electromagnetic mass spectrometer. (Courtesy of Consolidated
Electrodynamics Co.)

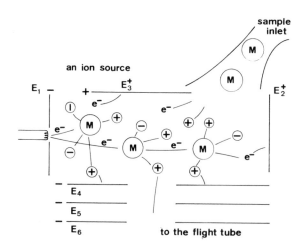

FIG. 99. Diagram of an ion source.

itive ions (+), negative ions (-), electrons (e⁻), and neutral molecules
may be formed. The positive species are separated from the negative species
by E_3 and E_4 which have a small potential of a few volts across them. The
positive ions are then accelerated down the tube E_5, E_6, etc., each having
several hundred volts applied to them. A total accelerating voltage of
2000 V is normal.

Consider the molecule $CH_3CH_2CH_2SH$. Suppose that a high-energy electron
strikes the molecule and transfers its energy to it. The diagram below
shows what can happen.

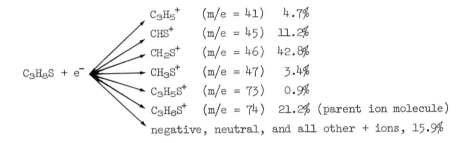

$$C_3H_8S + e^-$$

$C_3H_5^+$	(m/e = 41)	4.7%
CHS^+	(m/e = 45)	11.2%
CH_2S^+	(m/e = 46)	42.8%
CH_3S^+	(m/e = 47)	3.4%
$C_3H_5S^+$	(m/e = 73)	0.9%
$C_3H_6S^+$	(m/e = 74)	21.2% (parent ion molecule)

negative, neutral, and all other + ions, 15.9%

The percent composition obtained depends upon the energy of the impinging
electrons.

The above system works well for organic compounds, but high melting
solids and alloys are not affected. A high-voltage (100,000 V), high-
frequency (800,000 Hz) spark is produced between two electrodes made from
the sample as shown in Fig. 100.

Analyzers

The ions, accelerated in the ion source, are then separated. In the
electromagnetic instrument, the separation of ions of different mass-to-

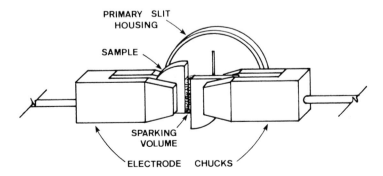

PRIMARY SLIT
HOUSING

SAMPLE

SPARKING
VOLUME

ELECTRODE   CHUCKS

FIG. 100. Electrode arrangement during sparking [30].

charge (m/e) ratios is accomplished by a magnetic field at right angles to the flight path of the ions. The lighter ions are deviated more than the heavier ions so separation occurs. (Note: A vacuum of about 10^{-6} torr is always applied. The reason for this is that once the positive ions are produced, you do not want to neutralize them prematurely by collision with the other molecules.)

After the formation of ions in an electron beam, the ions are accelerated through a potential drop of V. In so doing, the ions receive kinetic energy, T, equal to

$$T = \frac{mv^2}{2} = eV \qquad (40)$$

where

m = mass of the ion in g

v = velocity of the ion in cm/sec

e = charge on the ion, 4.8×10^{-10} esu

V = the voltage used to accelerate the ion

Upon entering a magnetic field H, the ions will take paths that are arcs of a circle with a radius R equal to

$$R = \frac{mv}{eH} \qquad (41)$$

Combining Eqs. (40) and (41) and rearranging gives

$$\frac{m}{e} = \frac{H^2R^2}{2V} \qquad (42)$$

The angle of deflection (radius) is usually fixed for a given analyzer tube, so that to focus ions of given (m/e) values on the detector system, either H or V must be varied.

Example calculation: Consider an electromagnet-type mass spectrometer having V = 2000 and R = 7.00 in. What must be the magnetic field to focus the CO_2^+ ion (m/e = 44) on the detector? Use Eq. (42). Here R is in cm and V is in erg/esu. Two conversion factors are necessary: 300 practical volts = 1 erg/esu and $esu^2 \times 9 \times 10^{20} = emu^2$.

$$V = \frac{2000}{300} = 6.667 \text{ erg/esu}$$

and

$$R = 7.00 \times 2.54 = 15.78 \text{ cm}$$

$$H^2 = \frac{2V(m/e)}{R^2}$$

$$H^2 = \frac{2 \times 6.667 \times (44/6.02 \times 10^{23})}{(15.78)^2 \times 4.80 \times 10^{-10}} \times 9 \times 10^{20}$$

$$= 7.33 \times 10^6$$

$$H = 2708 \text{ gases}$$

Detectors

The detector is an electrode onto which the positive ions fall. Connected in series between this electrode and ground is a resistor. Electrons from ground rush to neutralize the positive charge on the collector. Current across the resistor causes a potential drop that is proportional to the current flow (Ohm's law), so that by measuring the voltage, the number of ions of each type can be determined.

As early as 1943, Cohen used an electron multiplier in a mass spectrometer (Fig. 101). The principle is the same as was described for photomultiplier tubes in a previous section. The detector has a high sensitivity and a rapid response. Multiplication factors of 10^5 and 10^6 are usual.

The Wiley magnetic electron multiplier (Fig. 102), 1956, employs crossed magnetic and electric fields to control the electron trajectories. As the individual groups of ions arrive at the end of the field free-flight tube (time of flight mass spectrometer), they collide with the plane ion cathode of the magnetic electron multiplier. The plane ion cathode is used because it eliminates ion transit time variations encountered with a curved ion cathode (Fig. 101). Each ionization produces a group of electrons, and because of the crossed magnetic and electric fields present, the electrons follow a cycloidal path down the dynode strips of the multiplier. In this manner a current gain of the order of 10^6 is obtained.

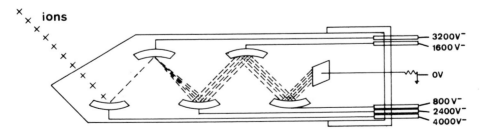

FIG. 101. Cohen-type electron multiplier.

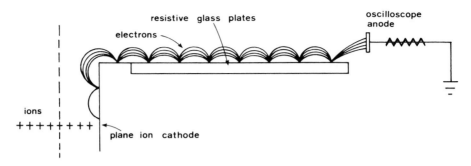

FIG. 102. Wiley electron multiplier.

A Typical Analysis

The work of Morrison and Kashuba using the spark source mass spectrometer for the determination of 60 elements in basalt rock will be used as an
example of what can be done and how it is to be done. Table 23 shows the
results of their work and how it compares with neutron activation analysis.
Notice that they used a double-focusing instrument and that they used indium
as an internal standard.

TABLE 23. Analysis of BCR-1 Basalt (ppm)[a]

Element	Mass Spectroscopy	Neutron Activation	Literature Values	No. of Labs.
Li	13	--	15	1
B	2.4	--	--	
O	41%	--	44.60%	1
F	460	--	485	1
Na	1.6%	2.46%	2.46%	--[b]
Mg	1.4%	2.21%	1.98%	--[b]
Al	6.3%	6.97%	6.97%	--[b]
Si	24%	--	25.4%	--[b]
P	1730	--	1610	--[b]
Cl	72	99	58-120	3
K	1.1%	1.4%	1.40%	--[b]
Ca	4.9%	5.0%	4.99%	--[b]
Ti	1.09%	1.4%	1.34%	--[b]
V	310	380	323-465	5
Cr	10.5	16	11-35	4

TABLE 23 (Continued)

Element	Mass Spectroscopy	Neutron Activation	Literature Values	No. of Labs.
Mn	1420	1380	1300-1600	6
Fe	7.5%	9.66%	9.44%	--[b]
Co	45	43	36-37	5
Cu	24	16	13-27	4
Zn	145	131	94.4-278	6
Ga	24	20	24	1
Ge	2.2	--	--	
Se	0.2	--	0.103	1
Rb	37	44	48.6-53	3
Sr	270	290	335-347	3
Y	39	--	--	
Zr	180	274	210	1
Nb	19	--	--	
Mo	0.9	1	2.9	1
Ru	(1)[c]	--	--	
Rh	(0.2)[c]	--	< 0.004	1
Pd	0.03	--	--	
Ag	0.02	--	0.036	1
Cd	0.3	--	0.067	1
Sn	3	--	--	
Sb	0.9	0.68	0.32-1.1	4
Te	(0.4)[c]	--	--	
I	(0.8)[c]	--	--	
Cs	1.1	1.0	0.91-1.5	5
Ba	730	840	650	1
La	23	23	22-23.7	3
Ce	45	43	46-53	3
Pr	8	--	--	
Nd	21	32	--	
Sm	6	6	5.5-7.4	3
Eu	1.5	2.0	1.95-2.3	2
Gd	6	5	--	
Tb	1	1	1.0	1
Dy	7	6	6.25	1

TABLE 23 (Continued)

Element	Mass Spectroscopy	Neutron Activation	Literature Values	No. of Labs.
Ho	1	1	--	
Er	5	--	--	
Tm	0.3	0.6	0.6	1
Yb	3.3	3.1	3.2	1
Lu	0.5	0.54	0.6	1
Hf	3.4	4.8	3.3-5.4	4
W	0.7	0.44	0.7	1
Re	<0.1	--	0.00084	1
Os	<0.1	--	<0.00001	2
Ir	<0.1	--	0.0007	1
Tl	0.3	--	0.36	1
Pb	13	--	13.56-29	3
Th	5	4.6	5.0-7.6	11
U	1.1	1.8	1.2-2.2	14

[a]From Ref. 30.

[b]Recommended value from Ref. 31.

[c]Values uncorrected for sensitivity factor, accurate to a factor of three.

Experimental

Mass spectrograph: The Nuclide Analysis Associates GRAF 2 double-focusing spark source mass spectrograph was used in this study.

Sample preparation: The diabase W-1 and the basalt BCR-1 samples were dried at $100°$ C for 1 hr. Two hundred and fifty ppm (wt) In as In_2O_3 was added as an internal standard. The mixture was blended with graphite (National Carbon Co. spectroscopic powder) or silver (Cominco American 5-9s grade Ag powder, lot HPM 7942). Mix ratios of rock-graphite of 1:1 and rock-Ag 1:9 were used.

Electrode preparation: Sample and conductor in the proportions given above were hand blended for 20 to 30 min in an agate mortar and pestle. A polyethylene slug of 11-mm diameter from the AEI pellet press was halved radially with a stainless steel blade. Sample-conductor mix was pressed at 5×10^{15} lb/in.^{2} to obtain a disk of 1- to 2-mm thickness. The disk was quartered axially with the stainless blade. The quarter disks were mounted in Ta electrode chucks as shown in Fig. 100 and presparked for a charge collection of 30 to 60 nC. The sparking occurred uniformly along the freshly exposed surfaces. No Fe, Ni, or Cr contamination appeared during analysis which could be traced to the press. Analysis of the graphite and silver powders was performed by visual estimation of line intensity. The analysis indicated that those trace elements present as a blank were also present in the rock samples at concentrations orders of magnitude higher, and they do not pose any problem in the rock analysis. The only exceptions were Ni and Cu present in relatively high concentrations in the silver; however, Cu was determined using rock blended with the purer graphite. Interferences precluded the determination of Ni.

SUMMARY

A brief discussion has been given of the various methods currently available for determining elements in trace amounts. It was shown that if a need arises, it is possible to determine most elements to the ppb range, and in many cases by more than one technique. It is also possible to determine these elements one at a time or several simultaneously. Great progress has been made toward examining very small volumes of material; however, we cannot yet get to as small a volume as a segment of a small cell which would be nice for toxicological research.

In the first few pages it was stated that the ability to detect the presence of the elements had far surpassed our ability to comprehend what the low levels actually meant. The analytical chemist has provided the toxicologist with the means to detect these elements; it is now up to the toxicologist to learn how to use these instruments and tell the world just what effect a few ppb of a particular element actually have.

REFERENCES

1. J. Dean and T. Rains, Flame Emission and Atomic Absorption Spectroscopy, Vol. I, Theory, Marcel Dekker, New York, 1969.

2. J. Dean and T. Rains, Flame Emission and Atomic Absorption Spectroscopy, Vol. II, Components and Techniques, Marcel Dekker, New York, 1971.

3. G. M. Hieftje and H. V. Malmstadt, Anal. Chem., 40, 1860 (1968).

4. D. J. Thompson, Trace Elements in Animal Nutrition, 3rd Ed., International Minerals and Chemical Corp., Skokie, Illinois, 1970, p. 25.

5. R. Kniseley, A. D'Silva, and V. Fassel, Anal. Chem., 35, 910 (1963).

6. P. J. Zeegers, Ph.D. Thesis, Utrecht, 1966.

7. C. S. Rann and A. N. Hambly, Anal. Chem., 37, 879 (1965).

8. J. Dean, Flame Photometry, McGraw-Hill, New York, 1960.

9. J. A. Dean and C. Thompson, Anal. Chem., 27, 42 (1955).

10. E. G. Pickett and S. R. Koirtyohann, Anal. Chem., 41, 29A (1969).

11. A. Walsh, Spectrochim. Acta, 7, 110 (1955).

12. J. W. Robinson, Atomic Absorption Spectroscopy, Marcel Dekker, New York, 1966.

13. J. Hwang, C. Mokeler, and P. Ullucci, Anal. Chem., 44, 2019 (1972).

14. M. T. Glenn, J. Savory, S. A. Fein, R. D. Reeves, C. J. Molnar, and J. D. Winefordner, Anal. Chem., 45, 203 (1973).

15. R. C. Weast (ed.), Handbook of Chemistry and Physics, Chemical Rubber Co., Cleveland, Ohio, 1970.

16. K. E. Zacha, M. P. Bratzel, Jr., J. D. Winefordner, and J. M. Mansfield, Jr., Anal. Chem., 40, 1733 (1968).

17. W. Kirsten and G. Bertilsson, Anal. Chem., 38, 648 (1966).

18. M. B. Denton and H. V. Malmstadt, Anal. Chem., 44, 1813 (1972).

19. R. M. Dagnall, G. F. Kirkbright, T. S. West, and R. Wood, Anal. Chem., 43, 1765 (1971).

20. V. A. Fassel and R. N. Kniseley, Inductively Coupled Plasma-Optical Emission Spectroscopy, Iowa State University, Ames, 1974.

21. R. W. Kniseley, V. A. Fassel, and C. C. Butler, Clin. Chem., 19, 807 (1973).

22. W. H. Wahl and H. H. Kramer, Scientific American, April (1967).

23. S. S. Nargowalla and E. P. Przybylowicz, Activation Analysis with Neutron Generators, Interscience, New York, 1973.

24. Energy Research and Development Administration, Californium-252 Progress, 13, (1972).

25. H. H. Willard, L. Merritt, and J. Dean, Instrumental Methods of Analysis, 5th Ed., Van Nostrand, Princeton, 1974.

26. P. J. Ouseph and M. Swartz, Topics in Chemical Instrumentation, J. Chem. Educ., 51, A139 (1974).

27. Energy Research and Development Administration, Californium-252 Progress, March (1974).

28. R. Rudman, J. Chem. Educ., 44, A99 (1967).

29. W. McCrone, Choice of Analytical Tool, Amer. Lab., April (1971).

30. G. H. Morrison and A. T. Kashuba, Anal. Chem., 41, 1842 (1969).

31. F. J. Flanagan, Geochim. Cosmochim. Acta, 33, 81 (1969).

31

BRITISH ANTILEWISITE (BAL),
THE CLASSIC HEAVY METAL ANTIDOTE

Frederick W. Oehme
Kansas State University
Manhattan, Kansas

The medicinal effect of natural and synthetic detoxicants is a well-established therapeutic principle. With further refinement of pharmacological measures, the development of biologically effective antidotes based upon prior knowledge will become of increasing importance. The purpose of this report is to trace the experimental process that resulted in the application of basic biochemical principles to the development of the heavy metal antidote, British antilewisite (BAL).

THE CHALLENGE

The toxic action of gases used in chemical warfare during World War I stimulated research concerning their mode of action. The arsendichlorides, obtained by chlorination of arsenoxides, proved particularly dangerous. Lewisite ($ClCH:CHAsCl_2$) was the most vesicant member of this series and produced lesions of the epithelium of the skin and respiratory system that were not reversible by any treatment then known. The work of Peters and others in the years before and during World War II met the challenge presented by these toxic compounds and eventually provided an effective antidote.

EARLY RESEARCH

Although described in the past as a general protoplasmic poison, arsenic is not an active protein precipitant. This suggested that its effect was on the functional activities, that is, the enzyme systems, rather than

on the structural factors of living cells. The effects of arsenicals indeed
proved highly selective to a number of enzymes, the pyruvate oxidase system
of the brain being especially inhibited by low concentrations of arsenic.
This particular action of arsenic was very similar to that of iodoacetate
[4] and led to the investigation of possible similar mechanisms.

The demonstration that iodoacetate reacted readily with thiol groups
in cysteine, reduced glutathione, and other proteins [5] led to the general
view that inhibition of a biological system by iodoacetate was due to reaction with the thiol groups present and necessary for that system's normal
functioning. It was thus expected that arsenic also exerted its toxic action by combining with the thiol groups of certain enzymes.

Employing monothiols, such as glutathione and cysteine, the effects of
arsenicals could be abolished [1]. Other experiments made clear that an
excess of simple thiol compounds was able to protect various biological
systems against toxic effects. This protection was only partial, however,
and in some instances physiologically inadequate. Regardless of the SH:As
ratio, eventual death was not prevented, although temporary response occurred [6,11]. The limited effect of the monothiols in protecting specific
biological systems was much less complete against arsenite than against
arsenoxides. Further, even when present in large excess, monothiols failed
to protect the brain pyruvate oxidase system from the toxic effect of arsenic.

Dilute solutions of arsenoxide and glutathione were shown to be more
easily hydrolyzed and dissociated, thus effecting less protection, while
strong concentrations with an excess of thiol favored the formation of
thioarsinite and offered more complete protection [10]. The reaction that
occurred was

$$RAsO + 2R'SH \rightleftarrows RAs{\Large\langle}\genfrac{}{}{0pt}{}{SR'}{SR'} + H_2O$$

The final equilibrium depended upon the pH and concentration of the reac-
tants.

The importance of the stability of the arsenic-thiol complex thus became recognized. It became clear that to be effective the "arsenic acceptor"
in living cells must form a more stable compound with arsenic than any of
the previously used simple monothiols had.

PHARMACOLOGICAL APPLICATION

A series of experiments were then conducted, largely in the laboratory of Peters, which led in a logical and systematic fashion to the development of an effective lewisite antidote.

Stocken and Thompson [7] added lewisite to kerateine, a derived protein formed by the rupture of the disulfate bonds of keratin, until all SH groups had reacted. They then investigated the protein's stability. Arsenic was found to be present in a relatively firm combination with the thiol groups and not merely in nonspecific physical association with the protein. At least 75% of the arsenic in the lewisite-protein complex was in combination with two thiol groups, and it appeared that the arsenic combined with two SH groups on the same molecule to form a stable ring.

Ring compounds of the structure

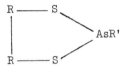

were more stable than complexes of an arsenical with two molecules of a monothiol of the type

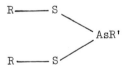

The high toxicity of the trivalent arsenicals was, therefore, hypothesized to be due to combinations with two closely situated SH groups on certain tissue proteins forming relatively stable arsenical rings.

It was reasoned that effective protection against such arsenicals would only be offered by the presence of competing dithiols capable of forming a ring compound at least as stable as the "tissue acceptor"-arsenical complex. Instead of arsenic producing an easily dissociable open-end compound with the previously used monothiols, the dithiols would hopefully prove more effective antidotes. Their SH groups would be close together in one molecule and would allow the formation of stable ring compounds which would permit one bond to hold firm if the other were temporarily split by thermal agitation.

Continuing studies investigated the protection afforded by simple di-thiol compounds [8]. It was considered that the suitable compound should have rapid skin penetrability, therefore small molecular size, and should form five- or six-member ring compounds with the arsenicals, for more easily obtained and more permanent stability. Hence 1-, 2-, and 3-dithiol compounds were selected. Several of these low-molecular-size dithiols were synthesized and tested in laboratory animals and humans, among them 2,3-dimercaptopropanol, later called BAL.

In a system at equilibrium containing equivalent amounts of lewisite oxide and a series of monothiols, dithiols, and thiol-proteins, the amount of lewisite combining with dithiols was greater than that combining with thiol-proteins, which was slightly greater than that combined with mono-thiols. The cyclic thioarsenites formed with dithiols were markedly more stable than the noncyclic compounds formed. All the dithiols investigated were nontoxic to the brain pyruvate oxidase system, and all either greatly diminished or completely abolished the enzyme inhibition produced by the arsenoxides and arsenite. These occurred when dilute solutions of the di-thiols were used. The 1,2- or 1,3-dithiol compounds, and especially 2,3-dimercaptopropanol (BAL), were shown the most effective arsenical antidotes when compared with compounds forming long-chained rings.

A mixture of BAL and lewisite was essentially nontoxic when added to the pyruvate oxidase system for 3 hr. The addition of BAL to the brain pyruvate system as late as 45 min after poisoning with lewisite markedly reversed the toxic effects; if added after only 15 min, complete reversal was attained. When added to rat skin slices, BAL gave complete protection against the effects of lewisite on skin respiration, while protein thiols and monothiols failed to protect.

Rats and guinea pigs with lewisite-contaminated skin were successfully treated with BAL, while the untreated animals all died. A high degree of recovery (88%) occurred, even when treatment was delayed as long as 2 hr and signs of toxicity had developed. Treatment with monothiols and hydrogen peroxide was much less effective. BAL was prophylactically effective for only short periods of time, however. Parenterally administered BAL also protected against intramuscular or topical administration of arsenicals. The protection was not complete but indicated a marked effectiveness under the conditions used. In human subjects BAL prevented arsenical skin vesi-cation as late as 1 hr after contamination. Olive oil and hydrogen peroxide were much less effective.

Toxicity studies of the dithiols were incompletely performed in rats, but gave promising results. An intramuscular LD_{50} of 113 mg/kg was determined for BAL. None of the other dithiols examined were found to be safer. The relative low volatility of BAL also favored this particular compound as a practical antidote. Subcutaneous injection of the lewisite-BAL complex indicated a toxicity one-fifth that of lewisite alone.

These studies revealed that BAL was an effective and practical arsenical antidote. There remained only investigation of its metabolism and fate to complete this compound's development.

THE FINISHED PRODUCT AND ITS METABOLISM

The synthetic product 2,3-dimercaptopropanol (BAL) had been shown to react with lewisite and other arsenicals to form stable ring compounds,

$$
\begin{array}{l}
CH_2SH \\
|\\
CHSH + RAsO \rightleftarrows \\
|\\
CH_2OH
\end{array}
\quad
\begin{array}{l}
CH_2 \!\!-\!\!\!-\!\! S \\
|\qquad\qquad\quad > AsR \\
CH \!\!-\!\!\!-\!\! S \\
|\\
CH_2OH
\end{array}
\quad + H_2O
$$

and to effectively protect against and reverse their toxic effect. Parenteral administration was possible and practical. The antidote was shown suitable for field use; its metabolism remained to be traced.

Arsenic was known to appear in the urine within a few hours after its application, and, depending upon its form, it might also be excreted in the bile and feces. Lewisite was excreted by the kidneys in amounts up to 20% of that applied, but elimination ceased after 1 week. Experiments were designed to determine the urinary and fecal excretion of arsenic with and without BAL therapy and to study the compound's metabolism [9].

Lewisite skin-contaminated rats treated topically with BAL after 15 min excreted 11-14% of the total applied arsenic in the urine during the first 24 hr; untreated rats excreted only 2 to 4%. If treatment was postponed for 1 hr, the percent of arsenic excreted in the urine rose to 27-33.5%. There was little difference in condition after 24 hr, regardless of treatment. BAL did not affect arsenic excretion in the feces, although diarrhea was completely prevented. After 48 hr the contaminated skin of the treated rats contained smaller percentages of the applied arsenic than did the control rats.

The biological fate of BAL was followed in subcutaneously injected rats and intraperitoneally injected rabbits, although intramuscular therapeutic administration was to be preferred in clinical patients. In both instances a transient diuresis occurred, accompanied by rapid urinary excretion of unidentified thiols. The disturbance of body thiol-disulfide equilibrium produced by the BAL injection was rapidly restored to normal by this mechanism. Excretion of the thiols began to fall after 3-4 hr and reached normal limits in 24 hr. The thiol excretion in rabbits was accompanied by a transient albuminuria, although no kidney damage was evident.

The rapid urinary thiol loss indicated the necessity of repeated BAL administration in clinical use. More recent information [3] indicates that the highest systemic concentration of BAL is reached 30 min following therapeutic administration. Absorption and detoxification are complete in 4 hr. A sharp rise in the urinary excretion of neutral sulfur accounts for 50% of the sulfur injected as BAL, and an increase in urinary glucuronic acid suggests that a portion of the BAL may be excreted in that form.

The present recommendations for the therapeutic use of BAL in acute arsenic toxicity are the intramuscular administration of single doses of 5 mg/kg of body weight every 4 hr for the first 24 hr. Thereafter the dose should be decreased and the interval between injections prolonged.

CURRENT STATUS

Although BAL has been effectively used to prevent and reverse the effect of various heavy metals on enzymes, metabolism, function, and growth, certain aspects of its application remain confusing.

Early research revealed that certain arsenic compounds mixed with thiols were as toxic as the original arsenicals [10]. That specific thiols were capable of potentiating the effect of arsenic inhibition of particular enzymes has also been defined [12]. While the mechanisms involved are unclear, it is assumed that the arsenical-thiol complex can more easily reach the functional SH groups because of increased lipid solubility. The formation of a tertiary arsenical-thiol-enzyme complex is also possible. The simple reduction of enzyme S-S linkages to SH groups in a region near the active site, and the SH group combining with the arsenical and thus interfering with the approach of substrate to the active site, has further been suggested.

The addition of substrate occasionally potentiates enzyme inhibition by an arsenical. This is explained as a reduction of S-S bonds to SH groups by NADH through FAD [12], much as glutathione reductase activity is

strongly inhibited by arsenite when NADPH is added. The susceptibilities
of metabolic systems may well depend upon the redox states of certain enzymes and hence on the supply of substrates and oxygen.

Recent investigations have also cast new light on the action of arsenite-BAL on electron transport and phosphorylation [13]. In liver and heart
mitochondria these processes are altered much more potently by equimolar
mixtures of arsenite and BAL than by arsenite alone. The complex is an
effective uncoupler of electron transport. It stimulates mitochondrial
ATPase activity more and causes greater mitochondrial swelling than arsenite
does. It affects oxidative phosphorylation by depressing oxygen uptake and
in certain concentrations causes a loss of respiratory control. Increased
penetrability of the arsenite-BAL complex is believed to be a factor in its
action, and a dissociation of the complex following penetration to the active site is thought to occur.

Not the least of the problems involved in the use of BAL is its own
toxicity, which requires that therapeutic administration be carefully man-
aged. When BAL is introduced in large dosages, it is believed to compete
with tissue SH groups and to interfere with cellular respiration, causing
tachypnea [2]. Competition for the metallic co-factors of metabolic enzyme
systems probably is also of importance. The administration of BAL to animals
with damaged livers results in toxic effects seen quickly and at low dosages.

Further investigations into the mechanism of action of BAL in all cellular systems seem warranted to clarify the problems currently presented.

SUMMARY AND CONCLUSION

Under the threat of poisonous gas warfare, studies to develop an antidote for lewisite intensified. Similarity in the effects of lewisite and
iodoacetate led to the view that enzyme thiol groups were the active site
of arsenical action. Studies with monothiols confirmed this, but administration failed to give adequate protection. Recognition of the need for
stable arsenic-thiol complexes stimulated investigations with dithiols of
low molecular size capable of forming five- or six-member cyclic compounds
with arsenic. The synthetic chemical 2,3-dimercaptopropanol (BAL) was
especially effective against lewisite's toxicity. BAL is rapidly metabo-
lized, but it still increased urinary excretion of arsenic and caused reversal of clinical signs. The toxic effects of BAL and the arsenic-thiol

and arsenite-BAL complex on certain biological systems present therapeutic cautions.

The logical and scientific development of this effective antidote to meet a specific need is a prime example of applied toxicological research.

REFERENCES

1. H. Eagle, J. Pharmacol., 66, 436 (1939).

2. G. T. Edds, Proc. Amer. Vet. Med. Ass., 149 (1950).

3. L. S. Goodman and A. Gilman, Pharmacological Basis of Therapeutics, 3rd Ed., Macmillan, New York, 1965, p. 933.

4. R. A. Peters, H. Rydin, and R. H. S. Thompson, Biochem. J., 29, 63 (1935).

5. L. Rapkine, C. R. Soc. Biol., Paris, 112, 1294 (1933).

6. F. O. Schmitt and R. K. Skow, Amer. J. Physiol., 11, 711 (1935).

7. L. A. Stocken and R. H. S. Thompson, Biochem. J., 40, 529 (1946).

8. L. A. Stocken and R. H. S. Thompson, Biochem. J., 40, 535 (1946).

9. L. A. Stocken and R. H. S. Thompson, Biochem. J., 40, 548 (1946).

10. W. I. Strangeway, Ann. Trop. Med., 31, 387 (1937).

11. E. Walker, Biochem. J., 22, 292 (1928).

12. J. L. Webb, Enzyme and Metabolic Inhibitors, Vol. III, Academic, New York, 1966, p. 645.

13. J. L. Webb, Enzyme and Metabolic Inhibitors, Vol. III, Academic, New York, 1966, p. 659.

A

Absorption, atomic, 4
Accumulator tissues, 17
Acromegaly, 759
Actinide elements, 607
Activity
  aminolevulinic acid dehydrase, 105
  grid crossing, 106
Adulterated product, 670
Albumin, 465
Alkali disease, 409, 446, 654
Alkaline earth metals, 553
  barium, 553
  beryllium, 553
  calcium, 553
  magnesium, 553
  radium, 553
  strontium, 553
Alkaline metals, 548
  cesium, 548
  francium, 548
  lithium, 548
  potassium, 548
  sodium, 548
Alpha particles, 893
Alternating current sparks, 871
Aluminum, 545, 594, 617
  absorption of, 594
  as a trace element, 30
Amaurotic epilepsy, 148
American Academy of Clinical Toxicology, 2
American College of Veterinary Toxicologists, 2
American Veterinary Medical Association, 2
Amino acids synthesis, 394
Amino-levulinate dehydratase, 650
Amino levulinic acid dehydrase, 156, 495

Analysis
  gas-liquid chromatographic, 4
  for mercury residues, 346
  neutron, 4
  neutron activation, 12, 14, 892, 895
  by public health officials, 175
  spectrographic, 544
Analytical limits, 4
Analytical methods, 4
Analyzers, 916, 919, 937
Analyzing crystals, 920
Anemia, 654
  hypochromic microcytic, 649
Anemia toxicosis, 648
Animal models, comparative studies of, 191
Animals, sentinel, 17
Anthracene compounds, 416
Antimony, 41, 601, 618
  body burden, 602
  stibine, 603
  in urban air, 602
Antimony hydride, 603
Antimony toxicity, 602
  occupational, 603
Argyria, 587
Arsanilic acid, 375-376
Arsanilic acid ingestion, 379
  clinical course, 381
  clinical signs, 379, 381
  pathologic changes, 384
Arsenic, 4, 9, 10, 30, 50, 52, 357, 450, 618, 654, 684
  absorption of, 70
  administration of dimercaprol, 72, 93
  biotransformation of, 71
  in blood, 366
  as capillary poison, 364

Part 1 comprises pages 1-515.
Part 2 comprises pages 517-952.

[Arsenic]
  carcinogen, 9
  differential, 368
  distribution, 70
  in drinking water, 362
  effects of selenium metabolism,
    654
  elimination of, 367
  embryocidal, 620
  excretion of, 71
  exencephaly, 620
  in food, 10
  formulations, 359
  inorganic, 619
  micrognathia, 620
  normal values, 367
  occurrence, 359
  organic, 620
  retention, 383
  safety margin, 360
  site-specific, 619
  with sulfhydryl, 364
  susceptibility, 359
  teratogenic, 620
  in tissue, 366
  toxic effects, 357
  uncoupling phosphorylation, 364
  urine content, 366-367
  in well water, 362
  whole blood content, 367
Arsenicals
  aliphatic, 357
  feed additives, 375
Arsenic poisoning, 359
  acute, 9, 360, 362, 366
  from arsenical dips, 363
  in children, 358
  chronic, 9, 360, 363
  diagnosis, 368
    Gutzeit method, 368
  histopathologic changes, 365
  in household pets, 358
  in man, 363
  nephrosis, 365
  pathologic changes, 365
  peracute, 362, 366
  percutaneous exposure, 365
  subacute syndrome, 360, 362, 366
  teratogenic effects, 364
  therapy, 369
    of large animals, 369
    of small animals, 369
Arsenic sources, 358

[Arsenic sources]
  arsenic trioxide, 358
  arsphenamine, 359
  copper acetoarsenite, 358
  dimethyl arsenic acid, 358
  dipping vats, 358
  disodium methanearsonate (DSMA),
    358
  grass clippings, 358
  insulation material, 358
  lead arsenate, 358
  medicaments, 358
  medicinal formulations, 358
  monosodium methanearsonate (MSMA),
    358
  paint pigments, 358
  pesticide, 358
  pyrites, 358
  ruminatorics, 358
  sodium arsenite, 358
  sulfides, 358, 654
Arsenic trioxide, 619
Arsenosis, chronic, 366
Arsine, 363-364
Ascorbic acid, 164
Ascorbic acid oxidase, 495
Atherosclerosis, 758
Atomic absorption, 825
  comparison of, 864
  detection limits, 822, 854
  flameless, 839
  interferences, 852
  sensitivity, 854
Atomic emission, comparison of, 864
Atomic fluorescence, comparison of,
  864
Atomic fluorescence signal, precision, 866
Atomization, 813
Auditory signal detection, 112

                          B

Background blood lead level, 158
Background emission, 815
Background tissue lead level, 159
  bovine, 159
  canine, 159
  equine, 159
  ovine, 159
  porcine, 159
  rumen contents, 159
  stomach contents, 159
BAL (dimercaprol), 372, 580, 605,
  607, 945
Bantu siderosis, 578

Baritosis, 558
Barium, 31, 557, 618
  absorption of, 557
Beryl, 543
Beryllium, 16, 31, 618
  absorption of, 543
  distribution of, 543
  in fluorescent lamp industry
      workers, 541
  as missile propellant, 541, 545
  soluble forms of, 543
  translocation of, 543
Beryllium alloys, 543
Beryllium disease, 541
  acute, 541
  case registry of, 542
  chronic, 542
  chronic toxicity, 543
  diagnosis of, 542
  diagnosis criteria
    clinical, 542
    epidemiologic, 542
  mechanism of, 542
  neighborhood cases, 542
  osteosarcomas, 544
  pulmonary granulomas, 544
  pulmonary tumors, 543-544
Beryllium oxide, 543
Beryllium phosphors, 542
Beta particles, 893
Bile, excretion by, 465
Binding sites, 69
Biological concentrations, quanti-
      tative analysis, 797
Bismuth, 32, 603, 618
  excretion, 604
  in urban air, 604
Bismuth telluride, 605
Blind staggers, 654
Bone decalcification, 205
Borax, 593
Boric acid, 593
Boron, 545, 592, 617
  dermal application, 593
  in food, 593
  industrial poisoning, 593
  oral administration, 593
  TLV values, 594
  as a trace element, 31, 56-57
  in water supplies, 593
Boron family, 592
  aluminum, 592
  boron, 592
  gallium, 592
  indium, 592
  thallium, 592

Boron hydrides, 545
Brain edema, 114, 155
Bremstralung, 917
British Antilewisite, 945
  therapeutic use, 950
Bromine, 32
Bromobenzene, 450
Bronchogenic carcinoma, 571
Burners
  diffusion, 806
  the flame, 808
  handling techniques, 808
  laminar, 806
  mechanical feed, 807
  nebulizer, 806, 835
  premix, 806
  total consumption, 806
  turbulent flow, 806

                    C

Cacodylic acid, toxicity of, 361
Cadmium, 32, 50, 52, 164, 454, 467,
      472, 618, 620, 633, 683
  accumulation of, 211
  acute, 10
  chronic, 11, 462
  cleft palate, 622
  clubfoot, 622
  content in tissues, 213
  daily intake of, 225
  detoxification by mercury, 656
  facial malformation, 621
  in food, 11
  in foodstuffs, 231
  geographical variation in, 229
  in grain, 11
  in Japanese foodstuffs, 226
  micrognathia, 622
  in night soil, 236, 238
  placental barrier, 621
  from polluted areas, 242
  as potent inhibitor, 620
  rib cage and limb bud defects, 621
  in rice, 217, 246
  in rice field soil, 222
  in shellfish, 230
  in silkworms, 245
  in wheat, 246
Cadmium content, in normal human,
  216
Cadmium salts, 411
Cadmium toxicity, 199
  characteristic symptoms, 200
  decreased inorganic phosphate, 200
  deformation period of, 209

Part 1 comprises pages 1-515.
Part 2 comprises pages 517-952.

[Cadmium toxicity]
  history, 200
  increased alkaline phosphatase,
    200
  incubation period of, 208
  Kamioka Mine, 203
  kitchen of patient, 204
  multiple fractures period of, 209
  osteomalacia, 200, 201, 208
  painful period of, 209
  renal dysfunction, 200
  sedimentation pool, 204
  sweet potato leaves, 206
  warning period of, 209
  x-ray photograph of, 211, 256
Cadmium uptake
  by rice, 247-248
  by wheat, 247-248
Cadmium and zinc, antagonism be-
    tween, 651
Cadmium-induced toxemia, pregnancy,
    656
Calcium, 110, 471, 649
  diets, 649
  EDTA (ethylenediaminetetraacetic
    acid), 157, 163, 506, 580
  environmental problems, 649
  microscopic deposits of, 400
Calcium metabolism, of rats, 248,
    250-254
Calcium phosphorus, 164
Calibration curve, 820
Cancer induction, 437
Canine distemper, 154
Carbon family, 598
  carbon, 598
  germanium, 598
  lead, 598
  silicon, 598
  tin, 598
Carbon rod furnace, 841, 843, 846
Carcinomas, 438
Cardiovascular hypertension, 11
Catalase, 461, 650
Cellular respiration, 951
Cerebrospinal changes, 157
Cerebrospinal fluid analyses, 183
Ceresan M, 331
Cerium, 32, 559
Ceruloplasmin, 461, 463, 492, 493-
    494
Cesium, 34, 549, 552
  absorption, 552

Chelating agents, 93, 506
Chelation, 853
Chemiluminescence, 814, 853
Chisso Corporation, 261
  acetaldehyde production of, 289
Chlorine, 33
Choppers, 846
Chromium, 15, 33, 50, 52, 56-57,
    545, 568, 689
  absorption, 569, 691
  birth effects, 695
  body burden, 569
  chemistry of, 689
  concentration in air, 569
  diagnostic uses, 696
  distribution, 691
  essentiality, 690
  excretion, 691
  glucose metabolism, 693
  growth, 695
  health effects, 693
  homeostatic mechanism, 569
  lipid metabolism, 694
  longevity, 695
  metabolism, 691
  protein synthesis, 695
  skin allergy, 570
  valence states, 568
Closed-field maze, 113
Cobalt, 33, 50, 52, 56-57, 456, 580,
    617, 696
  absorption, 581
  air concentration, 581
  cardiomyopathy, 581
  chemistry of, 696
  determination of, 700
  diagnostic tests, 699
  elevated B12 conditions, 702
  erythropoietic factor, 702
  essentiality, 697
  excretion, 581
  goiter, 581
  health effects, 699
  hyperglycemia, 702
  industrial exposure, 582
  malabsorption problems, 701
  metabolism, 698
  polycythemia, 581
Cobalt and iron, antagonism between,
    661
Collimating lens, 818
Collimators, 919
Collision, 814
Columbium, 566
Condensing lens, 815
Conditioned response behavior, 114

Congenital Minamata disease
  incomplete cases of, 289
  mental retardation, 289
  patients, mothers of, 276
Conjunctivitis, 542
Contaminated foods, 12
Continuous sources, 859
Coordination compounds, 69
Copper, 16, 34, 50, 52, 56-57, 60,
    455, 460, 462, 472, 491, 545,
    617, 622, 650, 684, 702
  absorption of, 464, 650, 654
  anemia, 708
  animal waste, 649
  bone formation, 709
  cardiovascular disorders, 711
  chemistry of, 702
  cuproenzymes, 707
  cuproproteins, 707
  dietary absorption, 662
  dietary factors, 496
  essentiality, 703
  excretion, 494
  fertility, 710
  health effects, 708
  heart malformations, 622
  interaction with cobalt, 491
  interaction with manganese, 491
  interaction with molybdenum, 491,
    504, 643
  interaction with sulfate, 491
  keratinization, 494, 710
  liver, 494, 503
  metabolism, 465, 494, 705
  in mice, 505
  neonatal ataxia, 709
  pigmentation of hair and wool,
    710
  physiological antagonism, 642,
    650
  in rats, 492, 505
  relation with inorganic sulfate,
    492
  relation with iron, 491-492, 504
  relation with Vitamin A, 494
  relation with zinc, 491-492, 504
  scouring of cattle, 711
  storage of, 646
  sulfate, 495, 504
Copper accumulation, liver lyso-
    somes, 503
Copper deficiency, 463, 491, 496,
    498, 660
  abnormal wool growth, 496
  amine oxidase, 497
  anemia, 496
[Copper deficiency]
  ascorbic acid, 499
  bone disorders, 496
  cardiovascular defects, 496-497
  cytochrome oxidase, 497
  depressed growth, 496
  desmosine, 497
  elastin, 497
  enzootic ataxia, 496
  falling disease, 497
  gastrointestinal disturbances, 496
  hair and wool depigmentation, 496
  heart failure, 496
  impaired reproductive performance,
    496
  neonatal ataxia, 496
  swayback, 496
Copper metabolism, lead interfer-
    ence, 662
Copper/molybdenum ratios, 498, 501
Copper-molybdenum-sulfate interac-
    tion, 495
Copper sulfate, treatment of teart,
    642
Copper thiomolybdate, 648
Copper toxicity, 466, 491, 493, 499,
    505, 648
  acute, 502
  analytical techniques, 506
  anemia, 491, 493-494
  aquatic vegetation, 506
  blood copper concentration, 502
  Bordeaux mixture, 501
  chronic, 502, 645
  copper chloride, 501
  copper-molybdenum imbalance, 500
  copper sulfate, 501
  dietary protein, 493
  dogs, 505
  fish, 505-506
  glutathione, 503
  hemoglobinemia, 501
  hemoglobinuria, 501
  hemolysis, 491
  hemolytic crisis, 500, 502-504
  hepatic necrosis, 491
  hepatogenous poisoning, 500
  icterus, 491, 501
  jaundice, 502, 504
  liver, 504
  Lupinus, 500
  methemoglobin, 503
  morbidity, 501
  mortality, 501
  nonruminant animals, 504
  physiopathology, 502

Part 1 comprises pages 1-515.
Part 2 comprises pages 517-952.

[Copper toxicity]
  postmortem changes, 502
  poultry, 504
  pyrrolizidine alkaloids, 500
  renal necrosis, 491
  retinol, 494
  in ruminant animals, 499
  serum enzyme, 502
  Trifolium subterraneum, 499
Corrections
  filler gas, 848
  hydrogen gas, 848
Crystal scintillation counters,
    901-902
Cutaneous adnexa, 411
Cyano (methylmercuri) guanidine,
    331, 345
Cysteine, 946
Cystine, 643, 645
Cytochrome oxidase, 492, 495, 650
  cytochrome c oxidase, 461, 464

                    D

Dancing-cat disease, 266
Decaborane, 545
Decaborane toxicity
  central nervous system signs, 545
  symptoms, 545
Deferoxamine, 580
Degeneration, axonal, 115
Delta-aminolevulinic acid, 156
Demethylation, 14
Demyelination, 115, 386, 497
  segmental, 115
Densitometer, 886
Dental fluorosis, 523
  degrees of, 523
Depletion region, 903
Dermatitis, 542
Desolvation, 811
Detection limits, 887
  activation analysis, 892
  for analytical techniques, 935
  of atomic emission spectrophotom-
    eter, 866
  of atomic fluorescence, 866
  mass spectrometry, 934
Detectors, 819, 939
  barrier layer, 904
  diffused junction, 904
  lithium-drifted, 905
  semiconductor, 902

[Detectors]
  x-ray fluorescence spectrometry,
    921
Dietary intakes, 7, 8
Dietary selenium, protective effect
    against mercury, 657
Diethylenetriaminepentaacetate
    (DTPA), 580
Dilution, 821
Dimercaprol (BAL), 372, 580, 605,
    607, 945
Dimercaptopropanol, 948, 949
Dimethyl mercury, 91
Dimethylselenide, 449
Diphenylselenium, 658
Direct current arc, 871
Discharge tubes, 872
Dispersion, 818
Dissociation, 812
Dithiols, 948
Dogs, bone lesions in, 182, 185
Dopamine-B-hydroxylase, 495
Doppler broadening, 833
Dose-response relationships, 98
Drift tube, 898
Dry material, ash in, 54
Double-beam operation, 847, 849
Duodenal mucosal protein, 650
Dysprosium, 34, 559

                    E

Effects
  mutagenic, 164
  organomercurials on genetic
    material, 321
  organomercurials on mammalian
    central nervous system, 324
  teratogenic, 164
Electroencephalographic changes,
    157, 182
Electron multiplier
  Cohen-type, 939
  Wiley, 940
Elements
  ballast, 29
  micronutrient, 28
Embryopathic effects, 164
Encephalomalacia, 451
Encephalopathy, 184, 194
Entrance slits, 815
Environmental concentrations, quan-
    titative analysis, 797
Environmental contamination, by
    industry, 654
Enzymatic blocking, 5

Epidemiological investigation, 18
Epilepsy, 759
Erbium, 34, 559
Erythrocuprein, 494
Essential biological proteins, 69
Ethylenediaminetetraacetic acid
    (EDTA), 157, 163, 506, 580
Ethyl mercuric phosphate, 625
N-(Ethylmercuri)-p-toluene sulfon-
    anilide, 331, 333
Europium, 34, 559
Excitation, 814
Exit slits, 819
Extraneous light, 819
Exudative diathesis, 451, 735
    chicks, 401
    lesions of, 401

F

Ferbam, 576
Ferritin, 650
Ferroxidase, 493
Fetal malformations, 11
Fish protein concentrate, 626
Flame composition, 815
Flame emission, 800
    detection limits, 822
    sample solutions, 805
Flashback, 804
Flow meters, 805
Fluorescence intensities, 858
Fluorescence principle, 857
Fluorescence radiation, 858
Fluorescence, x-ray, 916
Fluoride concentration
    fetal blood, 521
    maternal blood, 521
Fluoride sources, 519
    forage levels of fluorine, 520
    plant translocation, 520
    water, 520
Fluoride toxicosis, 517
    acute, 522
    chemical analyses, 537
    chronic, 523
    control of, 537
    diagnostic aids, 536
    factors of, 523
    general condition, 535
    lameness and stiffness, 532
    method of sampling, 532
    prevention, 537
    radiographic findings, 533
    structural bone changes, 532
Fluorides, 517

[Fluorides]
    beneficial effects, 519
    in bone, 526
    distribution in body, 520
    in fetus, 521
    gastrointestinal absorption, 520
    in milk, 534
    normal ingestion, 517
    organic, 517
    recovery from exposure, 534
    in tissues, 521
    tolerance, 536
    in urine, 534
Fluorine, 35, 50, 52, 517, 713
    aortic calcification, 716
    chemistry, 713
    dental caries, 715
    essentiality, 519, 714
    fertility, 716
    health effects, 715
    hematocrits, 716
    metabolism, 715
    osteoporosis, 716
Food additive, 670
Food contaminants, 3
    tolerances for, 671
Food and Drug Administration, 5, 10,
    13-15
    guidelines, 11
Foods
    of animal origin, 395
    content of, 14
Fresh produce, dry material in, 54

G

Gadolinium, 35, 559
Gallium, 35, 595
    absorption of, 595
    in drinking water, 595
    excretion, 595
    therapeutic use, 595
Gamma rays, 894
Gastrointestinal system, 143, 152
Geiger-Muller counters, 925
Geiger-Muller tube, 926
Germanite, 598
Germanium, 35, 598
    in drinking water, 598
    industrial hazard, 599
    in urban atmosphere, 598
Germanium toxicity, 598
Glucose tolerance factor, 690
Glutathione, 946
    metabolism, 417
Glutathione peroxidase, 397, 452, 660

Part 1 comprises pages 1-515.
Part 2 comprises pages 517-952.

Gold, 31, 588
Gold toxicity, 589
Grain, seed, and forage plants,
    percent ash of, 60
Granulomatous interstitial pneu-
    monitis, 542
Grating mountings, 882
Group IIB, 589
  cadmium, 589
  mercury, 589
  zinc, 589
Group IVB, 561
  hafnium, 561
  titanium, 561
  zirconium, 561
Group VB, 564
  tantalum, 564
  vanadium, 564
Group VIB, 568
  chromium, 568
  molybdenum, 568
  tungsten, 568
Group VIIB, 572
  manganese, 572
  rhenium, 572
  technetium, 572
Group VIII, 576
  cobalt, 576
  iron, 576
  nickel, 576

                    H

Hafnium, 35, 564
Hazardous containers, removal of,
    18
Heavy metals, 3, 669
  absorption of, 69
  biological effects, 2
  biological interactions, 2
  control points, 18-19
  decontamination, 17
  delayed teratogenic effects, 632
  digestive system, 70
  distribution, 69
  environmental contamination, 649
  environmental effects, 617
  epidemiological model, 5
  fate, 69
  perseverance, 2
  persistence, 1, 2
  physicochemical characteristics, 5

[Heavy metals]
  reactions with ligands, 69
  redistribution, 3
  teratogenicity of, 617-618
  threshold nature, 96
  toxic, 5
  translocation of, 93
Heavy metal intoxication, epidemi-
    ology, 5
Heavy metal toxicants
  safety measures, 16
  surveillance, 16
Hebb-Williams maze, 108
Hematopoietic system, 143, 152
Hemoglobin formation, 659
Hemoglobin synthesis, 493
Hepatic cancer, 430
Hepatic cirrhosis, selenium-induced,
    413-415, 442
Hepatic neoplasia, 413-415, 438
Hepatitis
  acute toxic, 411, 440
  chronic toxic, 411, 414, 440
Hepatolenticular degeneration, 505.
Hepatosis diatetica, 452, 736
Hip-pocket reactor, 900
Hodgkin's disease, 713
Holmium, 36, 559
Horses, grazing habits of, 175
Hunter-Russell syndrome, 273
Hydrogen selenide, 394
Hyperplasia, toxic, 411
Hypogeusia, 759

                    I

Inclusion bodies, 110, 148, 156
Inclusions, acid-fast intranuclear,
    157
Indicator plants, 629
Indium, 595
  absorption of, 596
Indium toxicity, 596
Industrial lead operations, 173
Infertility, 164
Initial lesions, 400
Inorganic arsenicals, 357
  uses of, 361
Inorganic compound, solubility, 69
Inorganic mercury, history of, 303
Inorganic tin, 600
Insoluble compound formation, 853
Interactions
  iron, 110
  lead, 143

Interferences
  chemical, 853
  physical, 853
  spectral, 853
Intoxications, food-borne, 3
Iodine, 36
Ion source, 936
Iraq, mercury compounds in, 624, 628
Iridium, 585
Iron, 457, 545, 576, 617, 649, 650, 721
  absorption of, 457, 493, 577, 654
  chemistry of, 721
  essentiality, 722
  excretion, 577
  ferritin in, 458
  health effects, 725
  inhalation exposure, 578
  iron-bind capacity, 725
  metabolism, 724
  serum or plasma iron decrease, 725
  serum or plasma iron increase, 725
  transferrin in, 458
  in urban air, 577
  in water, 577
Iron deficiency, 493
Iron metabolism, 659
Iron toxicity, 459
  acute, 579
Itai-itai disease, 11, 199
  animal experiments, 205
  case of, 210
  at endemic area, 221
  identification of, 208
  in mining districts, 206
  patients, distribution of, 224
  relation to agricultural damage, 202
  urinary findings, 222
  zinc and cadmium in patients, 215

J

Jaundice, 649

K

Kaschin-Beck disorder, 579
Kerateine, 947
Keratogenesis, 756
Kidney, 70, 157, 159, 185
  excretion, 70

L

Lactase, 495
Laminar neuronal necrosis, 155
Lamps
  electrodeless discharge, 859
  high density, 830
  hollow cathode, 859
  life of, 831
  multiple element, 831
Lanthanons, 558
  actinium, 558
  lanthanum, 558
  scandium, 558
  yttrium, 558
Lanthanum, 36, 559
Laryngeal paralysis, 150
Lead, 12, 39, 50, 52, 56-57, 101, 143, 462, 545, 618, 622, 633, 683
  absorption of, 72, 125, 181, 192
  accumulation of, 211
  air levels, 102
  analysis of, 158
  biotransformation, 73
  in blood, 156
  blood level, 127
  brain residue, 103
  chelating agents, 74, 132
  content in tissues, 213
  daily intake, 12
  delayed ossification, 623
  distribution, 72
  elimination, 156
  encephalopathy, 103-104
  in environment, 101
  excretion, 73, 125
  intrauterine growth retardation, 623
  metabolism of, 125
  neurological defects, 623
  neuropathy, 182
  from polluted areas, 242
  porphyrin metabolism, 130
  porphyrinuria, 73
  postnatal failure to thrive, 624
  rainwater residue, 102
  reproductive effects of, 163
  residues, 163
  in silkworms, 245
  tail malformation, 623
  therapeutic recommendations, 128-129
  tolerance of, 192
  toxic effects, 12

Part 1 comprises pages 1-515.
Part 2 comprises pages 517-952.

[Lead]
  treatment, 131
  uptake, 156
  uses of, 144
Lead analysis, hair, 158
Lead as inhibitor, heme synthetase, 94
Lead line, 154
Lead poisoning, 123, 161, 173, 179, 368, 467
  abortions in sheep, 154
  acute, 123, 134
    in adults, 134
  age relationship, 147
  analysis of blood, 157
  anemia, 156, 182
  anorexia, 114
  ataxia, 114
  bone marrow, 156
  cases of, 137-139
  cats, 145, 147, 188
  cattle, 145, 173
  central nervous system, 194
  in children, 103, 124
  chronic, 123-124, 174
  clinical signs, 114, 143, 152, 154, 182
  convulsions, 114
  delayed response, 114
  diagnosis, 127, 157
  dogs, 111, 147, 179
  ducks, 148
  equine, 145, 147, 173
  foals, 152
  hematologic changes in dogs, 182
  hyperactivity, 104
  lead shot, 148, 152
  mallards, 148
  pathologic changes, 155-157, 163
  primates, 114, 145, 148
  prognosis, 162
  seasonal increase in cattle, 145
  sheep, 112, 145
  susceptibility, 164
  treatment of dogs, 184
  urban, 147
  wildfowl, 145
Lead poisoning morbidity, bovine, 146
Lead poisoning mortality, bovine, 146
Lead poisoning susceptibility
  iron, 164

[Lead poisoning susceptibility]
  nicotinic acid, 164
  protein, 164
  zinc, 164
Lead residues
  in milk, 163
  in muscle, 163
Lead sources
  forages, 147, 149
  gasoline, 149
  grease, 149
  mines, 147
  motor oil, 149
  paint, 149, 181, 617
  pasture grass, 175
  petroleum, 150
  smelters, 147
  soil, 152, 175
  trash, 150
  vegetation, 174
Lesions, 155
  experimentally produced, 401
  gross, 384
  microscopic, 384
Lethargy, 114
Leucoencephalomyelosis, 148
Lewisite, 945
Line broadening, 832
Lipid peroxidation, 418
Lipid peroxides, 453
Lithium, 36-37, 50, 549, 630
  absorption of, 549
  in chick embryos, 630
  daily intake, 549
  excretion, 549
  in frogs, 630
  in mice, 630
  in mothers, 630
  in rats, 630
  therapeutic use, 550
  in toads, 630
Lithium toxicity, 550
Liver, 70, 157, 159
  as a body filter, 70
  as a detoxifier, 70
Liver catalase, 492
Liver necrosis, 452, 660
Lorentz broadening, 834
Lung cancer, 361, 571
Lupine toxicosis, 500
Lutetium, 37, 559

M

Magnesium, 545, 553
  absorption of, 554

[Magnesium]
  excretion, 554
  intoxication, 555
Mammary adenocarcinomas, 440, 442
Mammary cancer, 430
Manganese, 15, 37, 461, 545, 572,
      631, 647, 716
  body burden, 573
  bone growth, 719
  carbohydrate metabolism, 720
  central nervous system, 574
  chemistry, 716
  chronic nervous system effects,
      575
  dietary, 659
  essentiality, 717
  excretion, 573
  in guinea pigs, 631
  in hamsters, 631
  health effects, 719
  industrial toxicity, 574
  lipid metabolism, 721
  metabolism, 718
  neonatal ataxia, 720
  Parkinson-like syndrome, 575
  in rats, 631
  reproductive function, 719
  urban air, 573
  water supplies, 573
Mask, 815
Mass analyzer, ion microprobe, 932
Mass spectrometer, electromagnetic,
      936
Mass spectrometry, spark source, 933
Menkes kinky hair syndrome, 712
Mercaptans, 76
Mercurial fungicides, 331
Mercurialism, chronic, 13
Mercurial pollution, Niigata,
      Japan, 627
Mercuric salts, 405
Mercury, 35-36, 50, 53, 467, 618,
      624, 682
  absorption of, 74
  analysis of, 334
  behavioral emotionality, 624
  bioaccumulators of, 13
  biotransformation, 75
  in blood, 335
  in cats, 626
  cerebellum malformations, 625-626
  cerebral palsy-like disease, 627
  chelating agents, 77
  chemical characteristics of, 304
  cleft palates, 624, 626
  delayed rib calcification, 625

[Mercury]
  distribution, 75
  dithiols, 77
  in dogs, 626
  elimination, 345
  embryotic growth retardation, 625
  environmental considerations of,
      307
  excretion, 76
  fetal anomalies, 626
  in food, 15
  half-life of, 336
  in hamsters, 633
  kinetics, 77
  locomotor activity, 624
  miscarriages, 627
  neurons of brain, 624
  omphalocele, 626
  physical characteristics of, 304
  physiopathology, 308
  placental passage, 627
  poisoning, 332-334, 454
  residues, 332, 334, 337, 340, 344,
      346
  retention of, 334
  in sows, 626
  in tissues, 345
  uses of, 306
Mercury content
  in hair, 267
  in human organs, 267
  of Minamata Bay shellfish, 289
  in umbilical cords, 268
Mercury poisoning, 339, 658
  acute, 13, 334, 338
  in chickens, 344, 348
  diagnosis of, 310
  induced, 332
  New Mexico residents, 627
  pathologic changes, 344
  sheep, 338, 347
  signs of, 346, 353
  treatment of, 311
  in turkeys, 343
Mercury residues
  in chickens, 349
  in chicks, 352
  in hens, 352
  in sheep, 347
Mercury sources
  commercial, 305
  environmental, 305
Metabolic interactions among heavy
      metals, 662
Metal compounds
  long-term effects, 87

Part 1 comprises pages 1-515.
Part 2 comprises pages 517-952.

[Metal compounds]
  low-level effects, 87
Metalloids, 4
Metallothionein, 464, 651
  biochemical function of, 651
Metals
  competitive binding of, 473
  sources of, 173
  translocation of, 98
Metals in food, guidelines, 5
Metaphyseal sclerosis, 157
Metarubricytes, 183
Methionine, 643, 645
Methyl mercury, 13, 264, 624
  biological half-life of, 298
Methyl mercury compound, 264
Methyl mercury consumption, safe
    level of, 297
Methyl mercury dicyandiamide, 625
Methyl mercury poisoning, 270
Micromelia, 619
Micronutrients, 5, 15
Microprobe
  electron, 929
  ion, 931
Minamata area, neurological symp-
    toms of inhabitants, 285
Minamata disease, 261, 270, 624
  chronic, 290
  congenital, 276
  Hunter and Russell, 291
  Hunter and workers, 262
Minimum cumulative fatal dosage,
    174
Molybdate, in salt licks, 645
Molybdenosis, 37, 498, 642, 647
Molybdenum, 37, 50, 53, 56-57, 617,
    628, 726
  absorption of, 644
  anemia, 728
  chemistry, 726
  essentiality, 726
  health effects, 728
  metabolism, 727
  in newborn lambs, 628
  physiological antagonism, 642
  renal calculi, 729
  retention, 644
  urinary excretion, 644-645
Molybdenum excess
  achromotrichia, 497
  anemia, 497
  bone rarification, 497

[Molybdenum excess]
  degeneration of spinal cord, 497
  emaciation, 497
  hemosiderosis, 497
  liquid diarrhea, 497
  osteoporosis, 497
  swollen genitalia, 497
Molybdenum poisoning, 644-645
  chronic, 492
Monoamine oxidase, 463, 495
Monochromators, 818, 879
Monoethylmercury, 89
Monothiols, 946, 948
Murine pneumonia, chronic, 415
Muscular dystrophy, nutritional, 451
Muscular weakness, 114
Myelin, 495
Myocardial nutritional myopathy,
    lesions of, 399

                    N

Natural line width, 833
Nebulizer burner
  boling type, 838
  circular, 860
  lundegardh type, 836
  nitrous oxide type, 838
  ultrasonic nebulization, 860
Necropsies' results, 155
Neodymium, 38, 559
Neoplasia, percentage incidence of,
    438
Nephropathy, 193
Nervous system, 143, 152
Neurologic disorders, 154, 182
Neurologic manifestations, 103
Neuropathy, 384
Neutron activation, 10
Neutron activation analysis, sensi-
    tivity calculation, 914
Neutron generators, 896, 898
Neutron sources
  direct, 899
  isotopic, 898-899
Neutrons, 894
  thermal, 896
Nickel, 15, 38, 50, 53, 58-59, 545,
    582, 631, 729
  accumulation, 583
  body burden, 583
  chemistry, 729
  essentiality, 730
  health effects, 732
  metabolism, 731
  occupational carcinogen, 584

Nickel carbonyl, 583
Nickel itch, 583
Nickelous acetate, 631
Night soil, 234
Niobium, 38, 566
Nitrilotriacetic acid (NTA), 506
3-Nitro-4-hydroxyphenylarsonic
    acid, 375
Nitrogen family, 601
  antimony, 601
  arsenic, 601
  bismuth, 601
  nitrogen, 601
  phosphorus, 601
Noble metals, 587
  copper, 587
  gold, 587
  silver, 587
Nonaccumulator plants, 395, 629
Normal background levels, 158
Nuclear reactors, 896
Nucleated red blood cells, 154
Nutritional myopathy, 398
  clinical signs of, 399
  incidence of, 399
  lesions of, 399
  muscles affected, 399

                O

Occupational exposure, laboratory
    tests of, 136
Organic arsenicals, 375, 450
  absorption, 376
  clinical syndrome, 379
  excretion, 376
  metabolism, 376
  pathologic changes, 384
  route of excretion, 379
  tissue distribution, 379
  tissue residues, 383
  trivalent, 363
  urinary excretion, 377
Organic arsenical herbicides, 360
Organic chemicals, bioaccumulation
    of, 3
Organic mercurial, history of, 311
Organic mercurial ingestion, cases
    of, 312, 316
Organic tin, 600
Organomercurials
  in environment, 317
  toxicogenic mechanisms of, 320
Osmium, 585-586
Osmium tetroxide, 585
Osteofluorotic lesions, 526

Osteoporosis, 154
Osteosarcomas, result of beryllium,
    544
Oxidative phosphorylation, 71
Oxygen family, 605
  oxygen, 605
  polonium, 605
  selenium, 605
  sulfur, 605
  tellurium, 605

                P

Palladium, 16, 585-586
Panogen, 15, 331
Parakeratosis, 468, 649
Peat scours, 643
Pentaborane, 545
Peridontal disease, 736
Periodic table, 548
Peripheral neuropathy, 193
Peters, 945, 947
Phenylmercuriacetate, 658
Phospholipids, 495
Photographic plates, 880
Photon spread, 925
Phototubes, 880
Phytate, 471
Placenta, 156, 163
Plants
  geothermal power, 10
  selenium-accumulator, 10
Plasma, 873
  thermal isolation, 876
Plasma flame, 875
Plasma formation, 873
Plasma jets, 873
Platinosis, 586
Platinum, 16, 40, 585
Platinum-group metals, 584
  iridium, 584
  osmium, 584
  palladium, 584
  platinum, 584
  rhodium, 584
  ruthenium, 584
Poisonous substances, distinction
    between, 671
Polonium, 40
Posterior paresis, 381
Praseodymium, 40, 559
Pressure broadening, 834
Pressure gauges, 805
Prism mountings, 881
Promethium, 40, 559
Proportional counters, 927-929

Part 1 comprises pages 1-515.
Part 2 comprises pages 517-952.

Prostaglandin synthesis, 713
Protein-binding sites, 650
   competition for, 651
Protein precipitation, 69
Protoporphyrinemia, 94
Psoriasis, 713
Pulmonary granulomas, result of
      beryllium, 544

                    R

Radiation, white, 917
Radiative, 814
Radioactive atoms, 913
Radioactive decay, 912
Radioactivity measurement, units,
      893
Radiograph examination, 163
Radioruthenium chloride, 586
Radium, 40
Rare earths, 558
Rats
   behavior of, 108
   mental retardation of, 109
   paraplegia in, 107
Renal necrosis, 657
Resins, ion exchange, 853
Resolution, 815
Resonance fluorescence, 858
Resonance line, 800
Reversal, 806
Rhenium, 40, 576
Rhodium, 584, 586
   in embryos, 631
   micromelia, 631
Roaring, in horses, 152
Rotameters, 805
Rubidium, 40, 549, 551
   absorption, 551
   daily intake, 551
   excretion, 551
Ruthenium, 41, 584

                    S

Samarium, 42, 559
Sarcomas, 414
Sarcomere, 400
   degeneration, 400
Scandium, 41
Selenide, vitamin E as protector,
      417

Selenite
   dietary supplementation, 430
   high concentration, 433
   varying amounts of, 428
Selenium, 4, 15, 41, 50, 53, 446,
      617, 629, 660, 685, 732
   absorption of, 77, 396
   administration, 398
   annual release of, 395
   anticarcinogenic, 437
   antiinflammation, 405
   as an antioxidant, 417
   arsenic interference, 411
   bilateral club feet, 630
   biological use of, 396
   biologically active, 394
   biotransformation, 78
   blind staggers, 448
   in calves, 629
   cancer, 737
   as a carcinogenic agent, 415
   carcinogenic potential of, 413
   in cats, 629
   chemistry, 732
   chick embryo, 410
   as a cirrhotic agent, 415
   content in air, 395
   content in surface water, 395
   deficiency of, 451
   dietary concentration of, 396
   distribution of, 77, 403
   effects on reproduction, 404, 410
   electron transport chain, 417
   as essential element, 393, 733
   excessive amounts, 427
   excretion of, 79, 397
   excretory pathway of, 396
   feed efficiency, 402
   fertility, 736
   in foals, 629
   in foods, 395
   function, 418
   gastric cancer, 415
   in guinea pigs, 630
   health effects, 735
   heart disease, 738
   hemostatic mechanism, 416
   human cancer, 416
   in humans, 403, 630
   incidence of cancer, 440
   ingestion amount, 428, 430
   Islets of Langerhans, 630
   lethal dose, 407
   lipid therapy, 416
   in liver, 428, 430, 432

[Selenium]
  metabolism, 734
  methylation of, 92
  miscarriages, 630
  muscular dystrophy, 735
  neoplasm development, 440
  non-toxic amounts, 416
  nutritional requirements, 416
  pharmaceutical amounts, 412
  in plant soils, 398
  as protection, 397
  ration concentration, 430
  in rats, 629
  responsive diseases, 398
  responsive unthriftiness, 736
  restricted use of, 427
  in sheep, 630
  in skeletal muscle, 428
  sparing of, 402
  sterility, 404
  sulfhydryl, 79
  sulfur replacement, 78
  in swine, 629
  therapeutic response to, 400
  toxic concentration, 410, 412
  toxic exposures, 407
  toxicity, 446-447
  transportation of cadmium, 404
  valence state of, 393
  in yeast feed, 428
Selenium absorber plants, secondary,
    629
Selenium accumulation
  in muscle, 432
  self-regulating mechanism, 432
  self-regulation, 432
Selenium accumulator plants
  primary, 395
  secondary, 395
Selenium carcinogenesis, bioassay
    of, 413, 437
Selenium concentration, 396
  cancer, 433
Selenium deficiency, 398, 401, 438
  hypovascularization, 442
  in people, 403
  in rats, 402
  reduced viability of chicks, 405
  in turkey poults, 401
Selenium depletion regimen, 428,
    438
Selenium dioxide, 393, 658
Selenium/methyl mercury ratio, 14
Selenium poisoning, 656, 658
  accidental, 407

[Selenium poisoning]
  acute, 407, 654
  ancient cases of, 406
  blind staggers, 408
  cattle, 409
  chronic, 409, 654
  concomitant conditions, 406
  congenital malformations, 410
  lesions of, 407-408
  primary, 430
  protection, 397
  rats, 408, 410
  shoats, 408
  subacute, 408
  supportive therapy, 412
  therapy, 412
  toxic effects, 406
  toxicity criteria, 406
  vascular lesions of, 410
Selenium retention, 432
Selenium salts, pharmacologic and
    medical uses, 415
Selenium therapy, 404
Selenomethionine, 397
Seleno-trisulfide, 394
Sensitized fluorescence, 858
Shaver's disease, 594
Silicon, 41, 545, 739
  chemistry, 739
  essentiality, 740
  health effects, 741
  metabolism, 740
  urolithiasis, 741
Silver, 15, 30, 456, 467, 545, 587,
    618, 660
Silver acetate, 660
Silver nitrate, 660
Sodium, 38, 545
Sodium arsanilate, 375-376
Sodium arsenate, 654
  genitourinary abnormalities, 620
  hamsters, 620
  skeletal malformations, 620
Sodium arsenite, 619, 654
  lethal dose, 360
Sodium thiacetarsamide, 360
Soluble selenates, 393
Spectra
  band, 869
  gamma ray, 911
  line, 869
Spectral interference, 819
Spectrograph, 880
Spectrographic analysis, 200, 544
Spectrophotometer, 880

Part 1 comprises pages 1-515.
Part 2 comprises pages 517-952.

Spectrophotometry, atomic absorp-
    tion, 11, 507
Spectroscopy
  arc emission, 868
  atomic, 11
  atomic absorption, 12
  atomic fluorescence, 856
  gamma ray, 909
  optical emission, 12
Spectrum, continuous, 869
Spermatogenesis, 404
Sphalerite, 590
Squirrel monkeys, 402
Standard addition (spike), 821
Stark effect, 834
Stippling, 154, 182
Stray light, 819
Strontianite, 556
Strontium, 42, 58-59, 556
Sulfate, 449
  inorganic, 646
Sulfhydryl groups, 69, 71, 412
Superoxide dismutase, 464
Swayback, 643
Swine
  deficiency syndrome of, 400
  selenium concentrations in, 401

                    T

Tantalum, 567
Tantalum strip technique, 841-842
Teart, 492, 641
Tellurium, 605, 618, 631
  in ewes, 631
  in human organs, 606
  in rats, 631
Tellurium toxicity, 606
Temperature changes, 152
Terata, 617
Teratogen
  nonspecific, 618
  site-specific, 618
Teratogenesis
  effects of heavy metal interac-
      tion, 632
  molybdenum with copper and sulfur,
      632
  special mechanism of, 618
Teratology, behavioral, 634
Terbium, 42, 559
Testicular necrosis, 11, 655
Tetraethyllead, 88, 135

[Tetraethyllead]
  dealkylation, 88
Thallium, 43, 596, 632
  absorption of, 80
  animal tissues, 596
  biotransformation, 81
  in chick embryos, 632
  diphenylthiocarbazone, 82
  distribution, 80
  excretion, 82, 596
  interference with sulfur, 81
Thallium toxicity, 455, 597
  acute, 597
  chronic, 597
  occupational, 597
Thiol groups, 946
Thiol-proteins, 948
Thiomolybdate, 648
Thiosulfate, 643, 645
Thorium, 607
Thulium, 43, 559
Tin, 15, 42, 545, 599, 741
  body burden, 599
  chemistry, 741
  essentiality, 742
  growth effect, 743
  health effects, 744
  inhalation, 601
  metabolism, 742
  in urban air, 599
Tin toxicity, 600
Tissue lead levels, 126
  in birds, 162
  in domestic animals, 159, 161
Titanicosis, 562
Titanium, 15, 43, 545, 561, 632
  in rats, 632
Toxicants
  metal, 145
  removal of, 17
Toxic element, dietary level, 641
Toxic mechanism, 5
Toxicology, 97
Trace element data
  reliability of, 45-47
  statistical analysis of, 47-49
Trace elements
  action levels of, 672
  background level of, 669
  beneficial effects, 689
  biological magnification, 674
  control of, 673
  establishing a tolerance, 673
  in fruits and vegetables, 52-53
  in grain, seed, and forage plants,
      56-59

[Trace elements]
  interaction among, 641
  level in edible tissues, 673
  mixing of food, 672
  need of, 641
  nutritional sufficiency of, 59
  regulations, 670
  regulatory aspects of, 669, 682
  regulatory policy, 669
  sources, 674
  surveys, 669
  tolerances of, 641
  translocation of, 675
  uniform national level, 669
  USDA control of, 675
  in wheat grains, 50
Triga Mark I reactor, 897
Trimethylselenide, 449
Tungsten, 571
Tyrosinase, 463, 495

U

Upper concentration limit, 866
Uranium, 43, 607
  acute renal damage, 607
  inhalation, 608
  TLV, 608
Uranium tetrafluoride, 608
Uranyl fluoride, 608
Uricase, 495
Urinalysis, 183
Urinary amino-levulinic acid, 156
Urinary thiol loss, 950

V

Vanadium, 15, 44, 50, 53, 58-59,
    564, 617, 745
  bone development, 751
  cardiovascular disease, 749
  chemistry, 745
  cholesterol metabolism, 748
  dental caries, 750
  essentiality, 745
  excretion, 746-747
  glucose metabolism, 748
  growth response, 746-747
  hazards, 565
  health effects, 748, 751
  metabolism, 748
  reproduction, 751
  respiratory disease, 566
  triglyceride metabolism, 748
Vascular endothelium, 405
Vascular hypoplasia, 405

Visual discrimination task, 113
Vitamin E deficiency, 660
Volatile vapors, 839
Volatilization, 811

W

Wastes, gold mining, 10
Waste water, poisoning from, 202
Wilson's disease, 505, 711
Wolfram, 44
World Health Organization/Food Ag-
    riculture Organization, 5, 7,
    10-11, 13-14

X

X-ray fluorescence spectrometer,
    918
  sources, 918
X-ray fluorescent, 10
X-rays, production of, 917
X-ray units, nondispersive, 921

Y

Ytterbium, 44, 559
Yttrium, 44, 559

Z

Zinc, 15, 45, 50, 53, 58-59, 60,
    456, 462, 466-467, 545, 590,
    617, 630, 649, 751
  absorption of, 468, 650
  accumulation of, 211
  anemia, 759
  bedsores, 759
  body burden, 591
  bone growth, 756
  cancer, 758
  chemistry, 751
  cirrhosis, 759
  colds, 759
  content in tissues, 213
  deficiency of, 470, 630, 649
  dermal toxicity, 592
  dialysis, 759
  dwarfism, 630
  essentiality, 752
  excretion, 591
  in foodstuffs, 231
  geographical variation in, 229
  health effects, 756
  industrial exposure, 591
  infections, 759

Part 1 comprises pages 1-515.
Part 2 comprises pages 517-952.

[Zinc]
   leg ulcers, 759
   metabolism, 753
   metalloenzymes, 754
   metalloproteins, 754
   in night soil, 236, 238
   ocular hazard, 592
   from polluted areas, 242
   reproduction, 757

[Zinc]
   retardation of brain growth, 759
   in silkworms, 245
   slow healing wounds, 470
   in urban air, 590
   wound healing, 756
Zinc content, in normal human, 216
Zinc oxide, 592
Zinc smelters, 238
Zinc toxicity, 471, 492, 649
   anemia of, 650
Zirconium, 45, 562